The Whole Foot

A Complete Program for Taking Care of Your Feet

Brett R. Fink, MD
Mark S. Mizel, MD

16
EasyRead Large

RHYW

Copyright Page from the Original Book

ISBN: 978-1-936303-24-3
eISBN: 978-1-617050-96-1

Acquisitions Editor: Noreen Henson
Production Editor: Michael Lisk
Compositor: Newgen
Printer: Hamilton Printing
Visit our web site at www.demoshealth.com

Medical information provided by Demos Health, in the absence of a visit with a health care professional, must be considered as an educational service only. This book is not designed to replace a physician's independent judgment about the appropriateness or risks of a procedure or therapy for a given patient. Our purpose is to provide you with information that will help you make your own health care decisions.

The information and opinions provided here are believed to be accurate and sound, based on the best judgment available to the authors, editors, and publisher, but readers who fail to consult appropriate health authorities assume the risk of any injuries. The publisher is not responsible for errors or omissions. The editors and publisher welcome any reader to report to the publisher any discrepancies or inaccuracies noticed.

CIP data is available from the Library of Congress

Made in the United States of America.
11 12 13 14 5 4 3 2 1

Contributors

k, MD, FAAOS, FAOFAS
urgeon
diana Orthopedic Center
IN

abrielson, MD, FACS, CWS, FACCWS
rgeon
ector, Hancock Center for Wound Healing
IN

nsoori, JD, CO

Orthopro, Inc.
lis, IN

. Mirowski, DMD, MD
logist in Private Practice and
Associate Professor, Indiana University School
tistry
polis, IN

S. Mizel, MD, FAAOS, FAOFAS
edic Surgeon
sor, University of Miami, Retired
n, MA

M. Ristow
rford College

TABLE OF CONTENTS

To my wife, Patric…
who love me desp…
colleagues at I…
Community and Ha…
teach…

To my father, Harold…
pursue…

ii

Brett R. Fin…
Orthopedic S…
President, In…
Indianapolis,…

Cameron G…
General Su…
Medical Dir…
Greenfield,…

Keon Ma…
Orthotist
Advanced…
Indianapo…

Ginat W…
Dermato…
Adjunct…
of Dem…
Indiana…

Mark …
Orthop…
Profes…
Bosto…

Celia…
Have…

TABLE OF CONTENTS

To my wife, Patricia, and daughters, Alexis and Laurel, who love me despite my faults. To my patients and colleagues at Indiana Orthopedic Center and Community and Hancock Hospitals who continue to teach and inspire me.

—BRF

To my father, Harold H. Mizel, who urged me to pursue excellence.

—MSM

Contributors

Brett R. Fink, MD, FAAOS, FAOFAS
Orthopedic Surgeon
President, Indiana Orthopedic Center
Indianapolis, IN

Cameron Gabrielson, MD, FACS, CWS, FACCWS
General Surgeon
Medical Director, Hancock Center for Wound Healing
Greenfield, IN

Keon Mansoori, JD, CO
Orthotist
Advanced Orthopro, Inc.
Indianapolis, IN

Ginat W. Mirowski, DMD, MD
Dermatologist in Private Practice and
Adjunct Associate Professor, Indiana University School of Dentistry
Indianapolis, IN

Mark S. Mizel, MD, FAAOS, FAOFAS
Orthopedic Surgeon
Professor, University of Miami, Retired
Boston, MA

Celia M. Ristow
Haverford College

Haverford, PA

Introduction

The foot is a wonderful and amazing organ. It contains 28 bones, 31 joints, countless ligaments, tendons, and muscles, all working in concert to allow us to run, balance, twist, turn, and jump. The foot is seemingly impossibly complex and small, but it performs a huge variety of high-stress activities throughout our long lifespan—from the endless pounding of running a marathon runner to the disciplined balance of a ballerina *en pointe,* the foot is capable of grace and resilience. It can walk on soil, asphalt, and rock without significant difficulty. Even through the more mundane tasks of the daily walking, lifting, and adjusting to a wide array of terrain, feet perform reliably.

Unfortunately, there are also an endless number of ways that the foot can develop problems. When the foot malfunctions, pain is often felt with every step. The pain can severely limit our ability to work, parent, and perform daily activities. Recreational activities that made life enjoyable can become intolerable. These problems can become disabling.

Diagnosis and treatment of these problems can also be confusing and frightening for the people that have them. Often the structures involved are not the ones covered in high school biology. The mechanisms that lead to foot problems are also complicated and unclear, but the foot is a mechanical device and can be understood by using the same mechanical principles that can be seen all around us. A clear understanding of the mechanics of the foot can help us to design methods of treatment.

Surprisingly, foot problems are often not understood by some of the very physicians that we go to in search of help. When graduating from medical school, the new doctor is fully capable of diagnosing heart attacks and diabetes. It is surprising how little time is devoted to musculoskeletal problems in general—and foot problems specifically—in most medical programs. Musculoskeletal problems are also not given high priority during a routine checkup when time is limited. The explanations and treatment strategies are often not well thought out or completely satisfactory.

A clear understanding of a foot problem is helpful not only in reducing the anxiety associated with a painful condition, but also in understanding the goals and methods of the treatment. Medical treatment should be an alliance between you and your physician. Without a clear understanding of the goal and rationale behind a treatment, it is difficult for anyone to completely invest themselves in a rehabilitation and treatment program. If there is no enthusiasm for the treatment, the program will likely be ineffective. Vague instructions are difficult to follow and lead to failure of the treatment.

WHY THIS BOOK?

Few people can retain more than one or two things that are told to them at any one sitting. It is not that they lack intelligence, but it is difficult in a 5- or 10-minute discussion to learn a whole topic that is largely unfamiliar to anything that you have learned previously. Learning is most effective when the information can be built on a foundation of basic understanding. We would have the same difficulty with remembering facts if someone tried to help us learn electrical engineering or to speak Arabic in fifteen minutes. We would forget much of what we had learned or heard immediately and remember even less of the information several hours or days later. The main goal of this book is to build this foundation of information.

One would think that the Internet would settle all of this confusion. People are *more* informed than they have been in the past. Whether this means that they are *better* informed is debatable. Although there are many good references on the Internet, there is also a lot of unproven, inaccurate, and, sometimes dangerous information. Place any medical diagnosis in a search engine on the Internet and you will get a number of "hits" most likely in the millions. Few determined online researchers have the patience to comb through more than the first few pages of the results of any Internet search. Many of the web sites have paid for the privilege of being within that first few pages. Most of the sites have some financial interest in selling you something—a new medication, a procedure, or a device. Although these things may have some reasonable use, often the claims made are unsubstantiated by any reliable scientific study and don't work. It is important to establish the effectiveness of any form of treatment to establish the risks and benefits so that we can determine whether using it is worth the risk, inconvenience, and expense. We have seen many treatments and devices come in and out of fashion like the latest clothing style as initial enthusiasm is replaced by a sobering and disappointing realization of the problems and practical real-life results of a technique. It is clear that treatments that have not stood the test of time and careful scientific method should be approached with caution.

There really is no substitute for an evaluation and discussion of medical problems with a caring and knowledgeable physician. Self-diagnosis doesn't always work. "Medical Student Syndrome" is a phenomenon where students learning about medical conditions begin to suspect that the disease that they are studying is one that they actually have. Brian Hodges[1] stated, "This phenomenon caused a significant amount of stress for students and was present in approximately 70 to 80 percent of students." This can happen even in people learning about medicine informally through the Internet or a book. It doesn't mean that people should be uninformed about their conditions, but it emphasizes that the critical job of the physician is to bring an objective viewpoint to the evaluation of a medical problem.

Another critical task of a physician is to identify other factors that may interfere with treatment. For example, various blood thinners may be prescribed for the treatment of blood clots, strokes, or heart attacks. Many times over-the-counter anti-inflammatory medications are suggested for the treatment of various types of pain. It may be dangerous to take these medications together. A doctor can identify this and modify the treatment plan appropriately to minimize the risk of this interaction.

Finally, certain more invasive treatments may be necessary in the treatment of some foot conditions. These treatments may need close supervision and monitoring by a physician. Ankle fractures may need surgery, or at the very least various forms of weight-bearing restriction or brace protection.

Perhaps it is unrealistic to expect a short visit to the doctor's office, even a leading expert in a field, to be able to give us all the information necessary to completely and efficiently understand our foot ailments. After all, each person has a differing appetite for this information. In addition, because of time constraints, barriers to communication and sometimes to the limitations of our physician's knowledge of our particular problem, the information is inadequate and unsatisfying.

Diet books and other self-help books are available by the score, but there are not many resources available on common foot and ankle problems that explain in depth the current misconceptions, treatments, and limitations. The crucial goal of this book is to fill in these gaps—to give the reader a clear understanding of how the foot works and how it can break. This book will explain the common foot problems in clear everyday language not "medicalese" and will give plain explanations of the underlying processes that cause foot pain and disability.

This book is not a substitute for professional examination and consultation for foot problems. Unfortunately, there is no substitute for a careful evaluation by a foot care professional. This book is meant to help prepare you for your visits with your doctor and to make you better informed. It is also meant to show you the breadth of nonoperative approaches to many foot problems that time constraints will not allow your doctor or therapist to familiarize you with completely.

HOW TO USE THIS BOOK

The initial section of this book gives some tips on how to select a foot care professional. Chapter 1 discusses one of the main principles of this book: many foot problems, including the most common chronic foot problems, are due to overload of the front of the foot. The overload is caused primarily by improper posture, conditioning, and poor flexibility. These principles will be referred to again and again throughout the chapters. In addition, although surgery is often prescribed for many chronic foot disorders, surgery does not address the underlying forefoot overload and may leave you prone to other problems if it is not addressed. Also, traditional physical therapy is not comprehensive enough to treat it to maximal effectiveness.

The second section of the book separates the foot into common regions of pain. It explains the common disorders of these regions by reviewing the anatomy and mechanics there. It is a good idea to read over all the section's disorders because sometimes the problem may be misdiagnosed or there may be other contributing problems that could be overlooked. If your foot hurts "everywhere," don't despair. There will be a discussion of the possible reasons for this kind of pain. We will illustrate these problems by discussing a reasoned approach used on patients who we have seen in our clinic. Although the people's names have been changed as well as some of the demographic information, these are real people. We have selected average individuals with typical problems. The discussion will include practical solutions and concrete instructions for initial treatment of common foot complaints, focusing on nonoperative approaches. This discussion should fill in the gaps of information and instructions that your doctor may not have mentioned. Many people will find this helpful in beginning the treatment of their problem and help reinforce and expand what your doctor has discussed.

The third section will look more closely at the effect that certain systemic problems and conditions such as diabetes and rheumatoid arthritis have on the foot. The effect of these problems is often on more than one area and anyone who lives with these problems should be aware of the potential consequences that they can have on the foot.

The final section has references and explanations of various methods of approaching foot problems. Rehabilitation and exercise therapy is effective in the treatment of many foot problems, especially the chronic ones. Rehabilitation has gotten a bad reputation, partially because it may not be executed properly and can be expensive even with insurance. With patience and proper instruction, rehabilitation can be successful in many situations. A well-organized therapy regimen in a properly educated patient should not require many visits. Even in situations when rehab is not ultimately successful, it is our belief that proper and continuous rehabilitative treatment can increase the effectiveness of surgery and prevent other foot problems.

We will review various commercially available and prescription shoe wear that is helpful in the treatment of foot conditions. In addition to this, braces and orthotics will be explained, and useful Internet resources will be reviewed and discussed. We will try to avoid using medical terminology. However, if this is unavoidable and confusing, look up the definition in the glossary.

Remember: Surgery for nearly all chronic foot disorders and many acute problems is not a first choice even though many may look to it for a quick and reliable fix. Surgery—especially the reconstructive surgery prescribed for most common chronic conditions—rarely leaves the foot absolutely normal. This fact is often overlooked, sometimes with a great deal of disappointment and frustration.

Surgery is almost always a trade off; lose one problem (such as pain) for another, hopefully, less troublesome problem. Common examples of the other residual problems are stiffness, numbness, and scarring. Surgery can also disturb the fine balance of a foot.

Even doctors sometimes fall into this illusion of surgery as an easy "fix." Nonoperative treatment is hard. First, the physician needs to be familiar enough with the problem to really understand it. Doctors have to be able to explain the problem, identify its cause, and develop a plan of action. The patient must live with these changes, challenges, and instructions. Development of this plan takes your physician's time, which is his or her most valuable resource. Isn't it easier to simply operate and fix it? Again, it would be nice if by fix it, we meant restore it to normal, but this is uncommon.

Nonoperative treatment is also complicated, often more complicated, in some ways, than surgery. This is because an operative plan is developed by the surgeon and executed by the surgeon. A nonoperative plan is developed by the surgeon or therapist, but needs to be executed by the patient, the one with the least experience and least education about the problem. No wonder it is so common to give up on a nonoperative plan prematurely. This book is your guide to nonoperative treatments of a variety of foot problems. Remember, it is not always successful, but if it is done right, it can frequently be successful.

We have included diagrams and illustrations to help explain things to you. They may also be helpful to your doctor during your discussions. You are an integral part of your health and recovery. Discuss ideas that you have to aid your recovery. You really have nothing to lose. Good doctors will be receptive to your suggestions and if they don't agree with them, they should at least be able to give a rational explanation for why. Perhaps you will think of something that had not occurred to your doctor. We often find that our patients are a great source of inspiration in the treatment of their own problems. Mark on this book and leave notes or highlight it so that you can discuss the points with your doctor. Look over the rehabilitation section. If your doctor feels that some of these exercises may be useful, make note in the margin about how often and how many you need to do.

Good luck on the resolution of your foot problem. Remember that you and your enthusiasm are the greatest resource you have in your recuperation. You can access more support and information at our website www.wholefoot.com.

NOTE

[1] Hodges, Brian. Medical Student Bodies and the Pedagogy of Self-Reflection, Self-Assessment, and Self-Regulation, JCT Rochester. *J. Curriculum Theorizing* 2004;(20):41.

1

Choosing a Foot Professional

Choosing a doctor is a daunting task. A great deal of information is available, but much of it, including that gathered on the Internet, is questionable. The trust that patients place in their doctor is truly remarkable. It has always been a source of pride to us that we can meet a person and 20 minutes later tell them that they need surgery. When we begin to explain the rationale, they calmly interrupt us and state, "I trust you, Doctor." (We often think to ourselves, "On what basis?")

The trust that people place in their physicians is so commonplace but so monumental. The tests that physicians run can cost even a "well-insured" person a lot of hard-earned money. All medications have potential risk. Surgery is expensive and the recuperation can affect you greatly financially, even if it goes according to plan. Surgery has also risk not only because it can lead to complications, but also the results may not always be what you expect. Essentially you are placing your life and livelihood in the hands of someone who you have known for a relatively short amount of time. It would be foolish to go into this without preparation. Preparation requires that a knowledge of your problem and a familiarity with your doctor, his credentials and, more importantly, who he or she is as a person.

ORTHOPEDIST OR PODIATRIST?

One of the most frequent questions that we encounter is, "Should I go to an orthopedist or podiatrist?" This is a touchy subject between the two professions and here is the answer in a nutshell. Simply, there are many more important things about choosing a doctor than the letters behind their name. We need to also mention that we are orthopedists so there might be bias in our answer to this question. We will be as objective as we possibly can. In short, everyone should seek out the best *doctor* that he or she can find. This may be skirting the subject, but it is more important than the initial question. Orthopedic surgeons and podiatrists are highly trained professionals who should have your best interests foremost and both are physicians. Both can do many operations and prescribe medications.

A fully trained podiatrist undergoes extensive training that, in many ways, is similar to the training of an orthopedist. The training begins with completion of a four-year undergraduate college degree. Prerequisite mathematics and science courses are necessary. There is a wide range, but the average grade point average of a successful podiatric school applicant is 3.3 on a 4-point scale,[1] which is a respectable level of achievement. Most podiatric school applicants take the

Medical College Applicants Test or MCAT to gauge their science and other academic knowledge.

The successful podiatric school applicant will then enter a college of podiatry and begin a four-year course of study. The subjects taken during this course of study include physiology, anatomy, pharmacology, and other medical studies. The classes are demanding and thorough.

After podiatric school, the podiatric graduate applies and enters residency. Residency can be two or three years. Many curricula explore emergency medicine including treatment of problems other than that of the foot and ankle, family medicine, and other medical subjects. The surgical rotations often include exposure to general and orthopedic surgery as well as surgical experience that is almost exclusively devoted to operative treatment of foot problems.

Orthopedic surgeons begin their training after an undergraduate degree with medical school. The average undergraduate grade point average for a successful medical school applicant is 3.67 (2010).[2] In medical school, the initial classroom work is nearly identical during the first year or two of medical school and in some schools, podiatrists and medical school students are in class together. The later clinical work is much broader with more required rotations in general surgery, pediatrics, and internal medicine. Other elective rotations are more variable.

The medical school graduate interviews with and subsequently goes on to a residency, a period of specialty training. Orthopedic surgery is certainly one of the more competitive residencies. There are approximately 1.5 applicants for every orthopedic position and 98% to 99% of positions are filled every year.[3] The orthopedic residency program is five years in length, although some are six years. The first year is an internship, during which the resident rotates on various general surgical and specialty rotations such as urology, intensive care, and emergency care. After completion of the internship, the resident trains in the orthopedic department rotating among the subspecialty areas such as spine, hand, sports, and total joint replacement surgery. Surgical responsibilities and participation is gradually increased until at the completion of training the resident should be nearly independent. Although foot and ankle trauma and reconstruction is a part of many rotations, it is possible that the graduate of an orthopedic residency program may not go through a rotation dedicated to foot and ankle surgery during his or her training. The average orthopedic resident spends about 30% of his training time involved in the treatment of foot and ankle conditions.[4]

After residency, an orthopedist may decide to do an extra year of training, called a fellowship, which focuses specifically on foot and ankle surgery. The fellowship is usually spent with a mentor or small number of mentors who individually coach and instruct the fellow on the finer points of foot and ankle treatment, both surgical and nonsurgical.

The most important part of the training of any surgeon, whether a podiatrist or orthopedic subspecialist, is after residency and fellowship. During the early years of practice, the personal responsibility involved in practice quickly helps individual physicians to mature and develop their own practice style and discipline. It also helps to develop judgment and a sense of what their personal and professional limitations should be. To a great extent, the training and learning process never stops, as there are a large number of clinical problems in foot and ankle medicine that are not adequately solved yet and are unique to an individual.

So, which professional is better and more qualified to treat you? The answer really hinges on which, whether podiatrist or orthopedic surgeon, is the better doctor. There are qualities that make a good doctor that are not dependent on a college grade point average, MCAT score, the name of the school on the diploma, or the letters behind the name. There is little correlation between scores on standardized tests or grade point averages and methods of assessing success in clinical practice. However, having high scores on these tests does not make you a bad doctor or out of touch with others. The two qualities are just not closely related. The talents involved in actually examining, diagnosing, and successfully treating people are different than those required to ace an examination or write a flawless essay. No one has a monopoly on common sense or surgical skill. There is no physician who has not had amazing successes and catastrophic failures. In short, there are good and bad orthopedists. There are good and bad podiatrists. No physician wins them all.

WHAT MAKES A GREAT DOCTOR?

Most central to the selection of the doctor who takes care of your foot and ankle problem is their trustworthiness and how good they are at taking the information, making a correct diagnosis, and formulating a plan to successfully and reasonably improve the problem. Unfortunately, it is difficult to find a way to measure these skills. We have had the pleasure of meeting colleagues that were not particularly great students in the classroom, but had a great sense of the art of medicine and rapport with patients. We have also met people with amazing intellect and scholarship in the classroom who, in our opinion, should stay in the classroom or laboratory. All physicians technically have access to the same body of information and should read continually to educate themselves on developing techniques and research. All great physicians should possess a healthy skepticism when evaluating the literature and the discipline not to try anything new until it has been tested, and that the physician is comfortable with the technical aspects of the innovation. This takes a great deal of integrity, because the push to be on the cutting edge of innovation is important to physicians from a marketing standpoint, but can affect the patients negatively when the "real-world" results do not measure up to the hype. Although there are some differences in the approach of some podiatrists and orthopedists, most of them are really a matter of philosophy rather than the choice of one clearly inferior approach over a superior one.

So, how do you find a good doctor without the time-consuming chore of going from office to office in the hope that randomly you will hit upon one that meshes well with you? Your first resource is your primary care physician. Primary care physicians should have a working relationship with all of the physicians to whom they refer patients. They should have a general idea whether your podiatrist or orthopedist uses good judgment and what is the quality of their practice is.

Recommendations from friends are also helpful, but usually in terms of how your friend was treated and how well he or she could relate to the physician. Remember that your friend's problem is different from yours and may be easier or harder to treat. The most important part of the recommendation from friends is not whether they had a good result, although this is important. It is whether the physician communicated well with your friend. If there was a problem or concern, was it addressed and evaluated quickly?

Information on web sites that claim to rate or evaluate doctors is somewhat useful. However, it should be kept in mind that angry patients tend to be the most vocal. There is sometimes a motivation that if patients feel wronged in some way, they strike back at their doctor. In practice, a reason for this may have little to do with the quality of their care. Conflict between a doctor and a patient could include suggesting that chronically narcotic-dependent patients seek evaluation by a pain specialist instead of getting another surgery or be prescribed pain medication indefinitely. Another common reason is dismissing a patient for repeatedly missing scheduled appointments without cancellation or being excessively abusive to the physician's staff. It is not always in a patient's best interest for a doctor to give them exactly what they ask for. If, however, the review brings up specific issues—especially if they are recurrent and the physician is allowed to reply—it should be taken seriously and can be used to help make decisions.

The initial appointment with your physician specialist should be essentially a job interview. Doctors are the applicants and you are the employer. The first impression is often telling. Do they listen? How well do they understand your problem? You should get some idea about this from the amount of time that they spend listening to you explain the problem. They should fill in any details you left out with pertinent questions. They should take an interest in how the problem is affecting your life, hobbies, family, and livelihood. While the problem at hand is being discussed, you should be evaluating the physician for the qualities that you feel are most desirable in a doctor.

Initially, a good physician should be willing to allow you an amount of time to explain and describe the problem. You should be given enough time to tell your whole story. Constant interruptions or impatience is something of concern. In the beginning, the questions should be open-ended. "What hurts? When does it hurt? What makes it better or worse? How does it affect your day-to-day activity?" The physician should be filling in the gaps in the story. Finally, the physician may not know the diagnosis, but should know what the problem and what your concerns are, and should be creating a mental list of the potential possible diagnoses that may be present. Any other important medical problems and history should be reviewed as appropriate.

A complete physical examination of the involved area and any other adjoining areas is also expected. A physician who concentrates only on the problem toe and does not examine the rest of the foot and, possibly, other parts of the body might not understand the environment that the toe is operating in and may miss important points that may contribute to the diagnosis and should be addressed at the same time. Another red flag is the "doorway examination," in which a brief and cursory examination is performed. A complete examination includes testing motion, strength, sensation, circulation, and a thorough careful identification of tenderness throughout the entire foot. The patient who has tenderness in only the heel presents a different problem than the patient who has pain in the heel, but also in the shin, ball of the foot, ankle, and back. In the first case, various heel problems can be assumed to be present. In the second, other problems that may be more generalized should be suspected.

Often, but not always, x-rays are ordered and reviewed. A good physician should review and explain any abnormalities that are present. Usually it is necessary for the physician to directly view and be able to personally interpret the tests ordered to be able to truly understand them.

Finally, try to draw out from your doctor what his or her impression of your problem is and to describe his or her thought process. Physicians should explain what they knows and do not know about your foot. An airtight definite diagnosis is not always possible on the initial visit, but a discussion should be undertaken regarding the various potential problems that may be occurring. A plan should be outlined, if necessary, to find out what the problem is if the diagnosis is in question. This may involve further radiographic or laboratory test. You should understand what information is being obtained by the test and why it is necessary to obtain it now and what decision is being made with the test. If the test is positive, are you ready for surgery? If not, do you need the test?

Be cautious of any doctor who orders tests without an explanation of how these tests will be used to treat you. Tests should be never be ordered for curiosity's sake. There should be a definite decision hinging on the results of any test. It may be used to exclude a potentially dangerous problem like cancer, occult fracture, or infection, or it may be used to help plan for surgical treatment. For most problems, like the initial treatment of many fractures, tendonitis, or neuritis, nonoperative treatments can be safely begun without sophisticated tests such as MRIs, CT scans, or nerve tests. Often these tests can be delayed until nonoperative measures have failed because a definite diagnosis is just not necessary at the early stages of treatment.

Unless there is no other reasonable option, most problems—especially problems not caused by trauma—should be initially approached nonoperatively. Exceptions to this are life- or limb-threatening problems such as cancer, infection, or arterial circulatory problems. Certain fractures and traumatic tendon injuries sometimes require surgery to realign and make the joints function properly, since they do not reliably heal without surgery. Most other common conditions, especially chronic ones, have reasonable nonoperative treatments that can be completely explored prior to the prescription of invasive or expensive treatments.

At the end of your appointment, you should be impressed with the knowledge and experience of your physician. You should feel that a serious assessment of your problem has been completed: a reasonable, clear, and well-considered plan is in place and you have taken the first steps on the road to recovery. Treatment of any condition should be based on scientifically proven information and experience. However, faith, trust, and enthusiasm are just as important to the success and execution of the treatment plan.

NOTES

[1] www.aacpm.org/html/careerzone/cz3_faqs.asp.

[2] https://www.aamc.org/download/161690/data/table17-facts2010mcatgpa99-10-web.pdf.pdf.

[3] Clark R, Evans EB, Ivey FM, Calhoun JH, Hokanson JA. Characteristics of successful and unsuccessful applicants to orthopedic residency training programs. Clin Orthop Relat Res. 1989 Apr;(241):257–64.

[4] Panchbhavi VK, Aronow MS, Digiovanni BF, Giza E, Grimes JS, Harris TG, Roberts MM, Straus B. Foot and ankle experience in orthopedic residency: an update. Foot Ankle Int. 2010 Jan;31(1):10–3.

2

Forefoot Overload

- There is evidence that high levels of pressure on the front of the foot can lead to many common foot problems.
- Forefoot overload can be caused by a number of things, including obesity, poor flexibility, poor posture, and walking habits.
- Many of these problems become more common with age.
- Treatment strategies that address these problems may be helpful in treating these common conditions without surgery.

The foot is a mechanical device, an amazing versatile mechanical device with the ability to repair itself, but still a device that functions in accordance to mechanical principles. Having a superficial understanding of these principles can help us to understand how the foot works and how it breaks. Let's briefly review just a few simple points.

Force is the capacity to move something. It does not actually have to move it, but it could, if given the opportunity. For instance, if you are standing on a floor, gravity causes your body to apply force to the floor. The floor is also applying an equal force to your body and so you remain stationary. If someone came and cut a hole in the floor underneath you, you would fall so the gravity/force would realize the capacity to move you and down you'd go. With the floor underneath you, however, the forces are balanced so you don't move. Other words that essentially mean the same thing as force are pressure, stress, push, pull, and drive.

Force that acts at a distance from a pivot point on a lever is called leverage or torque and can cause things to rotate about the pivot point unless counteracted by another force. The classic example of this is a seesaw. The farther from the pivot point the force is, the greater leverage the force is able to make. The mechanical consequence is that the force also has to act through a greater distance to cause the same degree of rotation. If no rotation is occurring, then all forces or sources of leverage are balanced. This is the reason that a small child can balance his father on a seesaw if his father is closer to the pivot point.

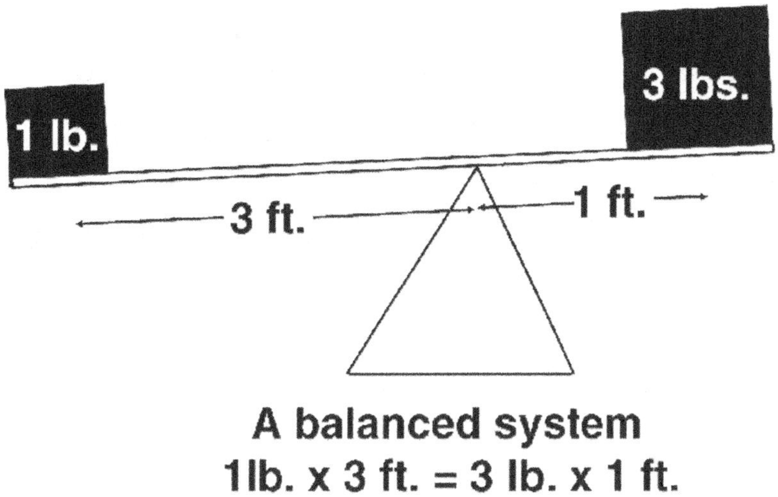

FIGURE 2.1 Equalized forces/leverage on either side of a pivot point.

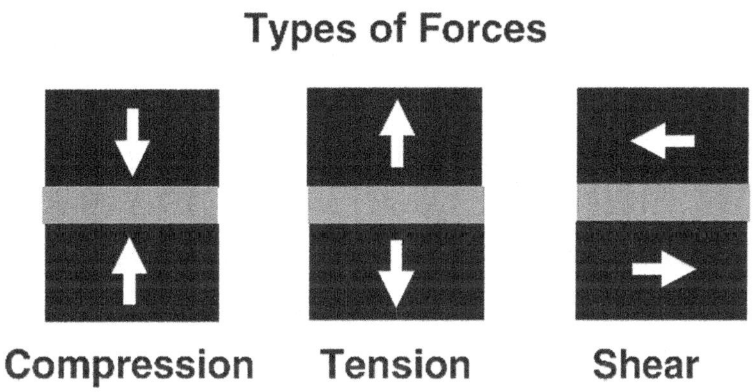

FIGURE 2.2 Types of forces affect the foot and other body parts.

Mechanical forces that affect the foot come in three varieties: compression, tension, and shear. It is important to separate these because the ability for tissues such as bone, ligaments, and cartilage to withstand these different types of forces is vastly different. Compression is a force that pushes something together. Compressive forces are well tolerated by bones and joint cartilage. A tensile force is a force pulling something apart. Within the body, tensile forces are usually controlled by connective tissues especially ligaments and tendons. Ligaments are structures that hold joints together and guide their motion. Tendons are structures that connect muscles, the generators of force within the body, to bones and joints. Bone is not able to withstand tensile forces nearly as well as compressive forces. Often when a bone breaks, it is the tension portion of the force applied to it that begins the crack within the bone. A shear force is a force that moves perpendicular to a surface. If you drag your feet on the floor, the friction that your foot feels with the floor is a shear force. Shear forces are not well tolerated by any tissue but are especially poorly tolerated by articular cartilage, the cartilage in the joint. Shearing forces, either directly or indirectly, are one primary cause for premature breakdown of joint cartilage leading to arthritis. The body in normal circumstances has developed amazing and ingenious techniques for minimizing shearing force that we will discuss throughout this book.

Many of the painful conditions that occur in your body are the result of a lifetime of usage. Your body, like any mechanical device such as a car or a kitchen mixer, wears out with time and use. However, unlike the nonliving mechanical devices, your body has the ability to repair itself. This ability to heal is limited, however. Some tissues like skin and bone can heal with minimal scarring and create tissue that is almost as durable and functional as the original, uninjured tissue was. Other tissues such are joint cartilage and nerve are so complex that the body has difficulty regenerating anything that comes close to being as useful as the original. Regeneration within connective tissues, such as tendon, ligament, and fascia is very slow, because there are few cells capable of repairing the injury. In addition, these tissues have a very small blood supply so that the oxygen, proteins, and sugars needed to power the repair process are not plentiful.

The way that we use our body can have a big impact on the rate and the way that our body wears, and on which structures wear. If a car's axle is out of alignment, the tires will wear more rapidly than if the tires are properly aligned. That is why we should regularly take our car to the mechanic to realign the wheels. In the same way, the stresses on the body can be misplaced and cause it to wear quickly or to overwhelm the body's ability to heal itself.

Improper use of your foot can cause undue stress and wear, which can develop into painful conditions. Overloading the forefoot, the area underneath the toes or "ball of the foot," is one common problem that will be explained in detail in this chapter. The pressure on the front of the foot is a combination of body weight and pressure from the large, powerful muscles in the foot used to control body weight during standing, walking, and running. There is considerable scientific evidence that overload of the forefoot can damage certain structures within the foot. It is our belief that it is pivotal in the development of many, but not all, common foot problems. The conditions with the most evidence suggesting this are plantar fasciitis or heel spurs, midfoot arthritis, and metatarsalgia, a painful condition in the ball of the foot. A great many other painful conditions such as posterior tibial tendonitis or "fallen arches," Achilles tendonitis, anterior ankle pain and arthritis, and many stress fractures may be caused by forefoot overload. The evidence is not yet certain.

Unfortunately, the hard evidence for the involvement of forefoot overload in the development of various foot pains, like in most criminal trials, is circumstantial. We are not able to prove this without a "shadow of a doubt," as is the case with many aspects of medicine. The evidence for any but the simplest questions is often low grade, indirect, and conflicting, and is likely to remain so for many years.

We must start with the most basic questions. What points to the involvement of the forefoot in development of these foot problems? There is evidence that people with conditions that are easy to measure such as lack of motion due to a stiff Achilles tendon and increases in forefoot pressure do have an increase in many of these painful foot problems. Increased forefoot pressure has been linked to great toe arthritis.[1] Achilles tendon contractures are a risk factor for plantar fasciitis,[2][3] and forefoot pain.[4][5][6]

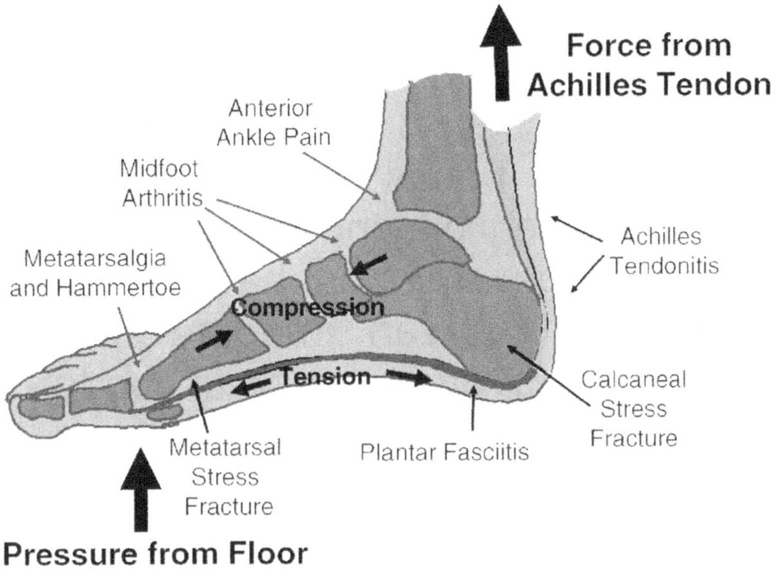

FIGURE 2.3 The major forces at work during walking and the areas that can break down as a result of them.

There is also some evidence that portions of the rehabilitation approaches outlined in these chapters are effective for some of the problems and that these interventions do limit forefoot stress. These approaches make conceptual sense and, therefore, constitute the most reasonable, effective, safest, and most comprehensive treatment for these problems with the available information today.

WAYS IN WHICH WE OVERLOAD OUR FEET

The most obvious ways in which we can overload our feet is to place too much weight on them. Obesity is an epidemic in the United States and it is spreading to many parts of the world. If a man, whose ideal weight is 160 pounds, weighs 200 pounds, it is essentially like he is carrying a 40-pound weight with him wherever he goes. Imagine, toting a backpack with 40 pounds of books with you everywhere, to work, into the shower, playing sports, jogging. In fact, carrying heavy bags such as backpacks can add to forefoot overload. You can imagine why this would cause fatigue and overwhelm your body's ability to withstand normal daily activities.

Although weight loss in an obese person is an important goal for relief of foot pain and for prevention many other injuries to the joints in the lower extremity that are being overloaded, it is a long-term goal. In fact, there is no truer saying in weight loss than "quickly off, quickly on." Healthy permanent weight loss is not achieved through short-term changes in diet, but by long-term changes in lifestyle. Fortunately, there are effective ways of combating foot pain even in the presence of considerable excess weight. Some tips for this are found in the resource section.

A second obvious concept is the relationship of foot pain with overuse of the feet in everyday activities such as a job. This is a common complaint that we hear in our clinic. "I work retail and I'm on my feet from the moment I come to work until I leave." "I stand at a cash register all day." "I work on concrete." This is a difficult contributing problem to eliminate. We all need to be productive and most of us need a job to make money and support ourselves and our families. So how do we eliminate this stress? Should a waitress quit her job? Should a store clerk sell dresses while sitting on a stool? In few situations is this practical. Fortunately, this is rarely necessary. This is most likely the least important part of foot overload. If you use your feet properly, they can withstand a considerable amount of use. With proper protection and rehabilitation, it is often possible to treat people successfully with these problems without asking them to take a prolonged leave from their job.

The body is remarkable in the way that it heals itself. Believe it or not, you damage the bones, tendons, and muscles of your body with every motion that you make. Every time that you get off the couch and get yourself a cup of coffee from the kitchen, little bits of damage occur in every structure that you use. In normal circumstances, the continual repair process that occurs can easily keep up with this.

In fact, if you increase your activity gradually, your body actually makes itself stronger—to a certain extent. This concept was articulated by Julius Wolff, a 19th-century German surgeon. Wolff's Law is one of the central concepts of orthopedics and physiology. For instance, a marathon runner or a soldier training in boot camp will adapt his or her bones, muscles, and tendons to become stronger and to withstand more stress every day. However, if people who are unused to these stresses are subjected to boot camp, the amount of damage that is likely to occur will overwhelm their body's ability to repair the damage and stress injuries will occur. This may be a stress fracture, tendonitis, or joint inflammation, depending on which is the weak link in the chain of structures in their body. The key to avoiding this is to keep a consistent level of activity, varying the types of activity that we do, and to gradually increase our activity level to achieve our target level of activity. These principles apply to athletics and also to every activity.

JOINT/MUSCLE FLEXIBILITY

The flexibility of our joints and muscles affects the way that stress is distributed throughout our body including the feet. The feet are affected by the flexibility and position of every joint from the head to the foot. The ankle being the closest to the foot is the easiest and most direct joint to use to illustrate this. One of the common problems that cause foot problems is an overly tight Achilles tendon/muscle.

The Achilles tendon is behind the ankle just above the heel. It attaches about halfway down the heel or calcaneus. The tendon extends almost halfway up the calf and connects two muscles in the calf to the heel and allows you to flex your ankle. Flexion is the action that you do when you press down on the gas in a car or stand on your tiptoes and push your toes into the floor. The two muscles are named the gastrocnemius and the soleus muscles. The gastrocnemius muscle begins above the knee, so the position of the knee affects how tight the Achilles tendon is.

If the Achilles tendon and its muscles are tight, then you may not be able to flex or extend your ankle easily. In extreme situations, the heel may not touch the floor during a step. This is called *toe walking* and is sometimes seen in adults, but more commonly in children. In more typical cases, the heel will not be on the floor a proper amount of time, which means that the front of the foot will have more weight on it, and the weight will be concentrated on the front of the foot for a greater percentage of the step than is normal. This causes damage and irritation to many structures in the foot that we discuss later in this chapter.

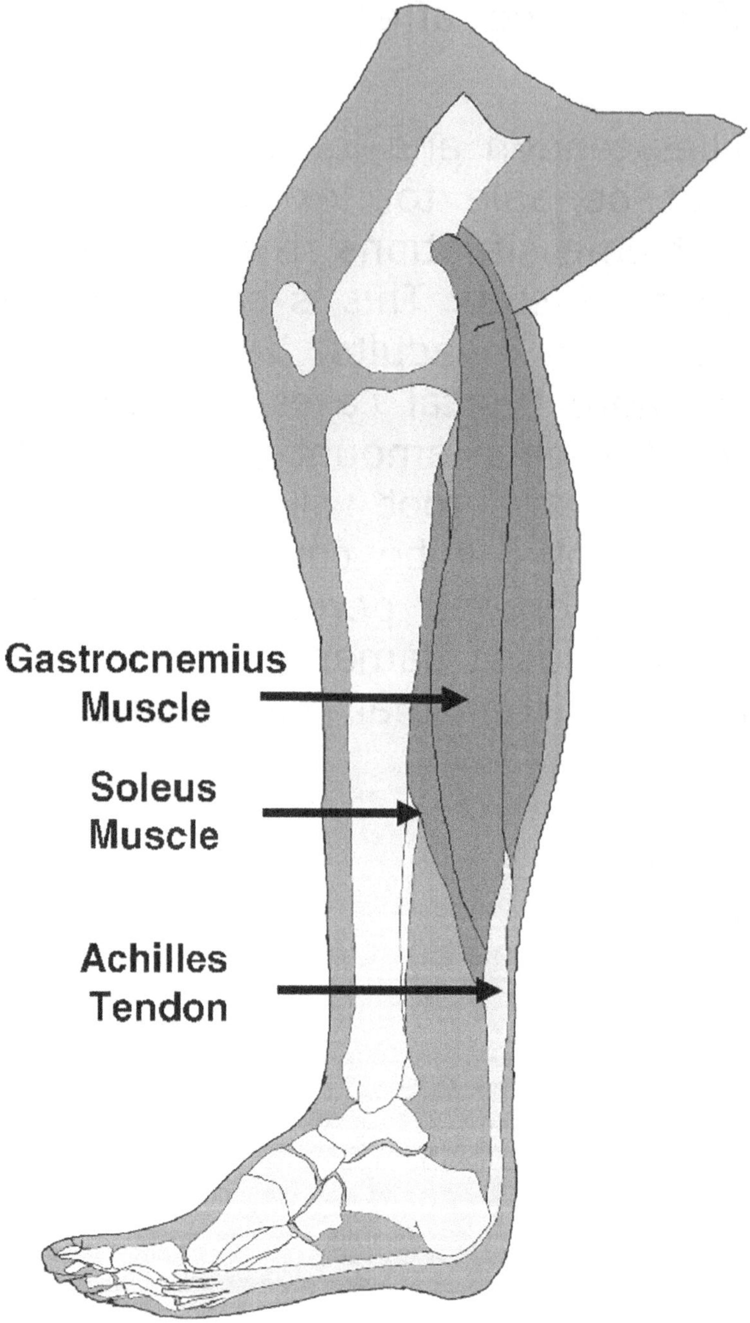

FIGURE 2.4 Illustration of the muscles (soleus and gastrocnemius) contributing to the Achilles tendon.

It is not immediately obvious, but lack of proper flexibility in other joints of the leg can also contribute to forefoot overload. Tight hamstrings or arthritic knees, if lacking full extension, can also shift weight to the forefoot. A weak gluteus muscle in the buttocks or a contracted hip can shift weight onto the forefoot. A compression fracture of the spine can curve your back into flexion, and shift weight forward and onto your forefoot. To illustrate the extra weight on your forefoot when these problems occur, try to walk while squatting slightly. In this position, the hip is slightly flexed, the knees cannot completely extend comfortably during gait, and the back is flexed or slouched. Where is the weight on your feet? Usually, it is shifted to the front of the foot. It may be difficult to place your heel on the floor.

POSTURE

Posture is the most important aspect of forefoot overload. Correct posture balances the center of body mass over the hip, knees, back, and feet. This occurs both when standing and while walking. Proper posture minimizes the amount of muscle action required to maintain a standing position and to walk and it equalizes the pressure across the foot so that ligaments, bones, joints, and tendons have minimum tension, stress, and work to do while walking.

Imagine a coat stand on a floor. When the load on the coat stand is centered on the axis, the pressure on the feet of the coat stand is equal. If we place a coat on the coat stand off to the side of the coat stand, the force on the feet of the coat stand will shift in response, decreasing the weight on one side and increasing it on the other. The farther out from the pole the coat is, the more weight will shift toward the coat until it falls over. In the same way, displacement of weight forward will shift weight from the heel to the forefoot.

What aspects of posture can cause us to overload the forefoot? Anything that moves the body weight forward. The most common cause is loss of tone in the abdominal muscles causing the typical "beer belly." Although this is usually associated with male obesity, it happens to women also. The root of this is loss of abdominal tone through inactivity and poor conditioning that allows the abdominal fat and intestines to protrude over the brim of the pelvis. A second cause is poor posture due to spinal deconditioning and, sometimes, poor habits. The shoulders, head, and the torso begin to roll forward. All of these problems displace body weight forward, weight that is counteracted by pressure on the forefoot. This pressure is applied by contracting the calf muscles on the heel. The constant contraction of all these muscles multiplies the pressure across the joints.

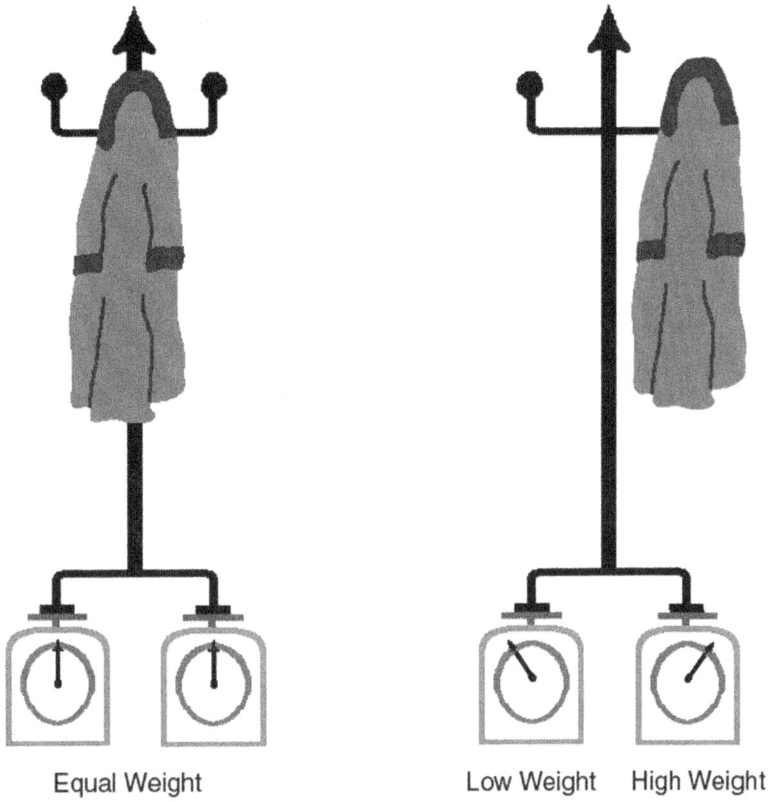

FIGURE 2.5 Illustration of how out-of-balance and uncentered forces affect their supporting structures.

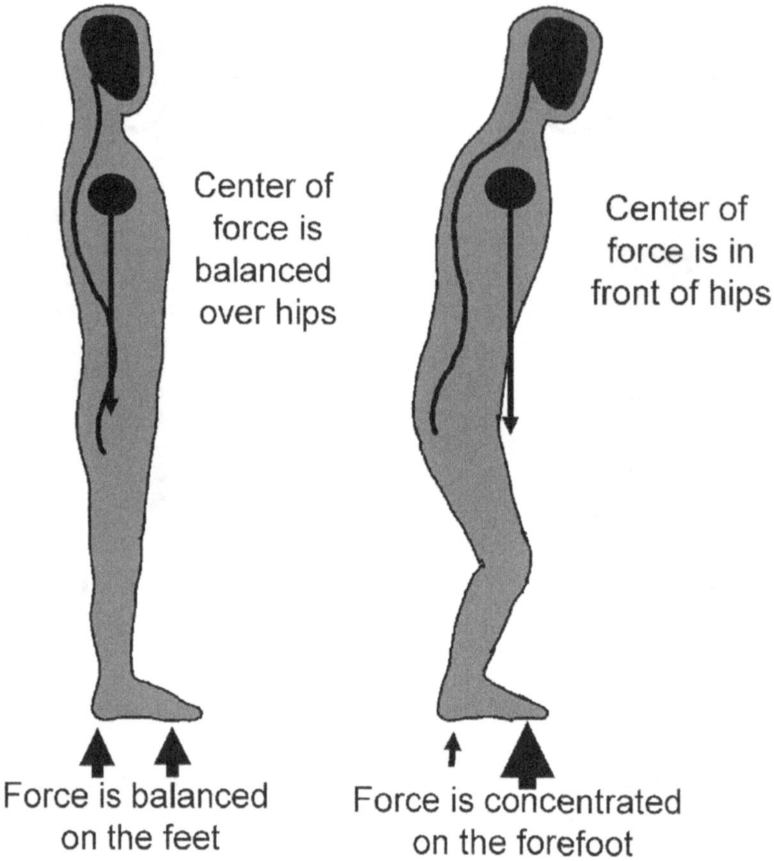

FIGURE 2.6 The forward shift of the center of weight with poor posture.

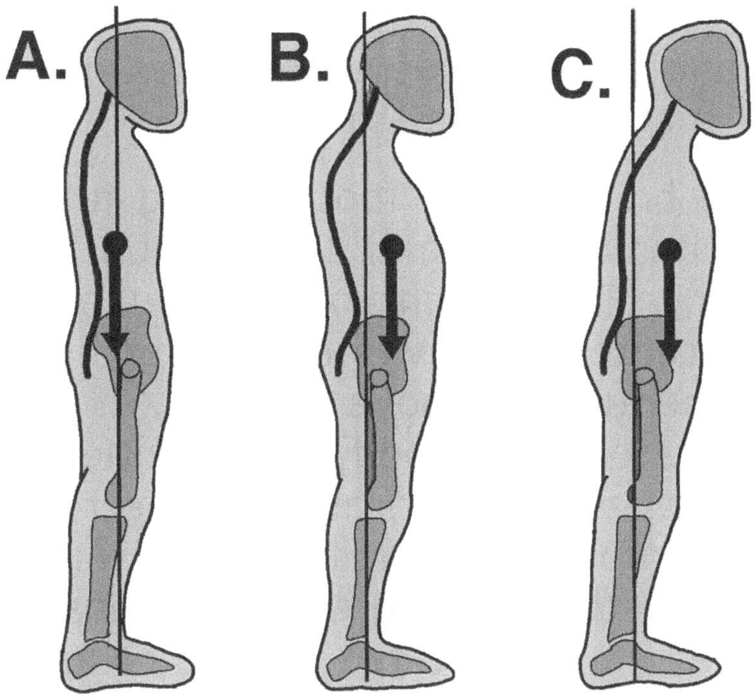

FIGURE 2.7 Comparison of center of weight between balanced posture (7a), poor posture due to abdominal and lumbar deconditioning (7b), and slouching (7c).

Although it is difficult to illustrate, posture is important when walking and even running. The posture problems mentioned above rotate the pelvis backward. This changes the position of the hip joint so that it is more difficult to fully flex the hip and take a complete step, placing the heel securely on the floor. The gait that results is shuffling or lumbering. Although many times a person's gait appears normal to the casual observer and the person walking may not be aware of it, a small departure from a healthy gait can have adverse effects on the foot over a long period of time. Contact between the floor and the heel decreases during the stride as a consequence. The length of time and the amount of pressure on the forefoot during the step increases and the forefoot experiences more pressure, which can make it prone to injury.

Additionally, bringing the foot and leg fully in front of the body when initiating a step, helps to propel the body forward. The weight of the leg and the slight drop in the center of gravity that occur helps the body use its momentum to move forward. If the center of mass is forward of our body, as mentioned earlier, a full step is not as easy because of the rotation of the pelvis. To compensate for this and for the loss of momentum, a thrust from the calf muscles through the heel may be substituted at the conclusion of the step. People who do this appear to spring at the end of the step. This is very stressful to the forefoot.

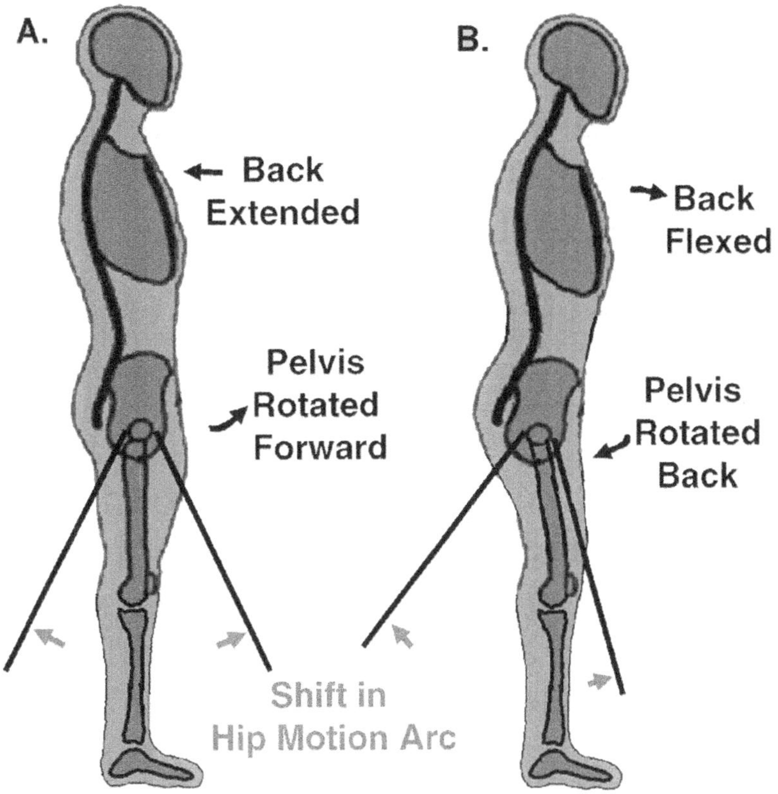

FIGURE 2.8 Fairly subtle loss of posture resulting from slouching, and rotation of the pelvis backward changes the position of the hip joint such that a full step is more difficult. The lines signifying the hip motion during a step are maintained in a constant position relative to the pelvis. Rotation of the pelvis with poor posture shifts the arc so that weight is borne by the forefoot more than with proper posture.

Finally, forefoot overload can occur by altering the cadence or rhythm of our gait. Often, people feel the need to walk much faster than is natural. The leg can be thought of as a pendulum. Every pendulum has a cadence that is related to its length, which causes it to swing at a specific rate. That is why Grandfather clocks are able to measure time. Any attempt to change the cadence of a pendulum requires extra energy. If one tries to hurry the steps in a gait, it requires extra work. This work is supplied by the large muscles in the leg and occurs in the end or "push-off" portion of the step. This extra force can overwork the connective tissue of the foot.

AGING, THE PLANTAR SKIN, AND FOREFOOT OVERLOAD

Changes occur in all parts of the body as we age. Some of the changes affect the foot and posture. General muscular deconditioning that occurs as the result of inactivity and aging can lead to worsening posture. The muscles that extend the foot up seem to become weaker faster than the larger muscles such as the Achilles that flex the foot down. This can worsen forefoot overload by altering the balance of these structures. This is not an inevitable part of aging, however, and can be treated through conditioning and training.

Several years ago, shoe companies began to market shoes that had air pockets within the soles to cushion the foot. Even today, running shoes are manufactured with air cushions. These air pockets become pressurized when loaded and help to distribute pressure across the sole and decrease the shock of initial foot strike. The inspiration behind this actually comes from the natural design of the skin in the sole of the foot. Fat globules within the sole of the foot are separated into compartments by connective tissue.

As the skin is pressurized, the globules of fat become rigid and distribute the weight more evenly across the surface of the foot. This process keeps the bones of the front of the foot from concentrating pressure directly on a small portion of the skin. In fact, the heel pad reduces the maximum impact to the heel about twice as well as Sorbothane, a common commercial shoe sole material. If the heel pad did not do this, the pressure under bony prominences would be very high and uneven directly underneath the bones of the ball of the foot and heel, causing pain and calluses.

Also, as the foot ages, the skin in the foot, as well as elsewhere on the body, thins. The fat directly underneath the skin also begins to waste away. This reduces the ability of the skin and the specially designed structures within the tissue to disperse weight and pressure, much the way that the shoe would not work as well if the air pockets developed leaks. The direct pressure on the bones in the front of the foot—especially the metatarsal heads in the ball of the foot—is not dispersed, increasing the pressure and stress on the bones and joints as well as sometimes causing painful calluses.

Aging connective tissues like ligaments and tendons are less able to resist repetitive stress and fail with less stress. Aging ligaments do not have as much elasticity or ability to store energy as younger ligaments. The natural stretch of a ligament allows the tissue to absorb energy more gradually in a younger person, much as a shock absorber on a car keeps it from transferring the energy from the bumps that you run over directly into the passenger compartment of the car. When the ligaments become stiffer, the energy is transferred more directly to the tissue and jars it suddenly. This increases the potential for injury, including repetitive-use injuries. This partially explains why the foot can handle poor gait habits when you're young, but not in the later years.

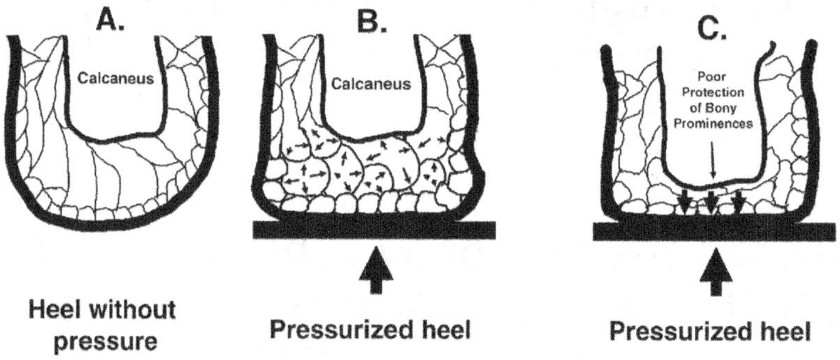

FIGURE 2.9 The effect of loss of fat under the skin lessens the ability of the sole of the foot to absorb and redistribute pressure. Although the heel is illustrated here, the same process occurs in the ball of the foot.

THE POSITIVE SIDE

Although this may sound gloomy, especially if it is your foot that hurts, the good news is that there are effective ways to counteract and treat many of these problems. Even though it is impossible to reverse aging and the damage that our lifelong activities have dealt to the structures within our feet completely, good posture and walking habits can reduce the continuing damage and pain. This can maximize our body's natural ability to heal and repair itself. In this way, we can effectively treat many types of foot problem.

In the rehabilitation chapter of this book, there are exercises and drills that, when done regularly, will help to develop healthy posture and walking habits. The alterations that occur when people change their posture, improves their flexibility, and become conscious of their feet and the way that they use them will get them on the road to recovery. Selecting shoes that reduce the stress to your feet can assist in this and is also covered in the resources. This is not a goal that can be achieved in a day. The problem developed over years of use. The exercises will lead to gradual improvement over a sustained period of time. Some new scientific evidence suggests that exercise may also help a number of other overuse problems such as low back pain, hip bursitis, and kneecap pain. It should be a start to a lifetime of excellent posture and pain-free feet and legs.

MARILYN'S STORY

Marilyn is a 58-year-old woman, a homemaker with a four-year history of constant left and right foot pain. The pain radiates throughout her foot from the heel to the ball of the foot. The top of her foot is so sensitive that she has difficulty wearing shoes with laces. She states that she is nearly unable to walk without a shoe with a "good arch." Lately, the front of her foot has been swelling on the left.

Marilyn has tenderness in the ball of the foot especially along the bottom of her second and third metatarsal heads as well as along the top of her arch area near the tarsometatarsal and naviculocunieform joints (two large joints near the arch). Her foot flexibility is otherwise normal. Both of her second toes slightly overlap the great toe. Stressing the midfoot joints in her arch causes her pain. When asked to stand on one foot, she sways and falls to the other side. When asked to bend over and touch the floor while keeping her knees straight, she is unable to place her fingertips beyond the midshin. She is tender on the lateral aspects of both of her hips and at the patellofemoral joints. She is otherwise moderately overweight with a protuberant abdomen.

The x-rays of both of her feet show mild arthritis along the top of the midfoot joints as well as having abnormally long second metatarsals (the toe bone in the ball of the foot that connects to the second toe) in comparison to the first and third. The slight tilting of the second toes are represented in x-rays but no further arthritis is seen.

Marilyn was instructed on the cause of her pain, forefoot overload syndrome, as well as the various problems that contribute to it. She was educated on selection of rocker-soled shoes and given initial stretching exercises. An inexpensive over-the-counter cushioning orthotic was prescribed. She was given a referral to a physical therapist who instructed her on some basic stretching and hip-, back-, and foot-conditioning exercises. In addition to this, advice was given on weight loss.

At four weeks, she was still working on the weight loss, but she felt that her pain was much improved.

Marilyn's clinical presentation is typical of forefoot overload with many separate areas of pain along the structures that support the forefoot when pressure is transferred in this area. She also has several other diagnoses common in people who have lost conditioning significantly. An initial surgical approach to these problems would be a disaster. Not only would it increase her tendency to concentrate her weight on the forefoot, because most people almost routinely do this postoperatively, it would treat the symptoms while leaving the underlying problem ignored. Even if initially successful, a further forefoot overload problem would be likely eventually.

NOTES

[1] Zammit GV, Menz HB, Munteanu SE, Landorf KB. Plantar pressure distribution in older people with osteoarthritis of the first metatarsophalangeal joint (hallux limitus/rigidus). J Orthop Res. 2008 Dec;26(12):1665–9.

[2] Riddle DL, Pulisic M, Pidcoe P, Johnson RE. Risk factors for Plantar fasciitis: a matched case-control study. J Bone Joint Surg Am. 2003 May;85-A(5):872–7.

[3] Irving DB, Cook JL, Menz HB. Factors associated with chronic plantar heel pain: a systematic review. J Sci Med Sport. 2006 May;9(1–2):11–22.

[4] Mickle KJ, Munro BJ, Lord SR, Menz HB, Steele JR. Foot pain, plantar pressures, and falls in older people: a prospective study. J Am Geriatr Soc. 2010 Oct;58(10):1936–40.

[5] Karadag-Saygi E, Unlu-Ozkan F, Basgul A. Plantar pressure and foot pain in the last trimester of pregnancy. Foot Ankle Int. 2010 Feb;31(2):153–7.

[6] van der Leeden M, Steultjens M, Dekker JH, Prins AP, Dekker J. Forefoot joint damage, pain and disability in rheumatoid arthritis patients with foot complaints: the role of plantar pressure and gait characteristics. Rheumatology (Oxford). 2006 Apr;45(4):465–9.

3

The Big Toe

Pain and problems with the big toe are some of the most well-known foot disorders. It is important to understand the main structures of the big toe before we discuss the potential problems.

ANATOMY

There are five metatarsal bones that compose the bony support of the forefoot that extends nearly parallel to one another from the arch to the ball of the foot. At the ends of these bones are the metatarsal heads that are the weight-bearing portion of the ball of the foot. Your big toe has two bones, the proximal and distal phalanx. The proximal phalanx of the big toe forms a joint with its metatarsal head called the metatarsophalangeal (MTP) joint. The tarsal bones are near the ankle and form a joint with the base of the metatarsal called the tarsometatarsal (TMT) joint.

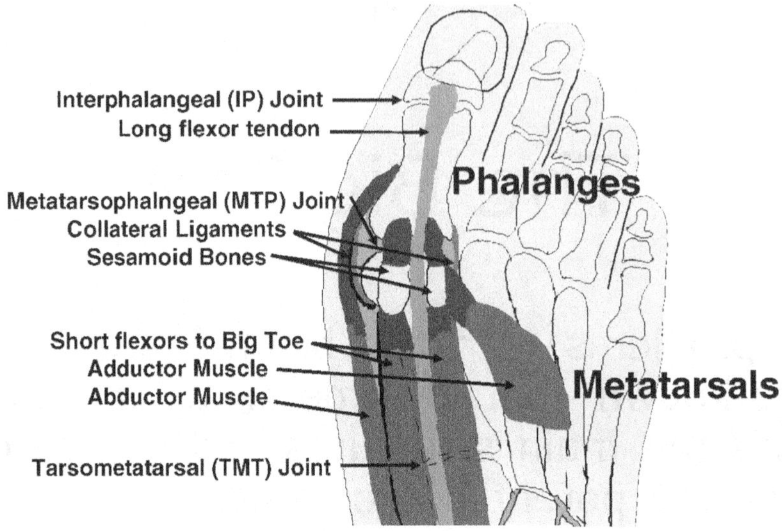

FIGURE 3.1 Major anatomical structures of the bottom of the foot.

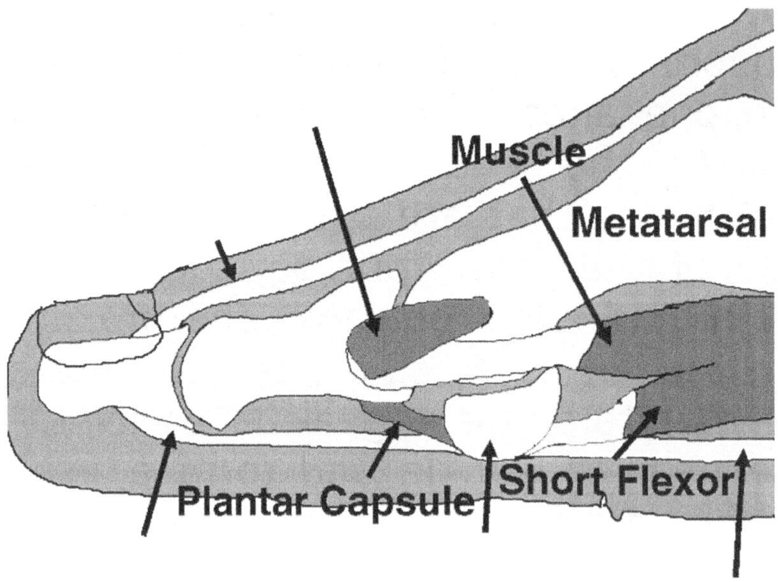

FIGURE 3.2 Major anatomical structures of the big toe.

Two bones are directly under the metatarsal head of the big toe called *sesamoid bones.* Each of these bones forms a groove-like joint on the bottom of the metatarsal head. The sesamoid bones are attached to a small muscle in the arch that act to move the toe toward the sole of the foot, the short flexor of the big toe. The relationship of the sesamoid bone to the toe is similar to the relationship of the kneecap to the knee. An additional muscle attaches to the outer sesamoid and acts to pull the toe to the outside of the foot. A muscle attaches to the inside of the proximal phalanx and counteracts forces pulling the toe to the inside, balancing the big toe on the end of the metatarsal head.

The tendons from the longer muscles of the big toe attach to the distal phalanx on the top and bottom of the big toe to flex and extend the end joint. Normally these tendons lie in the midline of the toe on the top and bottom. However, if the toe begins to drift off its axis, the tendons may deviate away from this centered position and become deformed.

BUNIONS

- A bunion is a bump on the inside of the big toe caused by instability of the big toe joint ligaments.

- Usually, the pain from a bunion is caused by pressure of the shoe against the prominence.

- Adolescent bunions develop in childhood. Other bunions can develop gradually in adulthood.

- Although little can be done to straighten the toe nonsurgically, choosing shoes that fit the width and shape of the foot and are flexible enough to stretch over the prominence can help with the discomfort of a bunion.

- Bunionectomy is a serious surgical procedure designed to correct the bunion. It has a significant recovery and a risk of complications. The decision to have a bunionectomy should be made based on significant pain and difficulty with comfortable shoe wear.

Bunions are probably the first things that most people think of when they think of problems around the big toe. When a bunion is present, the big toe looks like it has a big growth on its side. The prominence that you see on the inside of the foot is the end of the first metatarsal along with potentially some soft tissue irritation from rubbing on the shoe. Although "growths" of extra bone sometimes add to it, the most common cause for the bump is that the end of the big toe has slipped outward over the metatarsal, uncovering and projecting the end of metatarsal bone inward, toward the other foot.

Another term for a bunion is *hallux valgus.* Hallux is the medical word for the big toe. Valgus describes the toe position, drifting away from the midline of the body, a key feature of the bunion.

The most common pain caused from a bunion is felt along the prominence of the joint on the inside of the foot. If pain occurs in another part of the toe, another cause should be considered to explain the pain. The pain is usually greatest with shoe wear and the tighter the shoe, the greater the pain. Sandals, flip-flops, loose fitting shoes, or going barefoot may offer some relief.

Some people have had a bunion deformity since they were children. These are called *adolescent bunions.* These bunions are hereditary and form because the body's genetics have instructed the foot to develop a bunion.

Most bunions are acquired bunions. In an acquired bunion, the joint and the toe were, at one time, straighter and slipped out of place later. So why did this happen? Stable joints at both the TMT and MTP joints are important for maintaining proper alignment of the big toe. The ligaments supporting these joints need to be of proper length and tension to control the joints while allowing the joints to move freely. Age, medical problems such as rheumatoid arthritis, shoe wear, and improper usage can cause the ligaments to wear, stretch, and tear, disturbing this balance.

Bunions are more common in populations of people who wear shoes. Painful bunions occur in people who wear shoes that do not fit properly. Continual pressure from shoe wear contributes to molding the foot into a deviated position. Once this starts, it tends to worsen slowly over the years.

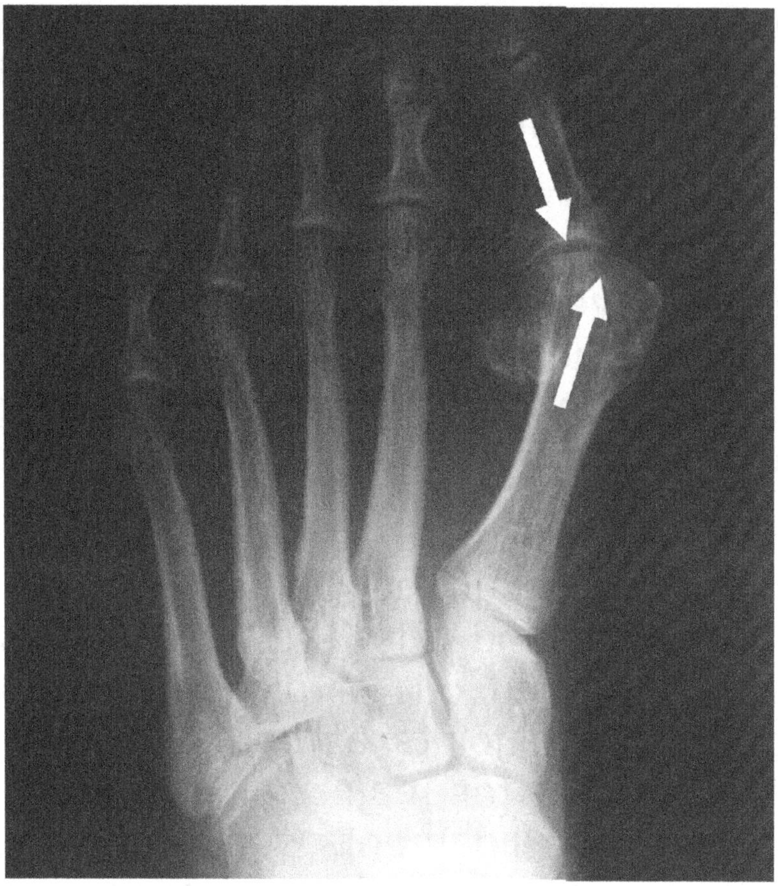

FIGURE 3.3 X-ray of an acquired bunion. This toe was once correctly aligned, but now the opposing surfaces of the MTP joint point in different directions.

Much of the risk of developing bunions is hereditary. A genetic predisposition toward the formation of bunions is common. People often say, "I inherited my mother's (or father's) feet." The inherited qualities that may contribute to the development of bunions include the architecture of the joints and the mechanical strength and resilience of the ligaments.

Women develop bunions more commonly than men. Although women's fashionable shoe wear is undoubtedly partially to blame, consider also that women develop deformities of the hands and other joints more frequently than men. The hormonal influences and other genetic differences in the bodies of men and women affect the ligaments of all joints causing a variety of joint-instability problems, including bunions and other foot deformities. Other underlying medical conditions that may lead to bunions such as rheumatoid arthritis and a host of other related inflammatory conditions that weaken the ligament are nearly all more common in women.

It is surprising how many people attribute their big toe pain to bunions even when no deformity is present. Even in the presence of a significant bunion, the possibility of other more subtle causes of pain around the big toe should be considered or any treatment directed toward the bunion may fail. Other things that can cause pain around the great toe are:

- Arthritis of the big toe joint.
- Irritation of the sesamoid bones.
- Gout.
- Other joint inflammatory conditions such as rheumatoid arthritis.

The most important part of nonoperative treatment is to put the bunion in perspective. The presence of a bunion does not mean that an operation is inevitable. Bunion surgery is a serious decision and many people who undergo the surgery are not prepared for the pain, and the lengthy and inconvenient recovery. Complications, dissatisfaction, and recurrence are common. If the bunion does become more severe, it is uncommon for the worsening of the bunion to obligate a significantly more involved form of surgical reconstruction. Surgery for bunions can therefore be safely delayed until it becomes a painful enough problem to warrant surgery. Changes in bunions usually form over a period of years and, therefore, aggressive treatment is almost never an urgent matter.

Many people are concerned that the bunion should be surgically corrected when they are younger because, as they get older, it may be more difficult to undergo the surgery. However, bunions usually become less of a concern with advancing age. Often, older people select shoes that are more comfortable and they are less active. Rarely does an infirm elderly person who is too sick or weak to undergo surgery have debilitating pain because of a bunion.

Central to the treatment of bunions without surgery is to find shoes that fit properly. Although the cause of a bunion may not be shoe wear, one key to making the bunion comfortable is sensible, comfortable shoe wear selection. Fitting an EEE foot into a D-width shoe is a recipe for pain. One exercise that is commonly recommended is to place a bare foot on a plain piece of paper and outline the foot. Then take the shoe and place it over the outline. Any portion of the foot that lies outside of the shoe imprint is going to have pressure on it and will be painful if pressed on long and hard enough. Shoes should be selected that fit the shape of the foot.

Flattened arches perpetuate some bunions. When the arch is flattened, the toe rotates so that the weight of the body weakens and stretches the inside ligament of the big toe. In people who have flexible but flat arches, an arch support is often helpful in lessening bunion pain. But arch support is not helpful the majority of the time. Usually, a noncustom, over-the-counter arch support is less expensive and nearly as effective as a custom arch support. The arch support should not be so high that it causes a lumpy sensation in the arch. When buying shoes, a better fit is possible if the shoes are fitted with the arch support. Most effective arch supports take some room within the shoe and this can make the upper of the shoe snug. It is helpful to select a style of shoes that has a liner or insert within the shoe that is removable, so that the liner can be removed to allow more room within the shoe for the arch support. The laces should be completely loosened before fitting the foot into the shoe after placement of the arch support.

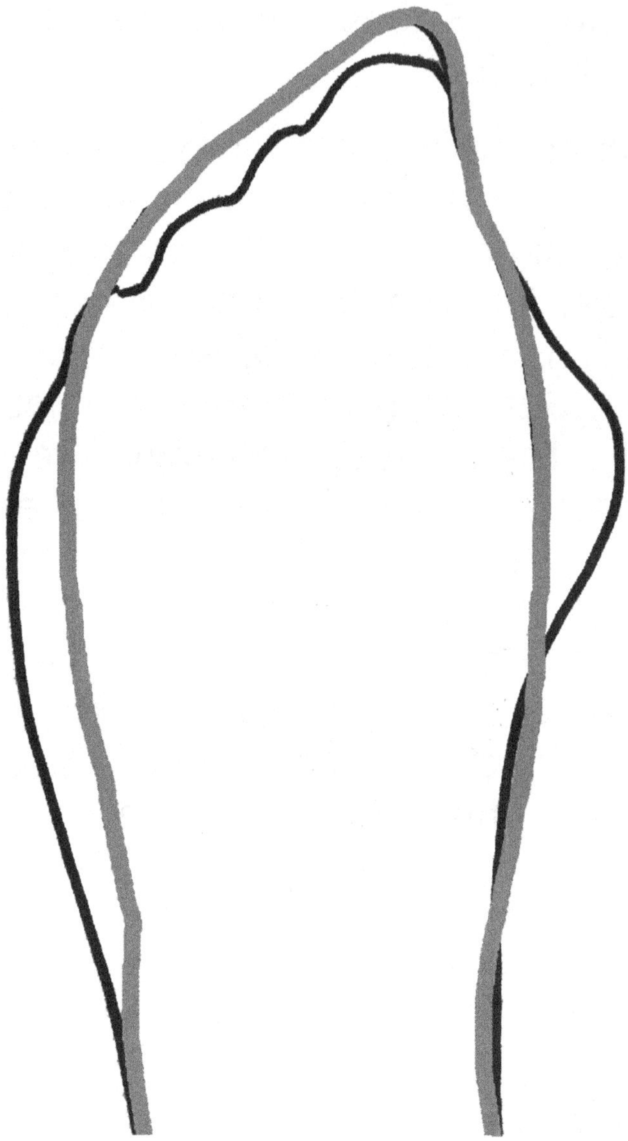

FIGURE 3.4 An outline of a foot (black) with a bunion superimposed on an outline of the shoe (gray). Note: The bunion prominence and prominence along the fifth toe must be pressed on in order for the shoe to accommodate the foot.

Many commonly suggested bunion devices do not help. Toe spacers are almost never effective in correcting the deformity. In a shoe that is already challenged with space limitations, the volume of the spacer generally makes the snug shoe tighter. The one time that spacers are helpful is in the treatment of painful corns from pressure between the big toe and the second toe.

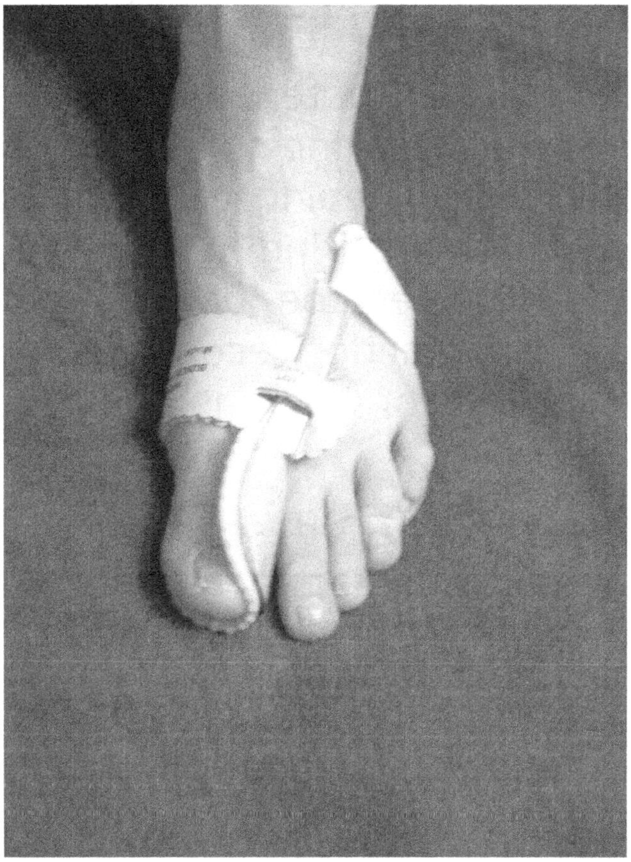

FIGURE 3.5 Commercially available bunion splints are generally ineffective and impractical for routine usage.

Numerous corrective splints, some of them quite creative, have been developed that, for the most part, are not practical or effective. Night splints are also of little help. Therapeutic exercises are of limited or no benefit.

The decision to proceed to surgical reconstruction should be based on the failure of nonoperative methods to control the pain. Although you need to look attractive and professional, very high heels or uncomfortable shoes are not required. Often changing to shoes made with extra width in the toe area, made with compliant leather material, with heels limited to one to one-and-a-half inch, should allow for an acceptable look while keeping the pain at bay. If pain is still present when wearing sensible pumps, switch to flats, and a roomier toe box may be necessary. Cosmetic or prophylactic reconstruction of bunion deformities or repair of bunions that are not painful is not advised.

There are more than 150 described operations in the medical literature to correct a bunion. Why so many? Because in planning a bunion correction, many factors have to be weighed to permit the best restoration of the joint, while minimizing the severity and complications associated with the surgery. Another reason is that none of the surgeries is without pitfalls.

We're not going to describe all 150 bunion operations, you should just know that most involve two steps. The first is to realign the metatarsal bone, MTP joint, and phalanges of the toe through osteotomy (cutting and repositioning the bone) or fusion (eliminating a joint and allow the bones on either side of the joint to heal together like a fracture does). Often metallic or dissolvable plastic fixation devices like screws, pins, and plates are used to stabilize the bony corrections while they heal. The second is to rebalance the ligaments especially around the MTP joint to reposition the toe. This is done by tightening the ligaments on the inside of the joint and loosening the ligaments on the outside of the joint.

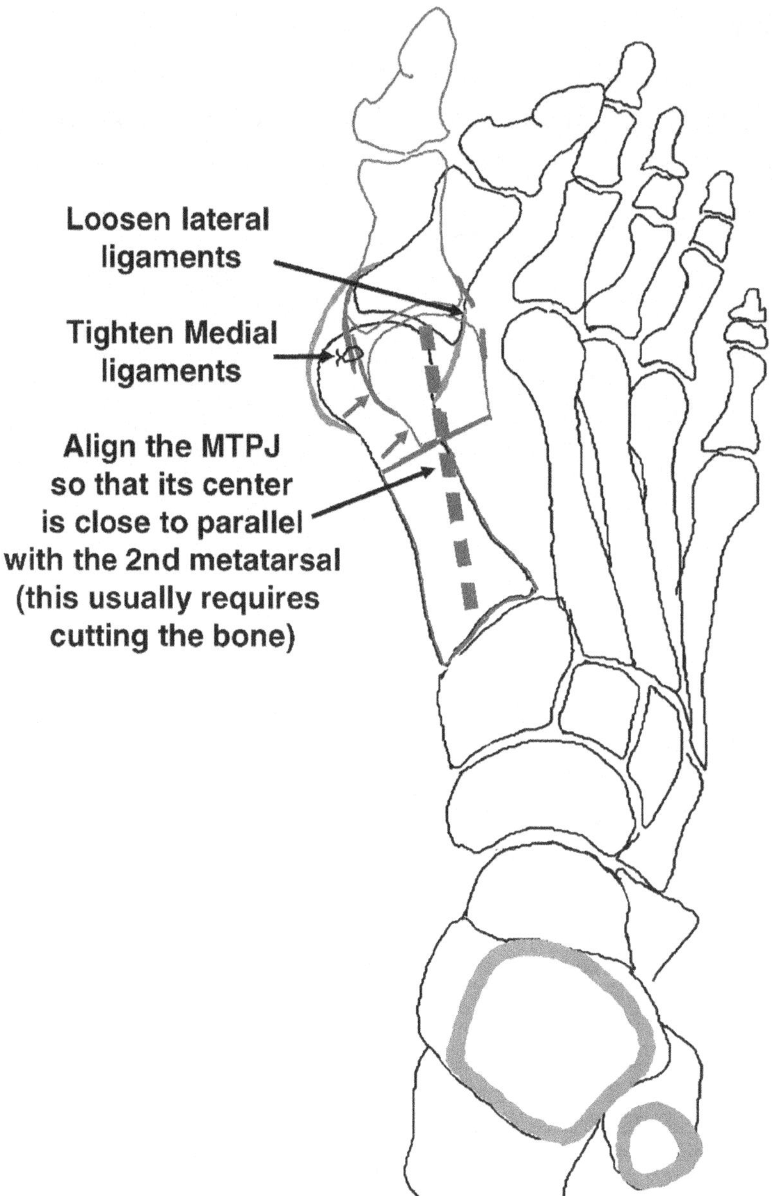

FIGURE 3.6 A bunion reconstruction involves repositioning the MTP joint so that it points in line with the foot and is a normal distance from the remainder of the foot. The ligaments around the joint need to be re-tensioned to accomplish this.

It is normal after surgery to have pain that requires narcotics. Swelling is one of the most nagging symptoms and can take months to gradually resolve. Wearing a shoe may be difficult during this time. Often the toe is wrapped for several weeks to protect the repair from stress or injury.

Even after successful reconstruction, it is common for the toe to lose some of its flexibility. Usually the loss of motion is mild but may be troublesome for athletes. Bunion surgery in avid long-distance runners should be considered carefully. Joggers may become frustrated giving the bunion a proper period of time to heal (sometimes four months or more) before returning to running. Areas of joint injury such as along the sesamoids on the bottom of the foot may remain uncomfortable even after successful reconstruction. The goal of bunion reconstruction is to allow comfortable wear of reasonable shoes. Even after surgery, heels may still be uncomfortable.

Sensory nerves lie at every quadrant of the big toe. Damage to any of these will lead to numbness, most commonly over the top and inside of the toe. Sometimes the damaged nerve can become intensely painful. Fortunately, this is rare and usually clears with time, but in a few cases becomes permanent and can be disabling.

MARLA'S STORY

Marla, a 52-year-old secretary, came into the office to discuss her bunion. She was wearing modest pumps and said that the inside portion of her big toe was becoming uncomfortable in her shoes. She had noticed prominences along the insides of her feet for years. Now, at the end of the day, she couldn't wait to get home and slip off her shoes. She was an avid recreational runner and had a slight amount of pain while wearing her running shoes. She had seen a doctor 15 years ago about her feet and surgery was recommended. However, the foot did not hurt much at the time and she was really too busy then raising her young children to have surgery.

Marla's feet are shown below. She has a big toe that tilts toward the outside of her foot. The metatarsal bone also points toward the inside. This creates an abrupt angular prominence along the inside border of her foot, which presses against the upper part of her shoe. She also has a hammertoe of her second toe, a deformity commonly seen along with a bunion.

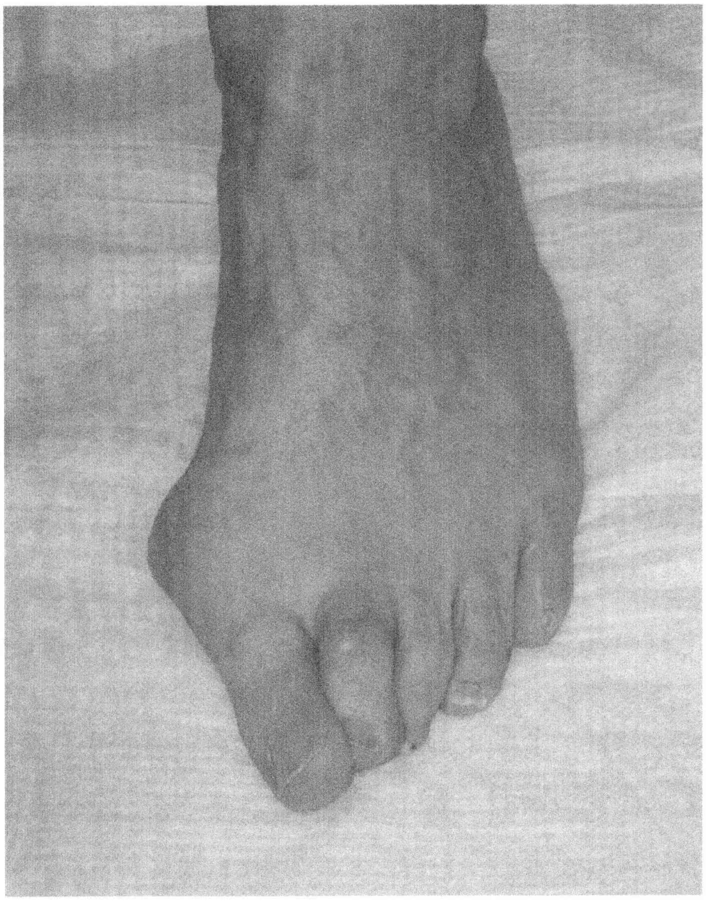

FIGURE 3.7 A photograph of Marla's bunion.

Marla said she was expected to present a professional appearance at work and felt obligated to wear fashionable shoes. She usually wore high heels, partly because she is five feet two inches tall and feels short in flats. She was also concerned with the possibility of the bunion worsening to the point that the surgery may be much more severe and that if she waited she would be "too old" to have the surgery.

We told her that many people continue to be unable to wear the snug, constrictive shoe wear often popular with business people (even men) after bunion surgery. We also discussed the stress that is placed on the front of the foot in a shoe with significant heel that may damage the healing bunion. After discovering the prolonged recuperation and swelling common after bunion surgery, Marla decided to delay surgery until the bunion became worse.

ARTHRITIS OF THE BIG TOE

- Osteoarthritis of the MTP joint is a common painful condition of the big toe.
- The joint characteristically wears on the top. This suggests that connective tissue contractures may act to shear the cartilage as the toe is extended at the end of the step.
- It usually causes stiffness especially in extension of the joint, tenderness, and a bump primarily on the top of the joint.
- Osteoarthritis of the MTP joint can be treated with rehabilitative exercises, stiff, rocker-soled shoes, and analgesics (such as Motrin or Aleve).
- A variety of operative options exist to treat the pain.

Arthritis means *inflammation of a joint,* but the term is used to describe a joint that is wearing out. The joint cartilage that gives the joint a smooth friction-free surface becomes worn and damaged. The most common type of arthritis is osteoarthritis, caused by wear and tear. Other types of arthritis such as rheumatoid arthritis and gout are different and are discussed elsewhere in this book.

The joint in the big toe that is most commonly affected by arthritis is the MTP joint, commonly thought of as the joint where the bunion occurs. Common signs of arthritis are pain, stiffness, and swelling. The symptoms are often confused with gout and bunions, the other big toe ailments with which many people are familiar. Often the pain occurs on the initiation of activity or with prolonged or intense activity. In general, arthritis progresses over a period of years, but the rate of progression is variable and the amount of pain is difficult to predict even after evaluating the x-rays.

In the big toe, osteoarthritis begins on the top portion of the joint, which eventually causes deformity and spurs that increasingly limit motion and enlarge the joint. As the problem progresses, the joint becomes increasing stiff and the pain increases. The pain is greatest at the end of the step when the joint is extended the most and weight is transferred onto the front of the foot. Some people begin to walk on the outside border of the foot to adjust to the limitation and pain at the big toe. This often causes the pain to seem to shift to the outside border of the foot. The stride of someone with big toe arthritis is frequently shortened to avoid coming up on the ball of the foot.

No one knows for sure why osteoarthritis of the big toe occurs, although there are many theories. Certainly, a great deal of the rate of wear is genetically determined, because it is often seen in both feet and many people who have osteoarthritis of the hallux and can remember relatives who had similar problems. Many genetic qualities about the foot can influence the development of osteoarthritis, including the shape of the bones of the joint and the mechanical qualities of the bone.

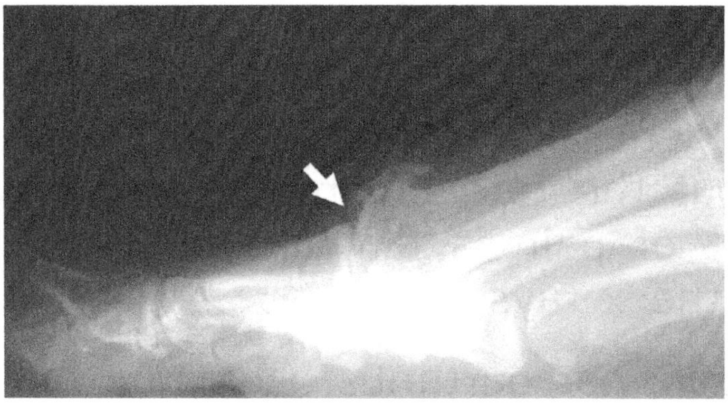

FIGURE 3.8 Lateral x-ray of arthritic MTP joint. The cartilage of the joint at the top of the toe is worn and a large spur has formed (white arrow).

The shape of the joint can limit the amount of play in the joint. If a joint is not able to move from side to side easily, then it is more likely to be damaged when everyday activities push the joint and shear the joint cartilage. Specifically, a flat or wedge-shape joint surface at the end of the metatarsal will limit the play within the joint and can cause damage when the joint is pushed to the side. This peculiar shape is a common finding in people with osteoarthritis of the big toe.

The hardness of the bone is another genetically influenced factor that likely determines how much the joint is beaten up and wears over time. A certain amount of sponginess protects the cartilage of the joint from sudden impacts. Certain people with congenital bone disorders that cause hard bones are known to have early arthritis in many joints. This has not been specifically studied in the MTP joint of the big toe, but we have seen many patients with MTP arthritis who have arthritis in multiple other joints.

Trauma can rarely accelerate osteoarthritis, but it is typical for arthritic joints to be prone to injury and, therefore, slight injuries are often blamed for the arthritis. The slightest overextension or abnormal twist of the joint can make an arthritic joint uncomfortable for a prolonged time. Small injuries that would not cause a nonarthritic joint to become painful might be very painful to a person in the intermediate stages of osteoarthritis. Although a fracture or ligament injury can begin a path toward a prematurely worn-out joint, this is probably uncommon.

Ligament or tendon tightness can also have an effect and may possibly be the most important underlying problem. The plantar fascia is a ligament that connects the heel of the foot to the base of the proximal phalanx on the bottom of the great toe. Although a specific defect has not been conclusively linked to the development of MTP arthritis, mechanical studies indicate that plantar fascial tightness may be a reasonable explanation for the wear pattern.[1]

Contractures of structures on the bottom of the MTP joint could cause restriction of extension of the joint. As a result, the proximal phalanx will dig into the cartilage at the top of the joint on the metatarsal head. This causes the cartilage surfaces to shear, destroying the cartilage leading to arthritis.

Other diagnoses should be considered when osteoarthritis is suspected. These other diagnoses are usually easy to differentiate from arthritis from the distribution of the tenderness and pattern of the pain. Other explanations for the pain in this joint include:

- Gout.
- Stress fracture.
- Bunion.
- Sesamoiditis, which is when the sesamoid bones—the two round densities overlapping the metatarsal head on the top view of the foot—are irritated.

Specialized diagnostic tests such as bone scans and CT scans are not usually necessary. If the radiographs are normal, then other types of joint damage may be suspected. MRI may be necessary to visualize these unusual problems and plan for surgical reconstruction. MRI is not usually necessary in cases of straightforward big toe arthritis.

Surgery is not the initial treatment of great toe arthritis. Antiinflammatory medication such as naproxen

(Aleve®), ibuprofen (Motrin®), celecoxib (Celebrex®), and other pain medications such as acetaminophen (Tylenol®) can effectively decrease the pain while they are being taken, but do not cure the arthritis. Oral medications composed of natural joint components such as glucosamine and chondroitan sulfate are shown in some studies to give temporary relief in the knee and have few side effects. No information is available specifically for the MTP joint of the big toe, but we would expect a similar mildly positive, pain-relieving effect in the MTP joint. Use of these medications should be discontinued unless considerable pain improvement is experienced within two weeks.

Osteoarthritis of the MTP joint is aggravated by any activity that forces the joint into extension. To decrease the pain, strategies that limit the motion of the joint are effective. One method of accomplishing this is to buy a shoe that limits this motion of the foot while walking. The simplest method is to purchase a rocker-soled shoe, also known as toners that are available in commercial shoe stores. The thickness of the sole makes it very stiff. The contour of the sole also allows the foot to roll over the toes without extending them. However, walking in rocker-soled shoes can often aggravate other parts of the body or make you feel off balance and you can even fall. If this is the case, using another less aggressive, stiff shoe may work. A steel or graphite stiffener can be built into another shoe and may change the use of the toe enough to make normal activity tolerable.

Heels of any height should be avoided because they will force the joint into extension. Simple noncustom arch supports are useful on occasion.

If the pain doesn't respond or flares in intensity, a physician could inject steroid medication into the joint. These are potent medications that can stop the production of inflammatory chemicals that the body produces when injured. Steroids give prolonged pain relief, but they also have a number of serious side effects. The improvement after steroid injection is usually temporary, as the injection does nothing to fix it.

Surgical treatment can be considered if you have tried many nonoperative measures first. The choice of surgical procedure is dictated by the degree of arthritis. Removal of the arthritic spurs on the top of the joint is called *cheilectomy.* It can free the motion of the joint and decrease the bulk of the joint. Despite the limited nature of this surgery, full recovery can take four to six months. However, you could be on your feet as soon as the pain allows.

More severe arthritis calls for more extensive intervention. The choices include an implant arthroplasty, resection of some of the bone, and fusion. In a fusion, the cartilage and hard bone immediately beneath the joint is removed and the surfaces are pressed together until they heal together. The metatarsal and the proximal phalanx are made into a single joint, eliminating the joint, the motion, and the pain. This requires stabilization of the bones with plates, screws, or pins. Healing can take 6 to 12 weeks. Avoiding ambulation and weight on the big toe is crucial during this period. Joint mobility at the MTP joint is completely eliminated, so that when buying shoes, close attention to heel height and room in the toe box is usually necessary to avoid pressure on the toe.

Resection arthroplasty is the removal of the arthritic joint and replacement of the joint with parts of the joint capsule or soft tissue from another area of the body. This preserves motion, but the pain relief is sometimes not reliable.

In implant arthroplasty or joint replacement, the joint is replaced with a metal or plastic device. Certainly, implant joint replacement procedures have been successful in the knee and hip. However, there has been some concern about loosening of these implants over time and a high reoperation rate has been reported recently.

Overall, approximately 80% to 90% of people undergoing these procedures report good results.

MARION'S STORY

Marion is a 58-year-old restaurant manager who developed pain in her big toe over the past two years. She noticed the pain especially when placing pans and dishes on the top shelves when she came up on her tiptoes or went up stairs or inclines. She also was unable to wear high-heeled shoes for the past year. She assumed that she had a bunion because of the enlargement of the MTP joint. She cannot move the toe in an arc of more than 20 degrees.

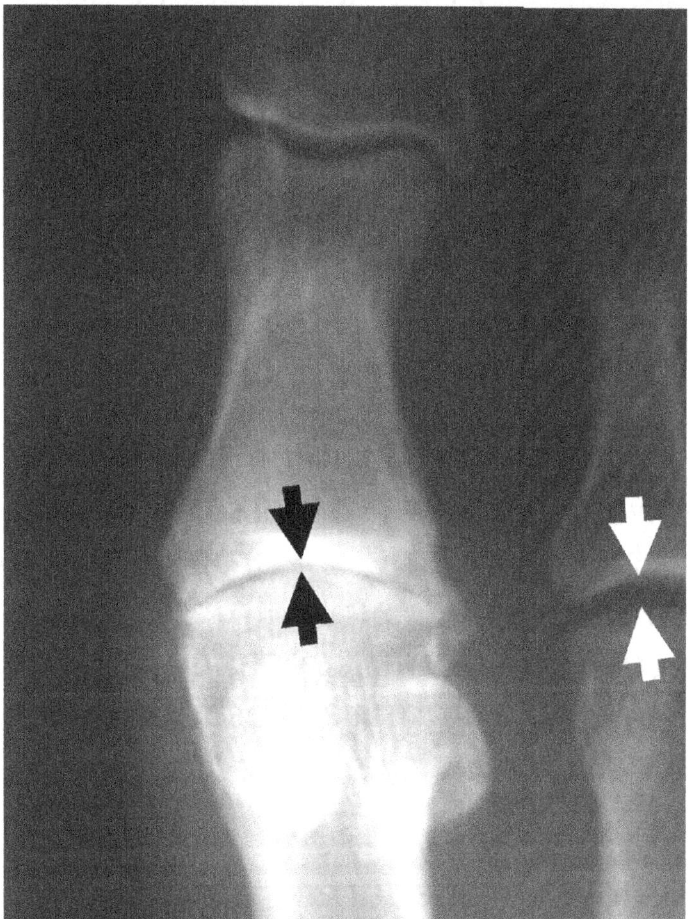

FIGURE 3.9 View of x-ray of big toe MTP arthritis from the top. The space between the joint surfaces of the big toe joint is narrow (black arrows) in comparison to the MTP joint of the second toe (white arrows). This suggests severe destruction of the cartilage in the joint.

X-rays showed the big toe MTP joint to be severely worn in comparison to the MTP joint of the second toe.

Simple stretching exercises to stretch the Achilles tendon and hamstrings were recommended to Marion. In addition, rocker-soled shoes were suggested. This helped immediately with the pain when we saw her four weeks later. Eventually, the arthritis may progress or become painful enough to warrant more aggressive surgical reconstruction. Surgery should be delayed this until the discomfort makes it necessary.

GOUT

- Gout is a disorder caused by the accumulation of too much uric acid in the body.
- The diagnosis is proven by the presence of uric acid crystals in joint fluid under microscopic examination.
- There is a strong genetic predisposition to gout and treatment of repeated gout attacks should be lifelong in the absence of an otherwise correctable cause.
- Initial treatment includes hydration, and anti-inflammatory medications such as colchicine, steroids, and nonsteroidal anti-inflammatory medications such as naproxen or ibuprofen. When properly treated, gout attacks should resolve within a couple of days.

- Long-term treatment involves slight dietary changes and medications that enhance the excretion of the uric acid or prevent its production by the body.

Gout is a disorder caused by the abnormal metabolism of purines, a component of DNA, the genetic material within our cells. When the body breaks down these substances, uric acid is formed and released in the bloodstream. Uric acid is a fairly nonreactive substance that can be excreted by the kidneys in normal circumstances. It is poorly soluble in water and blood or serum. Its solubility is even less when it is cooled. When the body's concentration of uric acid increases above its solubility, then it comes out of solution and crystallizes, much like a sugar or salt solution will crystallize as the water evaporates. The crystals can form in the soft tissues or in the joints where they can cause an inflammatory reaction, which can be extremely painful.

Gout typically has a relatively sudden onset, usually over a day or so. The MTP joint of the big toe is the most common joint affected. It becomes severely swollen. The skin usually has a shiny and reddened appearance and is exquisitely sensitive to touch. Often the gout resolves in about seven days and frequently the function of the joint returns to normal after the attack. Similar joint irritation can be caused by other inflammatory conditions such as psoriatic arthritis, rheumatoid arthritis, and infection.

The crystals that occur in the joints can initiate an aggressive inflammatory reaction. This happens because your body's white blood cells attempt to destroy the crystals like they do bacteria when you have an infection. During this process, the white blood cells release enzymes and other chemicals that your body's cells normally use to begin an inflammatory reaction to aid in fighting a bacterial infection. The swelling that results can look and feel nearly indistinguishable from an infection.

Gout involves the foot and hands more commonly than the knees, hips, and shoulders, which are usually warmer in temperature. It should be suspected if episodic swelling and severe pain are noticed in the foot especially around the big toe. Attacks of gout can last from two to four days, but some irritation can persist. During the attack, the toe is intensely sensitive to any movement.

Laboratory tests are necessary in the evaluation of possible gout. Identifying crystals within the joint fluid when possible is the most accurate way of diagnosing gout. Diagnosing it on the basis of joint swelling alone is not accurate, but is a common practice among doctors. Although the tests, including serum uric acid, are sometimes helpful in deciding whether gout is likely or not, serum uric acid levels can swing markedly during the inflammatory phase of a gouty attack and can decrease to normal or even low levels.

What causes gout? There are two ways that you can develop gout. The first is that you can create too much uric acid. This can occur by breaking down tissue that contains purines quickly or more commonly by eating things high in purines. The second reason is because the kidneys are not excreting the uric acid from the blood as fast as it is being made. It begins to accumulate within your system. This is the predominant reason for gout.

Gout tends to occur in men usually above the age of 30. People who are overweight or have diabetes are also more likely to develop gout. There are definite hereditary factors that predispose people to gout. If your mother or father has had gout, there is a 20% chance that you will get it as compared to a 0.8% chance in the general population.

Because uric acid is excreted in the urine, people with renal insufficiency can have increased uric acid in the blood. Dehydration causes increased resorption of water and electrolytes and other materials including uric acid that can result in an accumulation of uric acid in the blood. If not enough water is consumed, dieting can bring on an attack. Chemotherapy and surgery can also initiate a gouty attack by causing dehydration and increasing the amount of tissue breakdown. Genetic defects in the proteins that transport uric acid out of the serum in the kidneys have been identified in many people with gout and are the likely explanation for most people who develop gout.

Foods, which can contribute to gouty attacks, include beer, wine, and other alcoholic beverages, red meats, and oily fish such as anchovies. Although legumes such as bean and peas, mushrooms, cauliflower, broccoli, and asparagus contain high levels of purines, it is less certain that they can cause gouty attacks. Dieting can also be a cause.

Other problems such as osteoarthritis of the big toe, sesamoiditis, stress fractures and other joint injuries should be considered as alternative diagnoses when gout is suspected. The episodic pattern of gout, however, is fairly characteristic. Gout is most easily confused with infection. But infections usually get worse fairly quickly, and are usually accompanied by a sore or injury penetrating through the skin.

Although acute joint pain is the most common syndrome, there are other ways that gout can cause problems. Tophaceous gout is when uric acid deposits in the soft tissue. This can leave lumps under the skin that often look whitish. These lumps are full of chalky uric acid deposits embedded in connective tissue. The deposits can erode through the skin where the wounds that result can take a long time to heal. Gouty deposits in the joint can lead to erosion of the joints that can destroy them over time. Gout can also cause kidney stones and can lead to kidney damage.

The initial treatment of gout is directed toward blunting the body's inflammatory reaction, as well as improving hydration to help eliminate the uric acid.

Anti-inflammatory medications are the first line of treatment and can effectively reduce the pain from gout. Colchicine is another medication that is effective in treating gout attacks. Usually the pain can reliably be controlled and the attack stopped by using these medications. In resistant situations, taking oral corticosteroids can control gout. The steroids can also be injected directly into the joint.

Medications such as allopurinol or febuxostat (Uloric®) block the production of gout from other metabolites. Probenecid is a medication that promotes the excretion of uric acid through the urine. It is a useful in lowering uric acid levels. It is less effective if the kidneys are damaged. While these medications are useful in preventing gout attacks, taking them in the midst of a gout attack can make the problem worse.

Diets low in purines are suggested although the effectiveness of following these diets in lowering uric acid levels or preventing attacks has not been proven. Table 3.1 shows foods that are high in uric acid and foods that are generally recommended for the treatment of gout mostly through their effect on urine production. The recommended diet for someone with gout should be high in complex carbohydrates and low in protein and fats.

Aggressive, regular water intake is highly recommended because of the importance of urine production in the elimination of uric acid. Interestingly, even though caffeine is a purine chemical, people with high consumption of coffee seem to have a lower risk of gout than people who do not drink coffee. But, increasing your coffee intake during a gout attack can actually worsen the pain and inflammation. So beware.

TABLE 3.1 Dietary recommendations for people suffering from gout

Foods high in purines/Foods to avoid	Recommended foods to eat
Herring	Blue-red berries
Organ meats, liver, kidney	Carbonated beverages
Mussels	Coffee, tea
Smelt	Chocolate, cocoa
Sardines	High-fiber grains and wheat
Anchovies	Low-fat dairy products
Game birds	Water
Mutton	Drink fruit juices
Veal	Citrus fruits and peppers
Bacon	Pineapple
Salmon	Green-leafy vegetables
Turkey	Tomatoes
Scallops	Celery
Trout, haddock	Bananas
Goose breads and pasta	

Surgery is rarely necessary in gout. Only occasionally is a digit or extremity so painful and racked with tophaceous deposits that surgery is required. A high rate of wound problems is seen after this type of surgery because the gouty deposits interfere with healing.

High uric acid levels alone in the absence of gouty attacks do not require medication. Once medication for repeated or severe gouty flares has been begun, it should be continued indefinitely. Gouty crystals can take three to six months to completely leach out of joints and soft tissues. Recurrent attacks are common when medication is discontinued.

BILLY'S STORY

Billy, a 73-year-old man, a retired worker for an automotive assembly company, had had a surgery done to his lumbar spine. His recovery was unremarkable, but because he lived alone and was not able to cook and clean for himself, he continued his recovery at a rehabilitation facility. About one week after the surgery, he began to have excruciating left big toe pain and right wrist pain and swelling. His foot was swollen, especially around the big toe joint, warm and painful to any slight motion. He had been running a temperature of 100.5°F. He was sent to the hospital by the rehabilitation center due to concern for an infection in these joints.

Because of the concern for infection, the fluid within the wrist joint was drawn using a needle and syringe. As is usual, only a few drops of joint fluid were obtained. Microscopic examination of this fluid showed uric acid crystals within the fluid. X-rays of the foot were normal.

As happened in Billy's case, it is quite common to become dehydrated after surgery because of nausea and vomiting, blood loss, or simply not getting enough access to water from lack of mobility. Billy most likely has a normally high serum uric acid level, but it became much higher after surgery, prompting the attack.

Billy was given a nonsteroidal anti-inflammatory medication and colchicine to control his pain. As a result of the medication, he developed a mild case of diarrhea. After five days, the medication was stopped because the swelling and pain had stopped. Allopurinol was begun two weeks following the initial attack. The gout has not returned since this treatment.

PAIN UNDER THE BIG TOE/SESAMOID PAIN

- Sesamoids are little known bones located in the ball of the foot behind the big toe and under the first metatarsal.

- Sesamoids are contained within a muscle/tendon responsible for flexion of the toe. They help to improve the leverage of the tendon across the joint.

- Sesamoids can be a cause of pain through stress injury, fracture, and arthritis.

- Rehabilitative exercises and stiff-soled rocker-soled shoes help to reduce the stress on the sesamoid and allow it to heal. Foot pads and arch supports are generally not helpful.

- Surgical treatment rarely restores normal function and should be avoided unless prolonged nonsurgical treatment fails.

Although sesamoids are important and a common cause of pain around the ball of the foot, these bones of the big toe are not well-known. The sesamoid pushes the tendon of the short flexor away from the axis of the MTP joint. As a result, the short flexor muscle of the big toe has more leverage in its job of flexing the proximal phalanx of the big toe toward the floor due to the sesamoids. This allows the big toe to help us maintain balance and push off while running with greater force. They also act as the weight-bearing surface of the ball of the foot under the first metatarsal. These jobs place the sesamoid bone under a great deal of pressure, however, and this can lead to stress injuries in the sesamoid bone and joint.

When the sesamoid bones under the big toe are injured, the pain is felt directly under the ball of the foot under the big toe. As there are two sesamoid bones, the medial or inside bone and the lateral or outside bone, pain can be felt in either or both of these areas. Usually the pain becomes worse as weight is concentrated on the ball of the foot such as when you stand on tiptoe or at the end of a stride when running. Walking barefoot and walking in high heels often make it worse.

Pain around the sesamoids can develop for several reasons. Sesmoid pain can be due to tendinitis of the tendons that attach to the sesamoid. The bony tissue itself can begin to fail, eventually leading to a fracture. The joint beneath the sesamoid can become arthritic. The joint destruction can come about from wear and tear or it can wear due to change in the position of the sesamoids from a bunion.

Sesamoid bones sometimes do not unite into a single large bone. They can persist as two fragments developing into two-piece sesamoids. Although a two-piece sesamoid can form as the result of incomplete healing of an injury, they may be present from birth. The connective tissue that joins the fragments seems to be prone to injury. When injured, it can be quite painful and the pain may persist for a long time. It is also common for a two-part sesamoid to be completely pain-free. It is important when attributing pain to a two-piece sesamoid to ensure that the pain is located precisely over the sesamoid and that all other explanations for the pain have been excluded.

Other structures in the vicinity of the sesamoids on occasion can cause pain in this area. This can usually be identified by physical examination. The long flexor of the great toe passes in between the medial and lateral sesamoid and can become swollen in this area. Nerves are positioned along the inside of the medial sesamoid and outside of the lateral sesamoid and can become damaged.

If there is a great deal of pressure, a bursa can form. A bursa is sac that develops where the skin and underlying tissues rub against one another. The normal bursa allows the tissues to slide against one another without friction. An abnormal bursa thickens and fills with fluid until it becomes a painful lump on the bottom of the foot that is usually movable under the skin.

Sesamoid pain is almost always an overuse injury. Pressure on the sesamoid is applied both through the flexor tendon of the toe and through weight applied directly to the bone as a part of its job as the weight-bearing surface of this portion of the foot. Any increase in this pressure can overload this structure and lead to injury.

Any number of the factors discussed in the forefoot overload section (Chapter 2) can cause sesamoiditis, including loss of the plantar fat pad, changes in posture and gait. Other potential causes of big toe pain include:

- Big toe osteoarthritis.
- Ligament and joint injuries of the MT joint.
- Inflammatory arthritis of the MTPJ such as gout and psoriasis.

Bunions can irritate the sesamoids. As described earlier, the gradual change in alignment of the big toe will drag the sesamoids into a different position along the bottom of the big toe. The joints between the sesamoids and the bottom of the metatarsal head are tightly contoured and this shift in position coincides with erosion of the joint structures, resulting in arthritis of these joints. Realigning the joint through surgical bunionectomy only partial reverses and improves these changes.

Thinning of the skin is a common result of aging. The loss of skin thickness is most noticeable in the forearms and hands where the skin becomes prone to damage by bruising and tearing. Thinning affects the bottom of the foot also, where the loss of the padding exposes the sesamoids to more direct stress. Corns and calluses are common in this area of the foot and are often very painful.

Nonoperative treatment is without question the treatment of choice with sesamoid conditions. As a forefoot overload problem, the rehabilitative techniques outlined in the resource section are a successful method of treatment. The first step is to eliminate high-stress activities such as running and to substitute other strenuous, but low-stress exercises such as biking. Firm, rocker-soled shoes are also helpful. A rigid last, which can be built into the shoe or placed under the insert, also reduces the stress within the sesamoid area. By substituting the rolling action of the rocker of the shoe for the normal pressure on the ball of the foot, the stress of the sesamoid can be quite dramatically reduced. The motion of the big toe is also nearly eliminated. These factors usually reduce the pain significantly.

Arch supports can help to stabilize the foot. Supports that are fitted with a medial wedge in the heel can reduce stress on the big toe and medial forefoot and can be relatively inexpensive. Sesamoid pads are not well tolerated. Many people describe the use of sesamoid pads as feeling like a lump in their shoes.

Surgery for sesamoid problems is a last resort. Sesamoid surgeries have a reputation for having a low satisfaction rate and incomplete recovery. Prolonged attempts at nonoperative care are usually advisable. In situations in which rehabilitation has failed, the most conservative surgical approach is usually advised, retaining as much sesamoid tissue as possible. This includes repair or partial excision of the sesamoid bones and avoiding complete removal of the sesamoid when reasonable.

The potential complications of these surgeries are numerous. The weight-bearing surface of the first metatarsal is primarily the sesamoids. Approaching the sesamoids surgically involves disturbing the soft tissues of the bottom of the foot and may leave potentially painful scars. Removal of the sesamoids removes this portion of the weight-bearing surface, concentrating the weight on the other portions of the bottom of the foot. Calluses and corns can develop from the shift in pressure as a result of the sesamoid tissue removal. Nerves that closely follow the inner and outer border of the sesamoid bone supply sensation to the bottom of the foot. They can easily be injured, and scars can form on the nerve that can be very tender and cause numbness to the bottom of the big toe. Finally, if the mechanical function of the tendon that attaches to the sesamoid is compromised, the toe can drift away from the injured tendon causing a bunion or hallux varus, a condition in which the toe begins to point to the midline of the body making shoe wear difficult. If both tendons are weakened the toe can also elevate away from the floor causing a toe posture called a "cock-up" deformity. This deformity can make it difficult to fit into shoes at all.

Turf toe is an injury to the sesamoids and/or collateral ligaments that is an exception to the predominantly nonoperative approach advisable in sesamoid injuries. Turf toe is a traumatic injury or tearing of the ligaments of the MTP joint and possibly a fracture of the bones themselves. It usually occurs in situations in which the toe is forcefully extended or twisted to the inside or the outside of the foot. The injury is, as suggested by the name, usually a serious sports injury. Usually the completely torn ligaments do not heal well by themselves. Athletes specifically seem to have difficulty with persistent instability in the ligaments supporting the MTP joint. Severe injuries to the ligaments at the bottom of the toe and within the sesamoids will limit strength in the toe, which can profoundly affect most athletic activities. Also, varying amounts of joint damage are often present. Aggressive repair of the damaged structures is often necessary especially in the athlete and will often result in more normal function if performed early.

JOSHUA'S STORY

Joshua is an avid jogger and infantryman who began to notice pain under his big toe when getting ready for a deployment to Afghanistan. The pain was first present when jogging on a company run and felt like a "nail driven up my foot." It got a little better when he stopped running and after a couple of days he could walk on it well. However, every time he began to try to resume running, the pain returned. It had gone on for two months and his command was beginning to worry that he would not be able to be physically qualified for deployment.

Joshua's foot was tender directly under the ball of the big toe and the pain was increased with extension of the toe. Joshua's x-rays show that the lateral sesamoid bone was fracturing in several places.

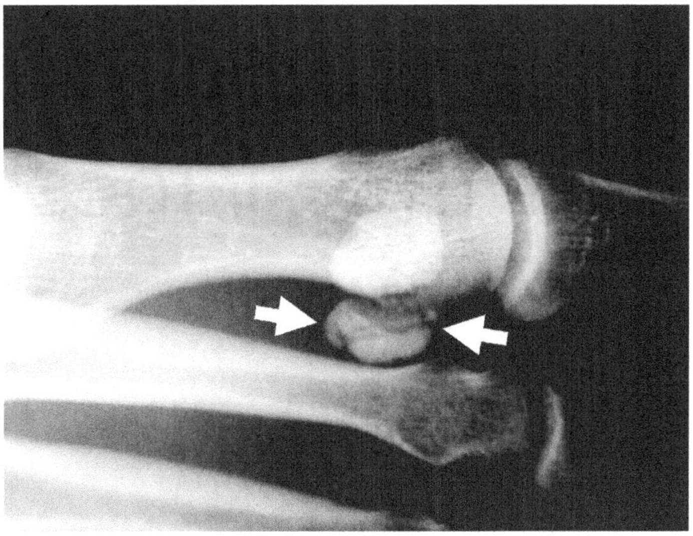

FIGURE 3.10 X-ray of the big toe showing a stress fracture of the lateral sesamoid.

There is no rushing the recovery from a sesamoid stress fracture. Joshua was told about nonsurgical treatments, including rocker-soled shoes and stretching and postural exercises. His pain gradually improved. Joshua rejoined his unit for deployment, after six months of treatment. He modified his boots with a steel last in the sole of the foot to stiffen the boots, but he didn't start running for a year.

NOTE

[1] Flavin R., Halpin T., O'Sullivan R. et al. A finite-element analysis study of the metatarsophalangeal joint of the hallux rigidus. *J. Bone Joint Surg Br.* 2008 Oct;90(10):1334–40.

4

The Small Toes

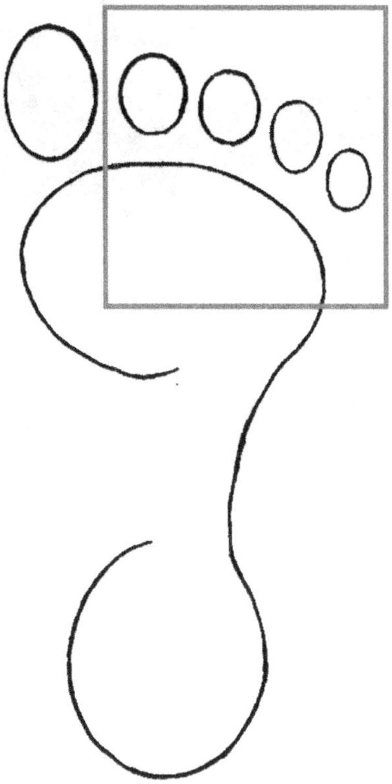

ANATOMY

Each of the smaller toes consists of three bones attached to the metatarsal. There are five metatarsals in the foot, which are numbered beginning with the big toe, one through five. The bones in the toe from base to tip are the proximal phalanx, the middle phalanx, and the distal phalanx. The joint between the metacarpal head in the ball of the foot and the proximal phalanx is the metatarsophalangeal joint, but we will call it the MTP joint. The other two joints, again from base to tip, are the proximal interphalangeal (PIP) joint and the distal interphalangeal (DIP) joint. Usually these joints are straight or slightly flexed. Flexor and extensor tendons control the toes and are powered by muscles in the arch and calf. Ligaments are connective tissues mostly on the bottoms and the sides of the toe joints that control posture and restrict motion around the joints.

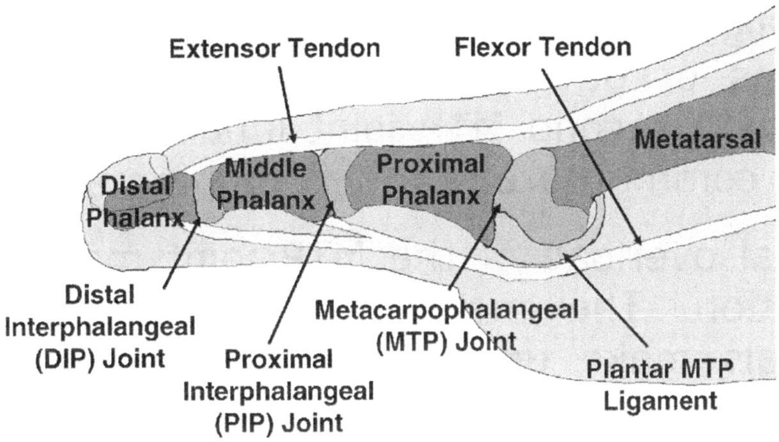

FIGURE 4.1 The major anatomical structures of the smaller toe.

METATARSALGIA, HAMMERTOES, AND OTHER TOE DEFORMITIES

Key points:

- Metatarsalgia is a term that means pain along the ball of the foot. Although it can be caused by a number of things, the most common cause is inflammation of the MTP joint.

- Often this pain spontaneously resolves, but approximately 50% of the time a hammertoe occurs.
- A hammertoe many times begins as a deformity of the lesser toe in which the MTP joint extends. The PIP joint flexes because of a change in the tendon tension.

Metatarsalgia is a medical term that describes pain under the front of the foot. Isolated swelling or irritation of the MTP joint is a common finding in metatarsalgia. It is not completely known what causes it. Bunions or other joint instability problems often coincide with second MTP joint inflammation, which is the most common area for this inflammation to occur.

Mechanical overload of the MTP joint may cause MTP inflammation. The metatarsal heads of all of the metatarsals make up the weight-bearing surface of the ball of the foot. If one of the bones is longer than the others, then the pressure will be concentrated on the long metatarsal at the end of the step as the heel is lifted off the floor. Because the second metatarsal is often longer than the adjacent metatarsals, it takes on more weight than the other metatarsal heads during walking and is the most common toe affected by metatarsalgia.

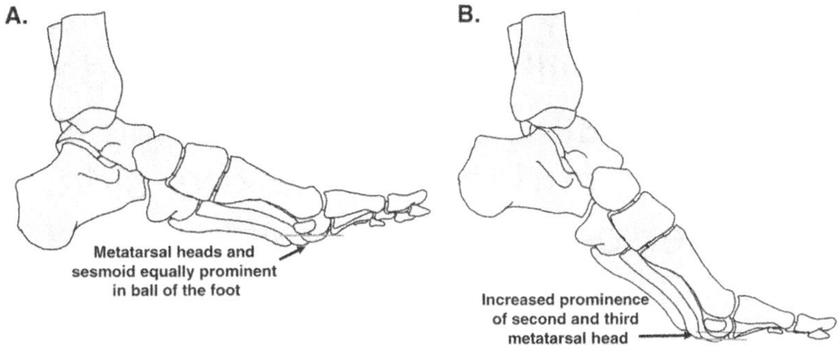

FIGURE 4.2 The relationship of the sesamoids of the big toe, the bottom of the second metatarsal head and the floor change with the position of the foot. When the foot is flat as it would be when standing (A), the metatarsal heads and the sesamoids are roughly the same distance from the floor. When the foot is flexed (B), the metatarsal head of the longer second toe is closer to the floor than the sesamoids and other metatarsal heads.

Contractures and tightness of the Achilles tendon or hamstrings also overload the ball of the foot. In addition, abnormal walking patterns, foot abnormalities such as abnormally high arches, or abnormal standing posture can contribute to pressure on the forefoot. Over time this will wear out the ligaments supporting the MTP joint.

Age can contribute to stress on the metatarsal heads. Atrophy of the fat under the skin is nearly universal with advancing age. The skin on the sole of the foot is affected in the same way. The shock-absorbing and pressure-distributing functions of the skin are decreased as the skin gets thinner. This concentrates pressure and accelerates wear on the MTP joints.

A hammertoe is a toe deformity that sometimes follows the development of inflammation in the MTP joint. Although many people define hammertoes in different ways, we will use it in its broadest sense as a term describing all deformities of the smaller toes in which the toes curl or tilt to the side. The most common hammertoe is a deformity of the toe where the PIP joint flexes. This causes the joint to be prominent on the upper surface. Often the knuckle pads on the tops of the toes are knobby or discolored from the abnormal position and the pressure from shoe wear.

Toe deformities at other joints are common. The most frequently associated deformity is an extension deformity at the MTP joint. This raises the toe, especially the PIP joint, against the shoe. The deformity can even progress to the point where the MTP joint becomes dislocated and the opposing joint surfaces at the base of the proximal phalanx and end of the metacarpal do not even touch anymore. A variant of the hammertoe in which the DIP joint is deformed into flexion and turned toward the floor like a mallet is called a *mallet toe.*

Complicating these deformities, any of these joints can turn to the inside or outside of the foot. In fact, one of the most common of these deformities is the "crossover second toe." In this deformity, the second toe completely overlaps the big toe. This can make it extremely difficult to fit into shoes. In addition, many people become embarrassed about the appearance of this deformity and avoid wearing sandals.

The most frequent complaint about a hammertoe is pain, which occurs in two ways. First, the hammertoe usually is a result of a rupture or tear of a capsular ligament on the bottom of the MTP joint. This pain will be sensed in this area where the tissue is damaged. Second, as the MTP joint starts to extend, the metatarsal head becomes more prominent in the bottom of the foot. We have heard some doctors refer to this as a *dropped metatarsal.* This most likely develops because of the local swelling from the torn structures on the bottom of the MTP joint and displacement of the normal protective fat.

Other problems arise when the toe hits the shoe. When a prominent corner of the toe from an acutely flexed PIP joint hits the shoe, a callus can form over the top of this bony prominence. Calluses or corns can also arise because of the different ways that the bones within the toes hit one another in between the toes. A callus or even a sore can form at the very tip of the toe when the toe is not flexible and the tip jams against the floor with weight bearing. The toenail can become deformed from this same pressure.

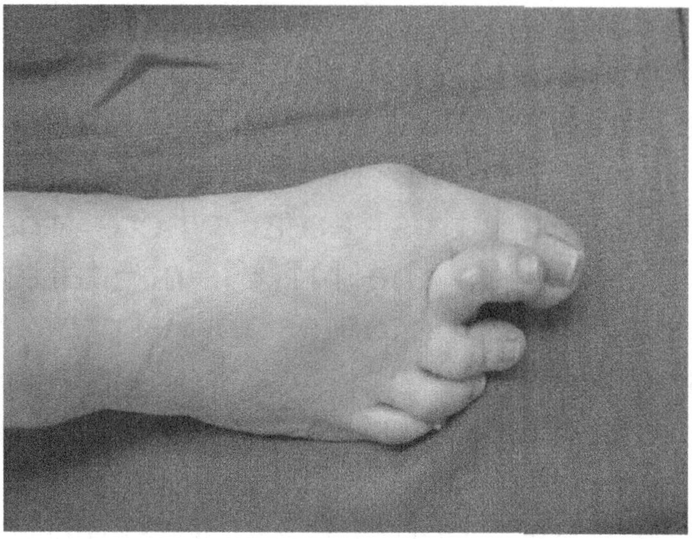

FIGURE 4.3 A foot with "crossover" second toe as well as a moderate bunion deformity of the big toe. A more typical hammertoe is seen on the third toe and fourth toe. The hammertoe on the fourth toe has led to a corn over the PIP joint from contact of the flexed joint with the shoe.

Whether the inflammation within the joint occurs before the ligament injury or vice versa is a little like arguing whether the chicken or the egg came first. The reality is that either problem can perpetuate the other. When the MTP joint becomes inflamed, the enzymes produced by the inflammatory cells can begin to digest the ligaments and they can tear. Usually the ligaments on the bottom of the foot become damaged, allowing the joint to extend, although the ligaments on the sides of the toe can also begin to tear so that the toe drifts toward the inside or outside of the foot. As the MTP joint starts to extend, the flexor tendons on the bottom of the toe begin to tighten and the extensor tendons loosen, flexing the PIP joint and DIP joint. Over time, the ligaments within these joints become so stiff that it is even difficult to straighten the toe manually with your hand.

Trauma can potentially initiate this problem. A direct blow such as stubbing your toes can injure the ligaments around any joint in the toe, just as it can in the hand when you jam your finger. This can lead to a hammertoe deformity that is often mistaken for a fracture because of the unusual alignment of the toe.

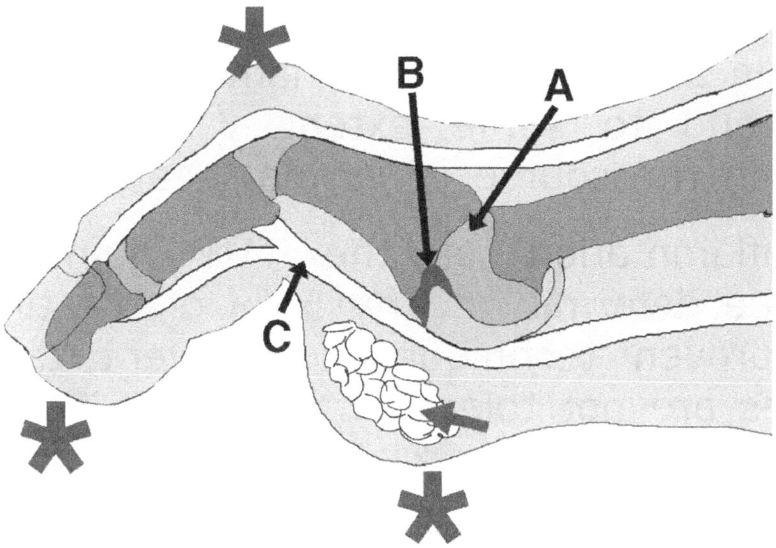

FIGURE 4.4 Stages in development of a hammertoe. The MTP joint becomes inflamed (A), damaging the surrounding ligaments (B). This changes the position of the MTP joint and alters the tension in the flexor and extensor tendon, causing the PIP joint to flex. The extension of the toe displaces the fat pad forward away from the weight-bearing surface in the ball of the foot (gray arrow). So you can see, the changes in position of the joints leaves areas of the toe prone to extreme pressure from the floor and shoe (asterisks).

Other problems that can cause pain in the lesser toes include:

- Interdigital neuroma or Morton's neuroma.
- Stress fracture of the metatarsal.
- Soft corn in between the toes.

When beginning treatment of any problem, the goals need to be carefully defined. Once a hammertoe deformity has occurred, there are no methods of reversing it nonsurgically. However, reduction of much of the pain associated with a hammertoe deformity is possible and to some extent will probably occur naturally in the course of normal healing.

Acute inflammation of the MTP joint leads to hammertoe deformity nearly 50% of the time. There are no proven techniques to prevent this. Taping techniques are not tolerated for long without pain or skin breakdown. Commercial devices that hold the toe down such as the Bundin splint or toe crests are generally only able to position the toe if the deformity is flexible and this is rarely the case. However, pads are often helpful in treating callus and corns that develop.

Forefoot pain—especially the pain in the ball of the foot—is effectively managed by wearing a stiff-soled shoe. The stiffness in the sole of a shoe that has a firm rocker sole or has been modified by inserting a steel support into the sole of the shoe will disperse the concentration of stress concentration in the ball of the foot. This decreases pain. Metatarsal pads placed into the shoe and metatarsal bars placed onto the sole of the shoe can disperse pressure and reduce pain. If one MTP joint is especially prominent, custom orthotics may be made to reduce pressure and pain under this prominence. Most off-the-shelf arch supports are not helpful otherwise.

Selecting shoes that have extra room in the toe box with an upper soft enough to avoid pressure can lessen pressure on deformed toes. If a shoe has a compliant upper, often a commercial shoe stretcher that can be purchased or accessed through a pedorthist or most shoe repair shops can loosen the fabric enough to reduce the pressure.

Steroid injections are relatively effective in decreasing the inflammation of the MTP joint. A doctor familiar with the technique can administer the procedure in the office. Overall, the degree of pain associated with this is relative mild. In our clinic 80% of patients report that the pain is only slightly more than a flu shot. Over the short run, over half of people note significant reduction of their pain. However, it is not a cure. It can be used to decrease the pain while it improves naturally or until a treatment program can be initiated. Side effects from steroid injections include injection site pain in about 25% that generally lasts for 24 to 48 hours. Some physicians have concerns about further damage to the surrounding ligaments from steroid injections, resulting in an increased chance of hammertoe formation. Well-controlled studies would be necessary to settle this question, but studies are not presently available. Until then, steroid injections for this problem should be used sparingly and judiciously.

Finally, rehabilitation programs are the key tool for the treatment of metatarsalgia. A graduated program is outline in the resources of this book for the reduction of forefoot overload. It is helpful in shortening the disability associated with this condition and avoiding surgery in the majority of cases. It will also treat the multiple other forefoot overload syndromes that commonly coincide with metatarsalgia.

Surgical treatment of MTP joint synovitis and hammertoe is directed to the overall deformity and the factors that may contribute to it. As with other forefoot overload problems, an aggressive rehabilitation program will help with recovery and should decrease recurrence of the pain. Surgical treatment must be tailored to the specific pains and issues with an individual foot. A surgical approach to metatarsalgia or a hammertoe may involve tendon and ligament releases or lengthening at multiple joints, the removal and fusion of joints, or the cutting and repositioning of bones. Fixation through temporary pinning of the joints may be necessary to allow the healing of the reconstructed ligaments and tendons. Restriction of weight bearing may also be necessary to allow the reconstructed bones to heal properly. If possible, the surgeon will preserve the joint surfaces to resection these joints or replace with silicone devices.

After an operation, considerable swelling may limit the types of shoes that you wear for months. Color changes (bluish, blackish, or reddish discoloration) will also be present for months. If the color is troubling to you, then a physician should evaluate them to ensure that the toe has proper circulation. Numbness is generally present to some extent after an operation because the sensory nerves around the toes are very small, numerous, and easy to surgically injure. After surgery, the toes will be stiffer and weaker.

The most common problem that occurs after the correction of a hammertoe is that it comes back. The most worrisome potential complication is the toe losing its blood supply and dying. Repositioning the toes from the deformed positions can stretch the arteries and nerves within the toe to the point that the arteries spasm for a considerable period of time. Persistent pain is common after hammertoe surgery. This can occur even when the surgery is technically successful.

Recently, innovative tendon transfer and ligament repair techniques have been introduced. Some techniques show the promise of returning the foot to more normal function. However, these methods have not really been stringently evaluated and published in the medical literature, so it is not possible to recommend them yet.

BRETT'S STORY

Brett's second toe on his right side had become very sensitive. The toe had begun as an ache more and more. The toe near the ball of the foot was painful with every step and had become so swollen that the veins were no longer distinctly visible on the top of the forefoot. He was having increased pain when he jogged, and he was limping. He had a longstanding bunion that had never bothered him. The alignment of the toe was otherwise normal.

He had a steroid or cortisone injection into his second MTP joint. In addition, he began the stretching and postural training program outlined in the resources section of this book. Rocker-soled shoes were used and the pain went away. Four months later, the pain and swelling partially returned. The toe also developed the deformity shown.

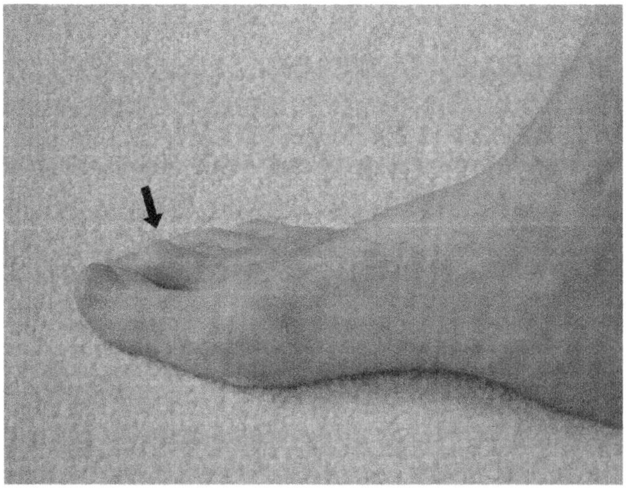

FIGURE 4.5 Brett's hammertoe that began four months following second MTP joint synovitis. The problem is now asymptomatic

although the deformity will be permanent. There's a bunion there that has been present since adolescence.

Two months following this recurrence the pain disappeared except for an occasional, nagging pain when he goes barefoot. Brett has since returned to all his normal recreational activities and has no limitations in what shoes he can wear.

BUNIONETTES

- A bunionette is a prominence of the fifth metatarsal head caused by the proximal phalanx sliding to the inside of the metatarsal head. It causes pain due to pressure against the shoe.
- Occasionally, prominences of the metatarsal head can also cause painful corns.
- Like a bunion, nonsurgical treatment centers on finding shoes that fit the shape of the foot or are flexible enough to adapt to the foot.
- Surgical treatment is directed toward realigning the joint.

The fifth (or smallest) toe is prone to a disorder similar to the bunions of the big toe. Although not as common as bunions, a bunionette is a prominence or knob that appears along the outside border of the foot where the small toe connects to the ball of the foot. Although it is not clear that fashionable shoes cause bunionettes, it is clear that they can cause them to hurt.

Many bunionettes have been present since adolescence. Sometimes, like when the fifth toe overlaps the fourth toe, these conditions are apparent even at birth. Some develop over time as the joints in the midfoot loosen slightly.

The key to treatment is to find shoes that fit the shape of the foot. To do this, look at the shape of the shoe and the shape of the foot. Ensure that the outline of the shoe roughly fits the shape of the foot. Shoe styles that come in widths can be helpful. In situations where the fifth toe overlaps the fourth, a significantly wider and deeper toe box may be necessary. This may be difficult to find without enlisting the help of a pedorthist, a specialist in fitting shoes. Choosing a shoe with an upper that is adaptable to the foot or stretchy material is also beneficial. Leather is capable of stretching and works well for this. Other synthetic foam materials can help in particularly difficult cases, but they are often not durable. Avoid designs with stitching over the prominent area of the foot, because seams do not stretch very well. Many shoe repair shops and nearly all pedorthotists have devices to stretch the shoe and can give further advice on particularly hard-to-fit feet.

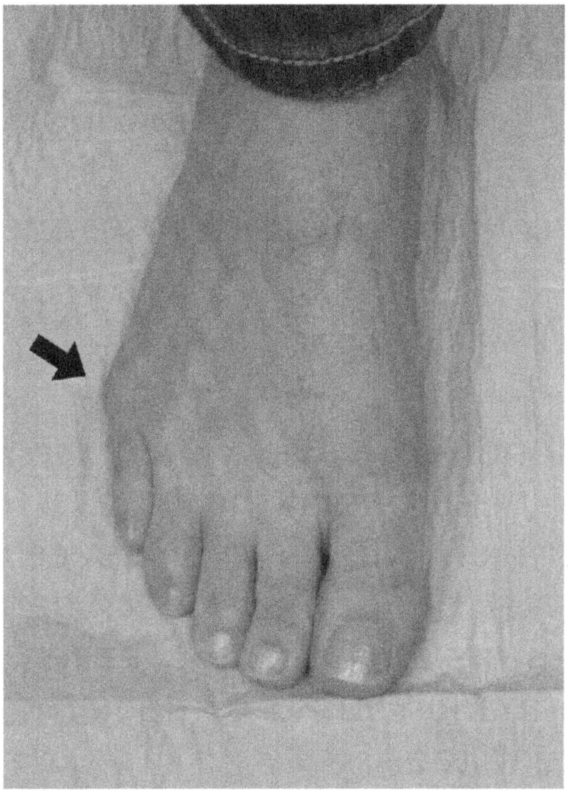

FIGURE 4.6 Bunionette deformity.

INTERDIGITAL NEUROMA/MORTON'S NEUROMA

- A Morton's neuroma is a compression of the interdigital nerve of the toe that causes pain and numbness in the toes.
- The most common nerve involved lies in the ball of the foot in between the third and fourth toes.
- Nonsurgical treatment centers on stabilizing the foot through rehabilitative exercises and supportive rocker-soled shoes. Steroid injections can give

temporary or permanent relief but do have some complications.

- Surgical treatment involves decompression or removal of the damaged portion of the nerve. Clear advantage of one approach over the other has not been proven yet.

The interdigital nerves travel within the space between the metatarsal heads near the bottom of the foot. As the nerves travel within the space between the metatarsal heads, they pass under ligaments that join adjacent metatarsal heads. These nerves carry sensation information on the medial side and lateral sides of adjacent toes.

An interdigital neuroma is an injury to this nerve in the ball of the foot. The most common symptom is pain directly in between the metatarsal heads. Usually, only one nerve is affected, although on occasion more than one nerve can be symptomatic. If more than one neuroma is diagnosed, other diagnoses should be considered carefully. The most common position for an interdigital neuroma is between the third and fourth toe, but neuromas between the second and third are sometimes seen. Squeezing the metatarsal heads together increases the pain from interdigital neuroma and occasionally causes a popping sensation.

The pain is most often described as feeling numb or burning and usually extends into the opposing sides of the toes, making up the web. The pain is usually worsened by activity especially running. Clicking while walking is common.

The term *neuroma* is used to describe tumors of the nerve. However, this is inaccurately applied to a Morton's neuroma. Tumors within the nerve are very rare. The nerve in a Morton's neuroma often appears normal although sometimes it is enlarged and scarred. It is more accurate to describe the problem as a repetitive injury or nerve irritation. The cause of interdigital neuroma is not definitely known.

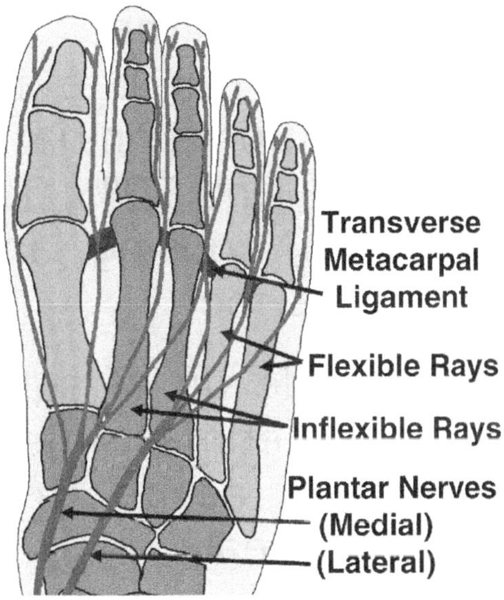

FIGURE 4.7 Branching of the posterior tibial nerve into interdigital nerves.

The most common condition that causes symptoms similar to Morton's neuroma is irritation of the MTP joint or metatarsalgia. The areas of tenderness for these problems lie close to one another. A stress fracture of the metatarsal is another important diagnosis to consider.

X-rays are usually normal but are often needed to exclude other problems. The nerves themselves are not visible on the radiographs. Although MRI and ultrasound may image the nerves, it is still unclear whether any particular abnormality such as increased size or local swelling is useful in confirming or excluding Morton's neuroma.

Various injections are used in the treatment of interdigital neuroma. Steroid injections can result in temporary improvement that is occasionally remarkable. Over the long run, the improvement may be more disappointing. Some initial improvement is reported at between 20% and 70%. The most common complication is local pain, bruising, and wasting of the fat on the bottom of the foot.

Sclerosing injections made up of solutions of ethanol or phenol are also sometimes injected around the interdigital nerves. Good results have been reported with this form of treatment. The orthopedic community, however, has been slow to accept them, probably because of the caustic and painful properties of these substances. Multiple injections (usually three to five) are typically prescribed. However, persistent and, potentially, increased nerve pain, soft tissue damage, and local pain have also been reported.

Surgery for Morton's neuroma is fairly straightforward. Usually, the interdigital nerve is identified through an incision either on the top or bottom of the foot, and then traced back into the tissue in the nonweight-bearing portion of the arch and cut. Unfortunately, any surgery may be unsuccessful in relieving the pain 10% to 20% of the time. This may be because the diagnosis is often difficult to establish with complete certainty. In some cases, people also develop painful areas where the nerve was cut, which can be difficult to manage.

STACY'S STORY

Stacy is a 36-year-old nurse who works in the intensive care unit of a hospital. Her job requires that she be on her feet for long periods of time. She has noted a continuous pain on the bottom of the foot that radiates into the third and fourth toes. It becomes worse and burns at night after work so much that it often keeps her awake. She has tenderness in the ball of the foot in between the third and fourth metatarsal heads and a click is appreciated when the ball of the foot is squeezed from the sides. All of her x-rays were normal.

Stacey started stretching and using postural exercises and stiffer rocker-soled shoes. At four weeks, her pain was only partially improved. An injection of a steroid was done into the third web space. Her pain went away.

STRESS FRACTURES

- Stress fractures are caused from repetitive forces on the bones that overwhelm the body's ability to repair itself.

- While osteoporosis is not a common cause of stress fracture, it should be excluded in recurrent stress fractures.

- The most common place for stress fractures is along the metatarsal shaft and it is heralded by unexplained swelling and pain in the front of the foot localized to the fracture site.

- Treatment and prevention of stress fracture is centered on shoe changes that lessen the load across the metatarsal involved. Rehabilitative exercises and postural training can also be helpful.

Most people are familiar with a traumatic fracture—when a force or blow is directed toward a bone breaking it into two or more pieces. However, bones can break in other ways. Every day, the wear and tear of daily activity on all tissue including bone causes injury that the body is continuously at work repairing. When the degree of injury overwhelms your body's limited ability to repair it, the injury begins to accumulate. This injury increases with your weight, activity level, and the shape of your leg.

Sudden changes in activity level such as when you begin a new exercise program or more physical job, can precipitate a stress fracture. If the pain that occurs with this process does not slow you down, then you will eventually completely break or fracture the bone. A minor twisting motion or normal step can break the bone in this weakened condition. Occasionally a sudden, painful crack is sensed. At other times, increasing pain or swelling is felt. Bleeding or bruising is often not seen in stress fracture.

The most common stress fractures are in the metatarsals, in the front of the foot (near the ball of the foot) and are commonly felt on the top. If the fracture displaces and causes you to shift weight onto your uninjured metatarsals, it can potentially cause the others to fracture, as well.

The stress that occurs with activity, both light activity and strenuous, causes small "micro-fractures," which normally the body can repair as they occur, begins to accumulate until physical breaking or a fracture happens. There are three ways that the micro-fractures can occur: the bone can be subjected to a greater stress than it is accustomed to through changes in activity level; the bone can weaken such as happens with osteoporosis; or the bone's mechanical environment can change.

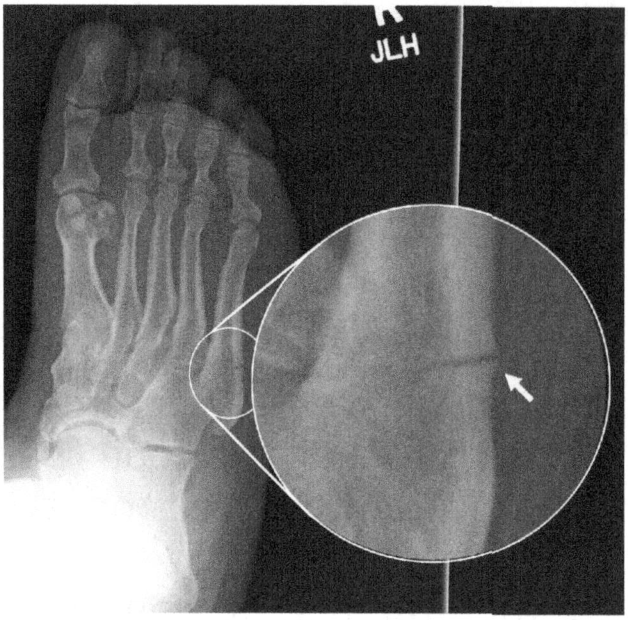

FIGURE 4.8 Fifth metatarsal stress fracture. Stress changes (white arrow) resemble a beak along the side of the bone and can be seen at the border of the fracture suggesting that this fracture was not the result of a single injury.

Another common method of overloading the foot is through loss of the protective thick padding of the plantar skin. This has been mentioned before, but bears repeating. As the skin on the ball of the foot thins (along with the skin throughout the body) with the passing years, the ability of this skin to dampen the pressure concentration through the bones of the foot is decreased. The repetitive stresses that occur through normal walking can overwhelm the body's ability to repair itself.

Other problems, which can mimic metatarsal stress fracture, are:

- Inflammation or synovitis of the MTP joint.

- Midfoot arthritis.
- Tendonitis of the extensor tendons.
- Morton's neuroma.

The specific area of tenderness and firm swelling along the metatarsal shaft is characteristic of metatarsal stress fracture. Stress fractures can occur in nearly every bone in the foot. Besides the metatarsal shafts, other common areas of stress fracture are the calcaneus, the navicular bone, the fibula shaft, and the sesamoid bones on the bottom of the big toe.

Treatment of stress fractures is centered on relieving the stresses that initiated the fracture. Therefore, careful protection and close follow-up of these fractures is often necessary. This may involve limitation of weight bearing or protection with a cast or cast boot. Occasionally a bone stimulator, a device placed outside of the skin of the leg that directs ultrasound or magnetic fields toward the fracture, can help speed the healing. There has been little quality evidence indicating what degree these devices help. However, the use of commercially available magnets has been shown to be of no use in the treatment of fracture (or anything else for that matter).

Therefore, careful protection and close follow-up of any fractures is often necessary. Even when a metatarsal fracture displaces slightly, judgment is necessary to determine whether realignment through surgery is worthwhile. The displacement may add pressure to other parts of the foot and may occasionally cause painful calluses, but often it is well tolerated with minor changes in shoe wear or orthotics.

Some stress fractures are particularly dangerous. Stress fractures associated with diabetes can progress to the point that the foot is misshapened, prone to ulceration, and does not fit into shoes. Fractures of the navicular bone in the midfoot just in front of the ankle can be disastrous if they displace. Surgery is sometimes recommended for these fractures.

There are two reasons that surgery may be necessary. First, some stress injuries have difficulty healing or may become recurrent because the person with the stress fracture places high demand on the bone or cannot risk the possibility of prolonged healing. This may be the case with an athlete such as a professional basketball player. The most common fractures that fit this description are stress injuries of the navicular and of the base of the fifth metatarsal. Usually, the surgeries involved in the stabilization of these injuries are quick, and people who have them recover quickly.

Second, surgery may be necessary when the fracture displaces so that there is little chance for pain-free function after healing. Highly displaced fractures of the metatarsals fit this description. When rehabilitation doesn't control the pain, realignment through recutting of the fracture and stabilization with a plate and screws is generally necessary.

LINDA'S STORY

Linda is a 53-year-old active stay-at-home wife and mother who had recently begun a workout regimen with several of her friends in anticipation of walking the Mini-Marathon, a popular prerace event before the Indianapolis 500. She began to experience swelling and increasing pain in her left foot approximately four weeks prior to the race. She noticed the pain was increasing and she had to miss several walks with her friends. Her foot became noticeably swollen and warm. Her second metatarsal was focally and firmly swollen along the neck of the bone, just proximal to the metatarsal head. Her x-rays were normal. Despite this, she was diagnosed and treated for a metatarsal stress fracture. Follow-up x-rays taken four weeks later when she was feeling quite a bit better confirmed the stress fracture.

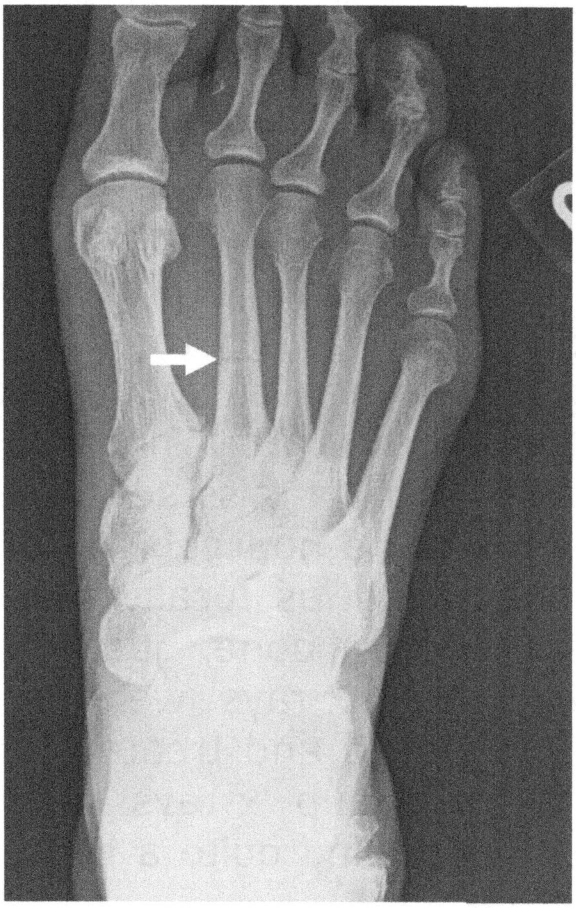

FIGURE 4.9 A transverse stress fracture of the midshaft of the second metatarsal, Four weeks after symptoms began. Initial x-rays did not show the fracture.

Upon initial diagnosis, Linda was placed in a prefabricated fracture boot. She was instructed to put off her walking regimen and to begin using a stationary bike or aqua-aerobic training program. She was feeling considerably better after four weeks, and at two months, she was allowed to progress to a rocker-soled shoe and started a stretching and conditioning program as outlined in the resources. She was gradually returned to a progressive walking program. We're sorry to say that she wasn't able to fully participate in the Mini-Marathon that year, but did complete it the following year.

TRAUMATIC FRACTURES OF THE FOREFOOT

• Fractures of the metatarsals and phalanges of the foot are among the most common fractures.

• Unlike the hands, exact anatomical alignment is not always necessary for good function.

• Fractures of the forefoot rarely require surgical treatment and generally heal in four to eight weeks. Functional use is sometimes possible much earlier.

Fractures of the metatarsals and the phalanges are some of the most common injuries in the body. The mechanism of injury is usually a jamming of the toes or a crush of the foot. The metatarsals can also be broken by a twisting injury similar to an ankle sprain. Although these injuries can be very painful, they are not usually dangerous and usually heal on their own.

Initial treatment is fairly simple. Assuming the toes appear to have good circulation, a trip to the emergency room is sometimes not necessary. A far more efficient and less expensive approach would be to call your family physician the following day and make an appointment. However, if the pain is severe, you should go to the emergency room.

First aid for fractures of the forefoot is easy. If the toe is in mild malalignment, you can leave it in its position. It is also reasonable to straighten it, but it will hurt of course. Ice is helpful in two ways. In the initial hours, it may reduce swelling. After the initial few hours, it is no longer required. It may be used to help with the pain by interfering with the transmission of nerve pain signals to the brain.

Walking is sometimes possible simply by shifting weight onto the heel, although this can be a slow and sometimes tiring gait. Walking is also possible through the use of crutches that can be purchased at most drug stores or grocery stores. Most insurances will reimburse this cost with your doctor's prescription. Weight may be placed on the heel for balance or to decrease the load on your arms. Choose a shoe that will allow for the swelling. Usually a sandal such as a flip-flop, a loose-fitting clog such as is made by Croc®, or a slipper/house shoe works well.

Anti-inflammatory medications such as ibuprofen and naprosyn and other over-the-counter analgesics such as acetaminophen work well for mild to moderate pain, but do little to control swelling. Antiinflammatory medication does inhibit blood clotting and can worsen bruising slightly. Elevation is really the only effective way of decreasing the throbbing that normally accompanies fractures of the foot. If a stronger pain medication is necessary, then emergent medical evaluation may be necessary.

Elastic wraps such as Ace wraps® do little to control swelling. Some people like the feeling of having their injury compressed, however, and so they may find it useful. It can also help to protect a fractured toe from getting caught on clothing with which it may come in contact. Casts and cast boots are usually not necessary for toe fractures, but can help with pain and walking in metatarsal fractures.

The rule of thumb for fractures of the toes is that if it fits in a shoe it is usually not necessary to fix or realign it. These fractures usually heal reliably and do not need to be frequently reevaluated by x-ray if the pain is lessening and if the alignment is acceptable. Fractures that involve the joint are somewhat more difficult to generalize. Physicians disagree on the need for realignment of these fractures, although surgically correcting these is tempting to improve the appearance of the radiograph. The end result is usually a stiff toe regardless of the treatment.

The main function of a metatarsal bone is to transfer weight from the arch to the metatarsal head. Assuming that the metatarsal heads are not out of alignment when evaluated within the ball of the foot, significant amounts of displacement are usually not of any consequence. If the metatarsal head is less or more prominent within the ball of the foot than normal, correcting this should be considered because pain and callus formation may result.

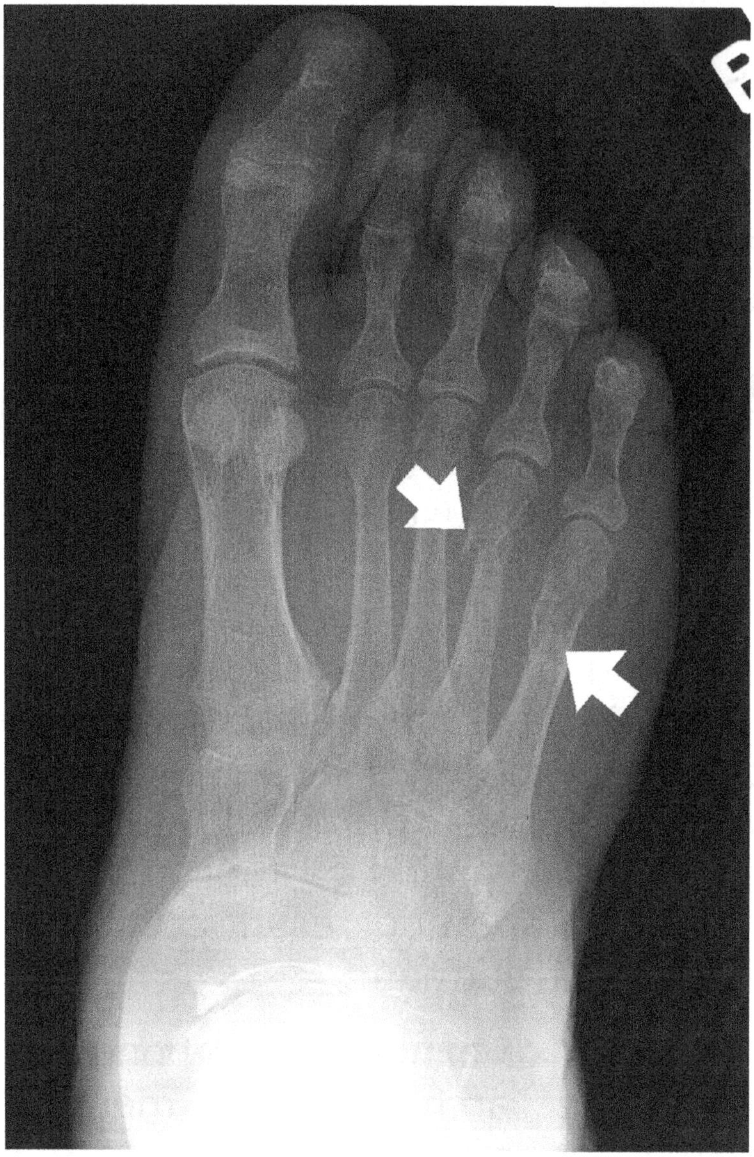

FIGURE 4.10 Fracture of the fourth and fifth metatarsal neck. Despite the mild displacement, the prominences of the metatarsal heads in the ball of the foot were normal. Weight restriction was all that was necessary to successfully treat this fracture.

Fractures of the base of the fifth metatarsal are fairly common. These fractures usually occur from twisting the foot and are called *Dancer's fractures.* They can be mistaken for ankle sprains. A variant of a basilar fifth metatarsal fracture can occur as a stress fracture. Usually, they can also be treated in a cast or cast boot. Certain fractures in this area can fail to heal and subsequently require surgery.

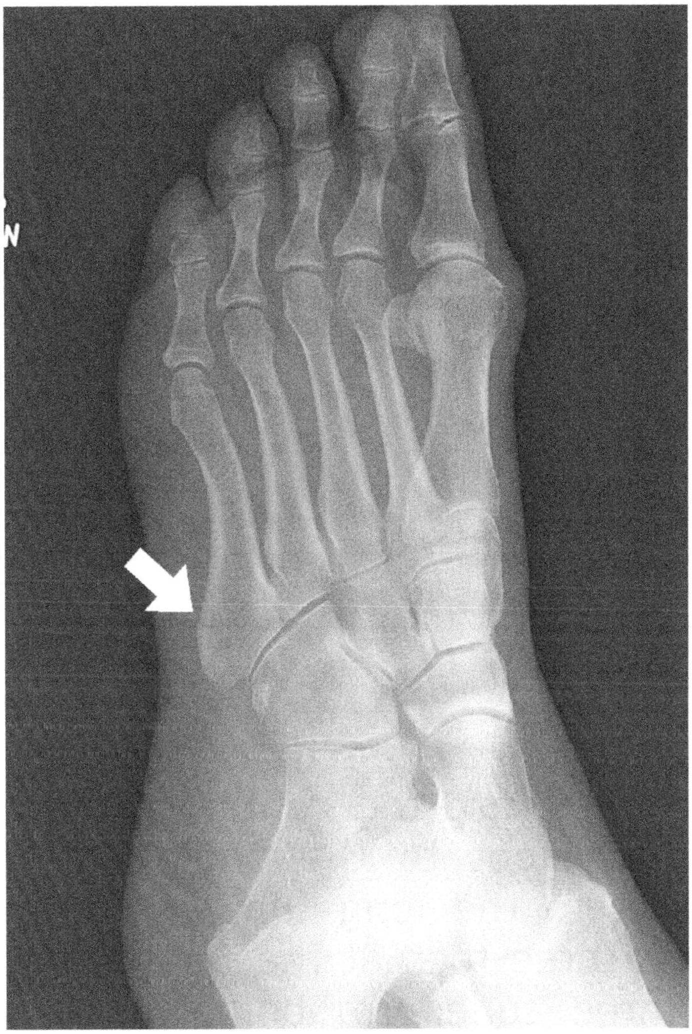

FIGURE 4.11 A common fracture of the base of the fifth metatarsal caused by a twisting injury of the foot.

5

The Midfoot

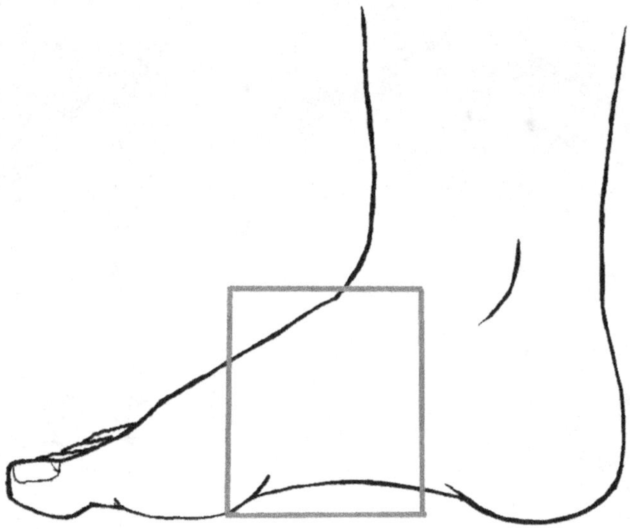

ANATOMY

Along the top of the arch are three bones, the cuneiforms, which are the center of the midfoot and connect the forefoot to the ankle and heel. These bones connect to the long tubular metatarsal bones from the first three toes at the tarsometatarsal (TMT) joint. The three cuneiform bones form a joint with the navicular bone near the ankle. The metatarsals to the fourth and fifth toes attach to the cuboid bone along the outer portion of the midfoot about halfway from the heel to the ball of the foot.

Strong plantar ligaments hug the bottom bony surface of the arch of the foot especially along the bottom of the midfoot. The plantar fascia also contributes to the stability of the arch. In fact, the plantar fascia protects the joint and bones of the midfoot from shear stress, preventing arthritis and stress injury.

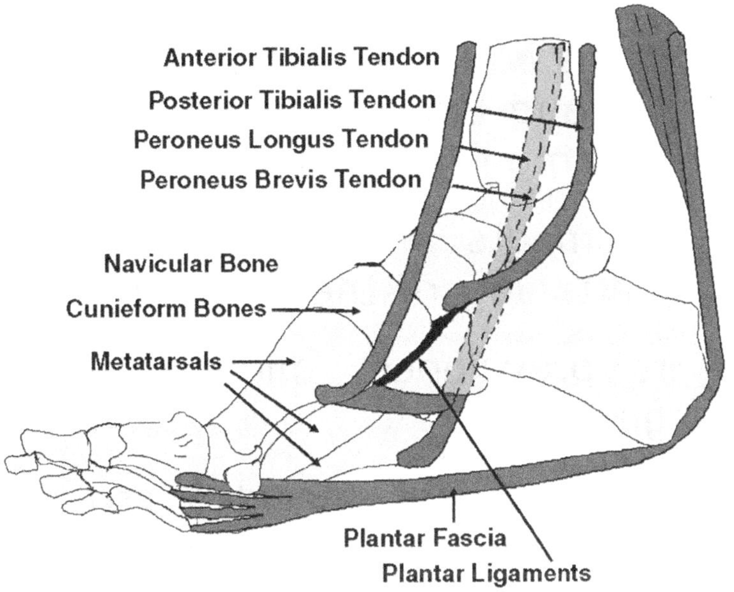

FIGURE 5.1 The major bones, tendons, and ligaments of the midfoot.

Tendons lie at every quadrant of the midfoot. The Achilles tendon attaches to the back of the calcaneus to draw the foot toward the ground or sole of the foot. The anterior tibialis pulls the foot toward the shin and attaches to the inside and lower side of the first metatarsal. The posterior tibial tendon attaches to the inside of the navicular bone to pull the foot inward and to accentuate the arch. Finally the peroneal tendons—both the brevis and longus—run along the back side of the fibula to attach to the base of the fifth metatarsal and underside of the base of the first metatarsal and cuneiforms. These tendons combine to draw the foot outward and to pull the first metatarsal downward.

MIDFOOT ARTHRITIS

- Midfoot arthritis is an extremely common condition in middle-aged and elderly people and seems to be much more common in women.
- As the ligaments and joints in the midfoot deteriorate, flattening of the arch can occur.
- Despite its prevalence, midfoot arthritis rarely requires surgery.
- Nonsurgical treatment includes stress reduction strategies such as rockersoled shoes, arch supports, and rehabilitative exercises.
- Surgical treatment usually involves fusion of the arthritic joints, a procedure that requires prolonged weight restriction and a significant risk of complications.

Pain, stiffness, and swelling are common signs of arthritis. Often the pain occurs on the initiation of activity or with prolonged or intense activity. In the foot, it can cause arch pain and the loss of the arch and bony prominences around the joints. In general, arthritis progresses over a period of years but the rate of progression is variable and the amount of pain is difficult to predict by simply looking at an x-ray.

Osteoarthritis is a wearing out of the joint through "wear and tear." In normal circumstances, the joints are very resilient. Midfoot arthritis is caused by damage and overload of the cartilage. This can occur through a single catastrophic event during trauma. A single high-intensity blow, twist, or fracture can damage fragile cartilage and their supporting ligaments enough to begin the deterioration that eventually leads to cartilage destruction. A hard enough blow can actually kill the cartilage, which, unlike many other tissues, does not repair itself well. The loss of the cartilage changes the tension of the ligaments, a little like letting the air out of a tire. This loosens the ligaments even more. This in turn can increase the rate of cartilage damage. Even a fairly subtle injury can lengthen the ligaments so that their ability to protect the joint cartilage for excessive stress is compromised. The overload of the joints initiates a cycle of cartilage damage increasing friction within the joint leading to more cartilage damage. This cycle is difficult to stop.

More commonly, the joint destruction is more insidious. Over long periods of time, fairly subtle factors can injure a joint. In the same way that a car with poor shock absorbers jars the passengers within, the cartilage experiences more intense jolts of pressure with normal activity if the bone is stiffer. Some people have a genetic predisposition to osteoarthritis in many joints.

Joint damage can also be a result of the design and use of the foot. The shape of the foot can cause uneven wear in some areas. This is the case in the "Morton's foot," when the second metatarsal is longer than the adjacent metatarsals. The length and prominence of this bone concentrates pressure on the second metatarsal. This overload is minimal in normal standing but is accentuated when the foot is positioned in a flexed position. The load from the second metatarsal is transferred into the joints of the midfoot, potentially leading to arthritis in the midfoot. The flexibility of the tendons and ligaments, and the posture that we use to walk and stand can also lead to increased pressure as it is transferred through the midfoot (See Chapter 2).

By far the most common cause of midfoot pain is osteoarthritis. Other things that should be considered include:

- Accessory bones.
- Crystal-induced inflammatory arthritis such as gout.
- Stress fractures especially of the proximal metatarsals and navicular bone.
- Tendon pain can also mimic midfoot arthritis especially along the insertions of the anterior and posterior tibial tendons.

Treatment of midfoot arthritis is generally begun without surgery. As this is a forefoot overload syndrome, treatment is started with rehabilitation and gait training and shoe wear changes such as rockersoled shoes. More information about all is in the resource section of the book. Arch supports help to support the midfoot and reduce compression and shear forces across the joint that usually help to decrease the pain. However, a high arch support is usually not comfortable in people with midfoot arthritis as the support pushes near to their arthritic joints and sometimes takes up much needed room within the shoe. This is especially important because arthritic spurs may form bumps on the top of the joint and be very tender.

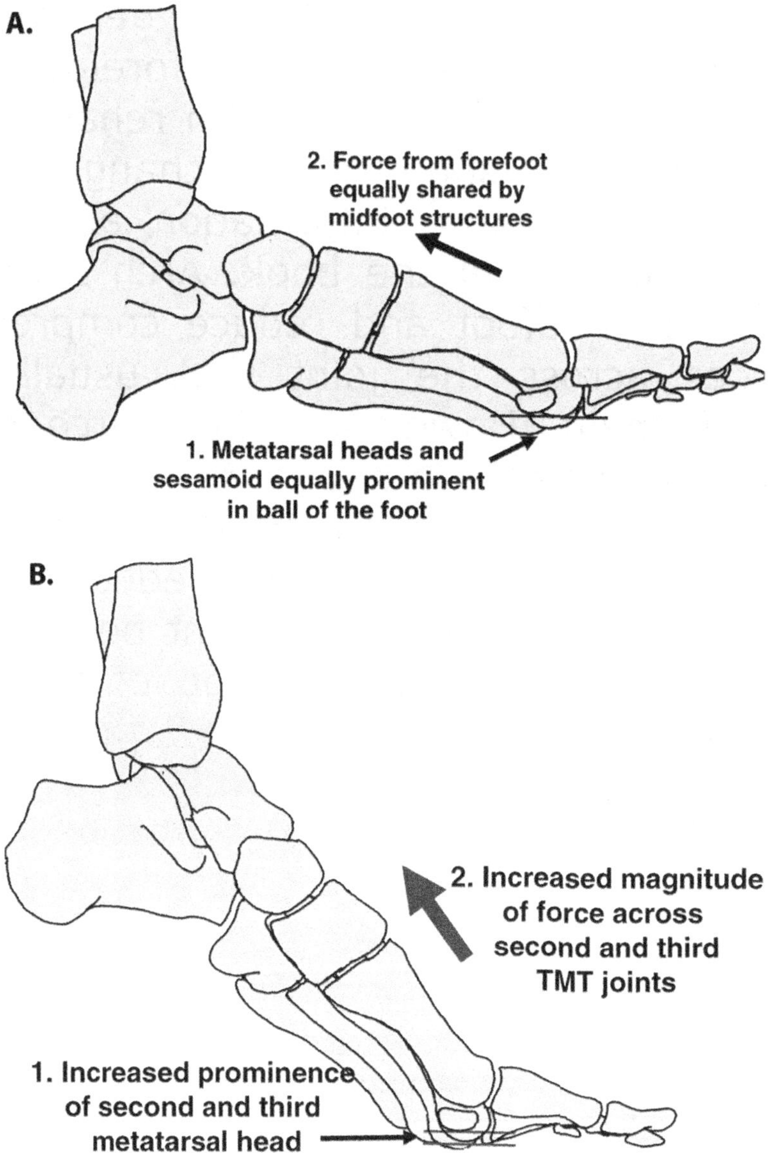

FIGURE 5.2 Force is transferred from the forefoot to the midfoot through the metatarsals (A) during walking. The more prominent and long the metatarsal is the greater the percentage of weight borne through that metatarsal. This becomes accentuated when the ankle is flexed and weight is transferred onto the forefoot (B).

Anti-inflammatory medication such as naprosyn (Aleve®), ibuprofen (Motrin®, Advil®), celecoxib (Celebrex®), and other pain medications such as acetaminophen (Tylenol®) can effectively decrease the pain while they are being taken, but do not cure the arthritis. Steroid injections may be done and sometimes can eliminate bouts of intense "flare-up" pain, but do not cure the arthritis. Injections and oral medications of natural joint components such as glucosamine and chondroitan sulfate have been thought to give temporary relief in knee arthritis and have few side effects. You can get these medicines at the drug store without prescription. The evidence regarding the effectiveness of them is still being explored.

In situations when this doesn't work or the pain continues to limit your ability to complete necessary activities, surgery can be considered. Simple removal of the spurs that occur on the top of the foot is usually unhelpful and can actually destabilize the joint and increase the pain. Surgery for arthritic midfoot joints involves removing the joint roughening up the bone underneath it and pushing the bones together until they heal across the joint and form one bone. This is called bone fusion or arthrodesis. It usually involves the insertion of plates and screws to hold the bones in proper alignment during healing.

The surgery is usually performed as an outpatient under local or general anesthesia. Depending on the complexity of the procedure, it may take one or two hours. The procedures are generally quite painful and narcotic pain medications are frequently needed for several weeks. A period of nonweight-bearing is required that will last between 6 and 12 weeks. During this time, a cast or cast boot is usually needed to hold the foot still to help with healing.

Complications include bleeding, infection, wound problems, numbness, and pain around the scar. A specific problem with this surgery is called *nonunion,* a condition in which the bones do not completely join together and happens about 10% of the time. This usually requires revision or redoing the procedure. Arthritis can develop in the joints next to the fusion because of overuse resulting from the lack of motion in the fused joints.

AGNES'S STORY

Agnes is a 63-year-old woman who works as a supermarket cashier. She has always been an avid walker. Over the past three years, she had noticed pain on the top of her arch that had been explained by a previous physician as spurs. The pain had increased recently and she was prescribed ibuprofen. Ibuprofen helped for a while, but the pain became worse. She began having difficulty going for her daily walks and going shopping and working even became uncomfortable. Then she noticed some sporadic swelling, and a bump on the top of the foot that started making her shoes uncomfortable.

Agnes's feet show firm bony bumps over the top of the midfoot. They cause a coarse grinding sensation in the midfoot, which is uncomfortable. She has fixed hammertoe deformities that are nontender and the ball of the foot is slightly tender with deep pressure, but, Agnes said, this does not bother her when she walks. Agnes wears deck shoes. She has fairly significant abdominal obesity. X-rays showed considerable deterioration of the naviculocunieform joint, a joint in the arch area.

Like many people with forefoot overload, other types of forefoot overload pain accompany the midfoot arthritis. In Agnes's case, she has a mild amount of metatarsalgia and hammertoe formation, both of which are likely to be caused by chronic overuse of the forefoot. It is not uncommon for people with forefoot overload problems like Agnes to complain that their whole foot hurts, a very confusing and frustrating complaint to evaluate and treat.

We suggested rocker-soled shoes and an inexpensive over-the-counter arch support. She was initially resistant to this as she was concerned about the extra weight of the shoes and the style. She was reassured that it could be worthwhile and was asked her to try a few different styles in the shoe store. We also suggested that styles with a Velcro closure might be easier on the prominence on the top of her foot. She began a program of postural training with stretching of the important Achilles, hamstring, hip, and back joints. We discussed the possibility of injecting the painful joints with a steroid, but decided against it. At two months, Agnes was quite happy with her shoes and the pain had decreased considerably and she was back to her fitness walk and was determined to go on to begin to lose the excess weight.

When Agnes came in, she expected that we would decide to remove the spurs. From her perspective, this was a simple and logical solution. After all, she had a painful spur; it only makes sense to remove the offending spur. In fact, this is rarely a satisfactory approach to midfoot arthritis.

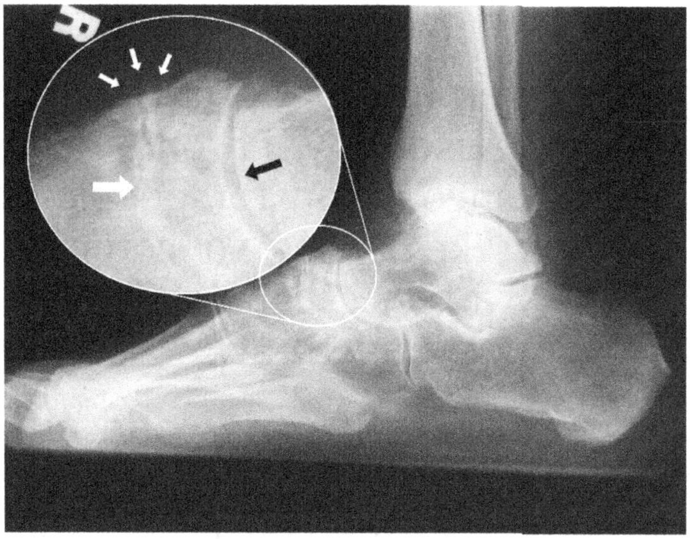

FIGURE 5.3 Deterioration of the naviculocunieform joint in a patient with osteoarthritis (white arrow). Compare this to the healthy joint to the right (black arrow). The spur (small white arrows) is faintly seen.

PAINFUL ACCESSORY OR "EXTRA" BONES

- Accessory bones can occur in several areas of the midfoot and ankle. Although usually they are not painful, they can be the source of discomfort.
- The source of the pain is from stress injury of the bone itself or from irritation of the connective tissue connecting the accessory bone to other structures.
- Initial treatment includes decreasing the stresses on the bone through immobilization and rehabilitative exercises.
- Surgical excision or fusion of the bony fragment is sometimes necessary.

A common variant of the development of the foot in childhood is the presence of "extra" bones. People who have a foot with this type of abnormality usually don't even know it, because usually the foot functions normally. These bones are often contained within the tendons and ligaments of the foot in areas of particularly high pressure and are similar to the sesamoid bones in the big toe that we have discussed previously. Their function is much like the kneecap in the knee. They improve the leverage of the tendon, protect the joints, and keep the tendon from experiencing pressure concentrations that may eventually wear it out. The most common of these bones are in the back of the ankle (os trigonum), on the inside (os naviculare), and outside (os peroneum) of the midfoot.

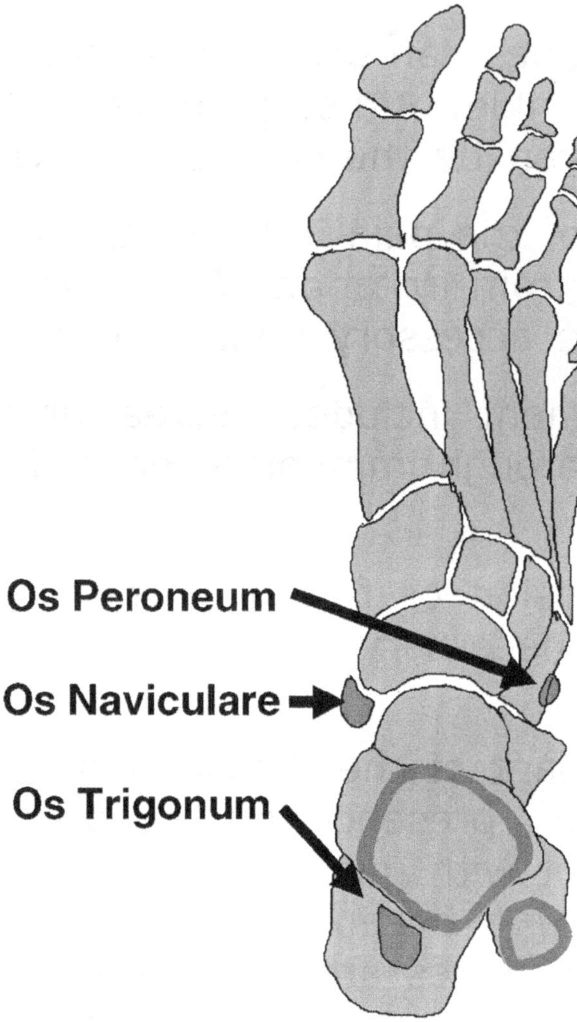

FIGURE 5.4 Common accessory bones in the midfoot and ankle.

Accessory bones are usually not associated with any pain, but sometimes they are very painful. Pain from an accessory bone commonly occurs after a traumatic event such as a sprain, but it can occur without any trauma at all. It can be seen at any age, but is common in the young or middle-aged athlete. A person may experience mild swelling and the pain usually becomes worse with increased activity. The pain is usually situated directly around the bones listed above. These three bones make up 95% or more of the cases of painful accessory bones.

The mere presence of these bones is not a problem, they are present in 2% to 12% of the population. Even in the people who eventually develop pain, the pain can begin after decades of pain-free usage of the foot. It is important to ensure that the extra bone is a painful condition and not just a nonpainful x-ray finding in the vicinity of another painful condition.

These bones generally form a joint with the larger bone that they are associated with. In the case of the os peroneum, the joint between the os perineum and the underlying cuboid bone has surfaces that slide against each other. The os peroneum is prone to a number of conditions including arthritis or joint cartilage injury and stress fracture.

The os naviculare and os trigonum are connected to their larger associated bone through fibrous and cartilaginous connective tissue that has the consistency of scar tissue. This connective tissue is, however, under a great deal of strain and has a limited blood supply. This means that this tissue is more likely to become injured and less likely to heal. The injury that occurs around these bones is similar to other forms of tendonitis in which the injured tissue simply fails to heal completely.

A painful os trigonum is a common problem with ballerinas. Because of the peculiar position that the foot of a ballerina maintains when *en pointe* or on tiptoe, an os trigonum can get pinched between the tibia and the calcaneus like a nut in a nutcracker.

It is important to eliminate other potential sources of pain, as these accessory bones are quite common and usually asymptomatic. Your doctor should be able to decide this through an examination. Other studies such as MRI and bone scan can be helpful in deciding whether the bone is symptomatic by the visualization of swelling and increased metabolism that is evident directly around these bones. Tendonitis or tendon rupture of associated or nearby tendons is a common problem that can be difficult to separate from painful accessory bone. Arthritis of nearby joints or stress fractures of larger associated bones is also another possibility that should be considered.

Like any stress injury, the first line of treatment involves a strategy of reduction of force around the injured structure. Immobilization techniques such as the use of a nonremovable casts or removable cast boots can reduce the stress around nearly any painful accessory bone to reduce the pain and potentially promote healing. Over time, the reduced stress may make the problem pain-free. An exercise program like the one in our resource section, may help promote healing over time. However, often the pain recurs after the resumption of activities.

Anti-inflammatory medications such as ibuprofen and naproxen can blunt the pain when used in concert with a comprehensive rehabilitation program. However, it is unclear whether they are helpful in curing the problem.

We have noticed that few athletes are able to resume competitive play after nonoperative treatment. This does not suggest that efforts at nonoperative treatment are futile or shouldn't first be attempted.

The surgical approach to painful accessory bones depends on the specific bone involved. It can vary from removal and repair of the surrounding structures to fixation with hardware to help the accessory bone heal to the associated larger bone. Sometimes, especially with os naviculare, an associated significant flat-foot deformity is present. If so, realigning the flat-foot deformity should be considered when the painful bone is removed.

ANNE'S STORY

Anne is a 58-year-old woman who injured her ankle in a supermarket parking lot. She went to the emergency room immediately and was told that her x-rays were normal and that she had sprained the ankle. The pain improved for one month, but then remained unchanged for the next three months. The remaining discomfort was enough to make it difficult to perform her job on a production line in a local factory. The primary care physician who initially evaluated her ordered an MRI. The radiologist read the MRI as a chronic tear of the lateral ankle ligaments with residual fluid within the ankle joint, and a tear of the posterior tibial tendon.

Anne had a mild degree of swelling. When stressed, her ankle ligaments seemed to be doing fine as the ankle joint did not seem to twist out of joint. Her tenderness was specifically located on the inside portion of the navicular bone. On reviewing the MRI, Anne had an os naviculare within her posterior tibial tendon with evidence of tissue injury between the os naviculare and the main body of the navicular bone.

In Anne's case, we placed her into a cast boot and instructed her to walk as much as she could tolerate. Many cast boots have a flat surface on the bottom weight-bearing surface of the boot. Anne's bone is intimately associated with the tendon that stabilizes the arch, so we added an arch support to the boot. Anne was able to keep the arch support on her foot by applying it directly to her foot and sock and pulling another sock or nylon over the top of this. She also began a rehabilitation program directed toward increasing the resilience of her damaged tendon and painful joint by gradually resuming her activities.

Unfortunately for Anne, although her pain improved, the treatment didn't cure the condition. This happens more than 50% of the time. In Anne's situation, her foot was operated on, which consisted of removing the bone and repairing the posterior tibial tendon to the navicular using a suture anchor. This is a device that is screwed or impacted into the bone. The device has an eyelet with sutures in it to allow the surgeon to sew or repair the tendon to the bone securely.

Anne was in a cast and was instructed to keep her weight off the leg for six weeks. After this, she was allowed to walk on her foot in her cast boot. Four months later, she had successfully resumed her previous activities and returned to her fairly strenuous job. This procedure is quite successful in younger patients, and should be considered if the child is extremely motivated to return to strenuous athletics.

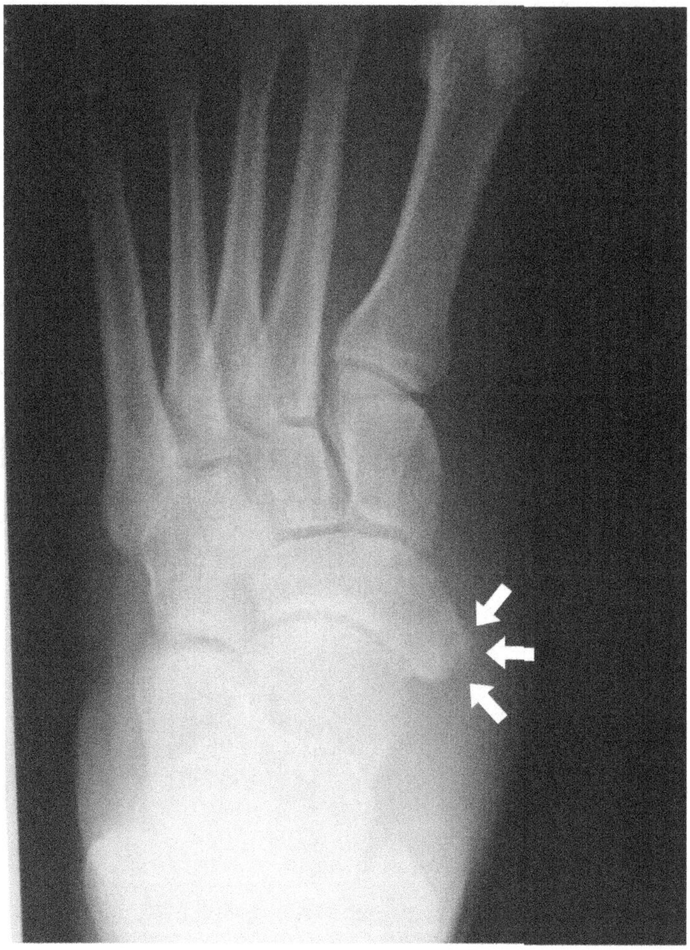

FIGURE 5.5 X-ray of os naviculare (white arrows), an accessory bone within the posterior tibial tendon near the navicular bone.

FLAT FEET

The posterior tibial tendon lies behind the medial malleolus, the bony prominence on the inside of the ankle. The tendon attaches to the lower portion of the bones of the inside midfoot, primarily to the navicular. When it is tensed, the foot begins to angle toward the inside of the foot. Essentially, it accentuates the arch. This is critically important as weight is transferred to the ball of the foot in the second half of the step.

Other ligaments along the bottom of the foot support the arch, especially the short ligaments directly below the midfoot joints, the talonavicular, the naviculocunieform, and the tarsometatarsal joint. The plantar fascia also acts to stabilize the arch by linking the ball of the foot and heel together. The bony architecture of the foot helps to provide stability, but strong ligaments are necessary to maintain its position.

FLEXIBLE FLAT FEET

- Most cases of flat feet function fine with a normal capacity for work, athletics, and other activities.

- Some flat feet will be painful. The stresses on a flat foot are different than the stresses on a foot with a normal arch and are prone to different painful problems.

- No good evidence exists that shoes, braces, therapy, or inserts have the capacity to keep flat feet from becoming painful or to aid in the development of a "normal" arch. Shoes, braces, therapy, and inserts may be helpful in the treatment of pain in a flat foot.

- Surgical treatment of the flexible flat foot is rarely necessary.

The height of the arch is often blamed for foot pain. The height, however, is variable between people and no particular shape of foot within this normal range is clearly better than another. Flat feet were for some time a cause for discharge from military service, but, for most people, their flat feet are not directly a source of pain. For those people and children who have a mild to moderately flat foot and do not experience pain, there is little cause for concern.

If you randomly examine feet, you will find that no two are exactly alike. None of these feet will be "the ideal foot." It isn't even clear what qualities the ideal foot would have. Some feet will naturally have a high arch and some will naturally have a low arch. Most naturally flat feet are more flexible than average. Most will never have significant problems related to the flatness of the foot. A very few will. Multiple studies looking at several factors—including ability to adapt to the rigors of military life, pain as an adult, and suitability for strenuous occupations—have failed to show a relationship with the amount of flatness in a normal foot and its durability, resilience, and tendency to be painful.[1] However, there are several painful conditions in the foot that can cause an unusual degree of flattening or a change in the flatness of the foot.

The majority of toddlers will have feet that appear to be flat because of a large fat pad present in the arch during childhood that regresses as the child matures. However, flat-footed adults usually begin as flat-footed children. Some of these toddlers will have flat-appearing arches that do not go away.

The use of an arch support in the treatment of flat feet in a child is controversial. When prescribing orthotics for children certainly price needs to be considered as it is rare for an insurance plan to cover them and prices can range from $100 to $400. An insert in a growing child will have to be changed after growing two shoe sizes, which may mean that a new one is necessary every four to six months during certain periods in the child's growth. Also, orthotic use will limit the style and variety of shoes, which may be important especially to girls. Most research indicates that custom orthotics have few advantages over cheaper over-the-counter orthotics in terms of satisfaction or comfort. There is also *no* evidence that orthotics will assist in helping to develop an arch as the child grows.[2] The height of the arch is primarily determined by genetics. It is a combination of the flexibility of the ligament and the shape of the bones.

There are studies comparing the shape of feet in people who grew up wearing shoes to those who did not wear shoes. It showed that the prevalence of flat feet dropped from 3.5% to 1.7% in people who did not begin to wear shoes prior to age 16.[3] This calls into question the widely held belief that flat feet can be treated by wearing "proper" shoes. Perhaps, the best shoe is no shoe. However, this isn't generally safe or practical in modern Western society. The issues concerning proper shoe fit are the same in flat-footed people as they are in a person with any other shape of arch: proper width and fit, appropriate heel height and a design appropriate for the intended activity.

If we have established that flat feet are not necessarily painful feet, what else could cause the pain? The answer is just about anything that causes pain in the foot. There are painful conditions that seem to be associated with flat feet. Tarsal coalition is an abnormal linkage caused from improper development of the joints in the hindfoot and is a common cause of ankle pain. We talk about this later in this chapter. Posterior tibial tendon rupture of failure is a common reason for the normal or flat foot to become considerably flatter. Painful accessory bones are another reasonable possibility for painful feet.

Irritation of the growth plates along the inside of the ankle, middle foot, and heel is quite common in children with normally aligned feet, but is probably more common in children with flat feet. The problem can be increased with tightness of the Achilles or hamstring muscles. This is common in growing children, because the length of the muscle sometimes needs to catch up to the bony growth.

The first step in treatment of foot pain associated with a flat foot is to determine if another diagnosis is to blame. If that has been eliminated, pain due to overuse of a flat foot can be effectively treated as a forefoot overload syndrome. Treatment would start with the use of an arch support, a rocker-soled shoe and a stretching and strengthening program as outlined in the resource section. In particularly severe or resistant cases, a short period of casting or immobilization as a prefabricated cast boot may be helpful. Physiotherapists can expand the therapeutic program.

A key principle is not to overtreat the flexible flat foot. The treatment should never be worse than the problem. Surgical treatment should not be considered until all other diagnoses have been ruled out and treatment options have been shown to fail.

A second key principle is not to treat the problem prophylactically. Prophylactic treatment is treating a condition before it is painful. An example of prophylactic treatment is to replace your car tires when worn before they blow out. Certainly, that sounds like a good idea for your car, but the human body is different. First, most invasive treatments have serious potential complications. Second, it is rarely possible to restore the problem to normal. Third, all invasive treatment has a cost, specifically, money, pain, and impairment/lost wages. These all need to be considered and rarely is there an advantage to treating a problem aggressively before it is symptomatic enough to require it.

If the pain is activity-limiting and all other methods of treatment have failed, surgery may be considered. Surgical treatments can be roughly divided into techniques that limit the bone motion (arthroeresis), that realign the bones by cutting them (osteotomy), and that fuse the joints and eliminate motion (arthrodesis).

Arthroeresis has been fairly well studied in children with some success reported. There is little good evidence that it is effective in the adult. Arthroeresis is a procedure in which a metallic or plastic screw is placed along the outside of the hindfoot between the calcaneus and talus. Although it is effective at improving the alignment of the heel and is less invasive than many other surgical alternatives, it should be reserved for situations in which all nonoperative measures have been tried and the pain continues to be severe and activity limiting over a period of at least six months. It is never the initial treatment of flat feet. Many uses of this implant are still considered experimental.

Arthrodesis and osteotomy take a longer time to recover from and complications are possible. Although effective at correcting certain malalignments, recovery time can be 6 to 12 weeks before walking can be resumed. Swelling to some degree can last for a year or more.

MICHAEL'S STORY

Michael is a 12-year-old boy who is very active in several sports offered by his grade school. His mother and grandmother have noticed that he has had flat feet since birth. Initially, the pediatrician said that he would grow out of it. When Michael's feet did not show any signs of "growing out of it" at age five, he was taken to a foot specialist, who placed Michael in custom orthotics. The orthotics cost $300 and were not covered by Michael's health insurance. Michael did not notice much difference in his feet after the orthotics because his feet rarely hurt him. He quickly stopped using them and has since outgrown them. He recently began basketball season and has noticed some mild pain around the heel after games especially tournaments. Several days ago, the same foot care specialist saw him and recommended surgically placing a screw in the outside of his ankle to correct the position, an arthroeresis. The family sought a second opinion.

Michael's foot appears normal when seated, having only some mild tenderness along the inside of his ankle near the medial malleolus and along the back of his heel. Normal motion is noted in all foot joints. However, when asked to bend over and touch his toes, he was unable to bring his fingers closer than six inches to his toes without bending his knees. On standing, the arch flattens significantly and the ankle leans to the inside, making the heel appear to jut out. When asked to stand on his tiptoes, the arch constitutes normally.

Michael has a flexible flat foot that is asymptomatic. He also has a profound hamstring contracture that may be contributing to his heel pain. The pain is due to an overuse injury of the growth plate on the inside of his ankle, probably aggravated by his flat feet and the traction placed on the ligaments on the inside of his ankle. Michael was prescribed an over-the-counter arch support and was started on a stretching program directed toward increasing his flexibility of his hamstrings and Achilles muscles. The pain improved especially after basketball season ended and did not return during track season.

TARSAL COALITION

Key points:

- Tarsal coalition is a genetic abnormality that occurs in a small portion of the population.
- Tarsal coalition is the incomplete separation of the bones in the mid- and back portion of the foot. It sometimes results in stiffness, abnormal alignment, and pain in the ankle and midfoot.
- While immobilization can cause the pain to regress, surgical removal of the coalition or completion of the fusion is sometimes necessary.

Tarsal coalition is a congenital problem in which the tarsal bones—those bones in the midfoot and hindfoot—do not completely separate. As a result, the joints do not completely form or move normally. Most commonly the area of the joint is not bridged by bone but by cartilage or scar tissue.

The majority of people with tarsal coalition do not even know it. One study that examined people at autopsy found that 12% had some degree of tarsal coalition. The number of symptomatic people is less than 1% of the population. People with tarsal coalition usually have feet with normal alignment, although a number of them will have very flat feet.

Usually, this problem becomes symptomatic during adolescence when the growth plates in the bones begin to close. It is likely that the abnormal areas that are joined by scar tissue also begin to solidify and become easier to injure. It is also common to develop pain as a young or middle-aged adult.

Pain from tarsal coalition often is confused with an ankle sprain. The calcaneonavicular coalition is located very close to the lateral ligaments that are usually injured during a sprain. It is only when the pain does not go away that the diagnosis is suspected. It is also quite common for the abnormalities to be missed on x-ray. They can be quite subtle, especially when the coalition is unsuspected.

Tarsal coalition is usually a genetic abnormality. It is transferred from parent to child through a dominant gene. This means that if you have a tarsal coalition, there is a 50% chance that your child will have the gene, regardless of whether that child is a girl or a boy. It is interesting that the coalition is not always in the same place between relatives.

The coalition is an abnormal link usually made of cartilage between the two bones. This is usually asymptomatic until a trauma or overusage injures the cartilage connecting the bones, which are probably normally under increased stress. Many times, if untreated, the cartilage will continue to be persistently painful. In many ways, the condition resembles painful accessory bones within the foot as described earlier. In the child, it is quite common to get various pains, usually associated with overstress of a growth plate cartilage.

Nonoperative treatment can be successful. This consists of reducing activity and immobilizing the area so that the tissue uniting the bones can heal. Pain medications such as ibuprofen and naprosyn can also reduce the pain during healing. Stretching exercises directed at the Achilles as well as the hamstrings are also useful. However, attempts to "loosen up" the stiff joints in the hindfoot will be unsuccessful and may aggravate the condition.

Although nonoperative treatment can commonly help speed recovery of the injured connective tissue linking the bones across the coalition, the tissue will continue to be prone to re-injury. Often when the pain becomes recurrent, athletic activity is not possible. In situations like this, resection of the coalition can predictably lead to resolution. The motion between the joints is often improved, but the alignment and function of the joint if abnormal is not usually changed after the surgery. In some instances, the coalition is so broad that there really is not enough normal joint to maintain stability if the linkage is removed.

ANGELA'S STORY

Angela is a 22-year-old young woman who came into the office for evaluation of pain along the outer portion of her hindfoot for the past eight months. Initially, she sprained the foot while playing soccer and it improved over the ensuing week. However, over the past several months, the ankle has become increasingly easy to aggravate and painful nearly all of the time. She gave up intramural soccer at the state university that she attends because of the pain.

Angela's foot appears to be slightly flat. Her motion from side to side is slightly decreased. Tenderness is along the area inferior and anterior to the distal fibula. When asked to raise her heel from a standing position, the heel does not invert.

X-rays show a connection from the anterior process of the calcaneus to the lateral navicular that is not completely ossified.

Angela was initially treated nonoperatively for four weeks in a short-leg walking cast. Although she was greatly improved initially, she re-injured the area two months later after resuming soccer. Because she was becoming frustrated with her progress and wanted to return to a high level of athletic competition, it was decided to remove the bar. The surgery was completed on an outpatient basis. She had considerable pain for about one week and then was progressively returned to full activity. She returned to full soccer play four months later.

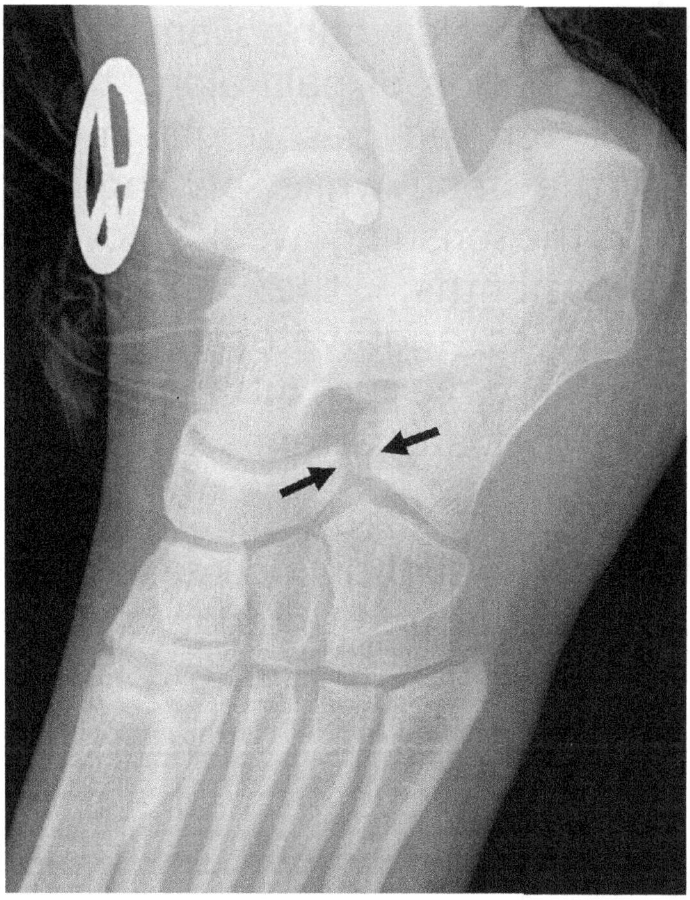

FIGURE 5.6 X-ray showing a fibrous calcaneonavicular tarsal coalition in Angela's foot. Note the broad connection between the anterior process of the calcaneus and the navicular, two bones that in normal circumstances do not touch together.

FALLEN ARCHES/ACQUIRED FLAT-FOOT DEFORMITY

Key points:

- Acquired flat-foot deformity is a change in the arch resulting in flattening and eversion of the foot. Although it can be caused by bone or ligament damage and arthritis, it most commonly involves tearing and loss of function of the posterior tibial tendon.
- People who have flat feet are more likely to develop acquired flat feet.
- Sometimes posterior tibial tendonitis will resolve with nonoperative treatment including immobilization and rehabilitative exercises.
- Once the deformity has developed, there is no nonoperative treatment that will reverse it.
- When bracing, inserts, and rehabilitative exercises fail to control the symptoms, surgical reconstruction should be considered. These procedures are extensive and recuperation from them is prolonged.

"Fallen arches" or loss of an arch, in a person who previously had an arch, is a sign of a problem. Many structures can be potentially to blame. The posterior tibial tendon, which runs behind the ankle and supports the arch can become inflamed and even rupture and cause the foot to lose the arch over a period of time. When the tendon begins to deteriorate or wear out, small tears form in the tendon. The tendon does not usually tear completely. It begins to gradually stretch out. Unfortunately, if the tendon stretches much, the muscle becomes much weaker because the muscle loses its tension. As the muscle is used less and less, it can permanently scar and waste away until it no longer has the capacity to recover. In this situation, even if the tendon were repaired, the strength would not return. Loss of the arch can also occur with the rupture of certain ligaments in the middle foot or ankle. Finally, certain types of joint arthritis within the midfoot can cause flattening of the arch. This is especially common when there has been nerve damage to the foot such as in diabetes.

Posterior tibial tendonitis is the most common cause for fallen arches. In the initial stages, it may be represented only by swelling and pain along the back and inside of the ankle. Sometimes, this pain is only temporary as it is often possible for tendonitis to resolve even without treatment. As the problem worsens, however, the foot can change shape. Comparing the injured to the uninjured foot, it may appear as if the inside of the foot is more bowed or scrunched together along the outside. The arch drops closer to the floor and the bones of the inner portion of the midfoot may become more prominent. The toes may appear to point away from the midline more than on the healthy side. When viewed from the back, more toes may be seen to the outside of the ankle on the injured foot than on the healthy foot. This is called *too-many-toes* sign.

It is fairly common for the pain to begin on the inside and back portion of the ankle. Often it radiates along the inside of the foot and into the calf. As the inside of the ankle bows, the bones of the outside of the ankle can compress, crushing the joint surfaces. The pain from this is usually felt in the front and lateral portion of the ankle.

Weakness and imbalance in muscle strength in the arch causes the flattening. The weakness can also cause a sense of instability and often people with posterior tibial tendonitis will fall easily. When examining people with posterior tibial tendonitis, there is usually weakness or even an inability to turn the foot to the inside or invert it.

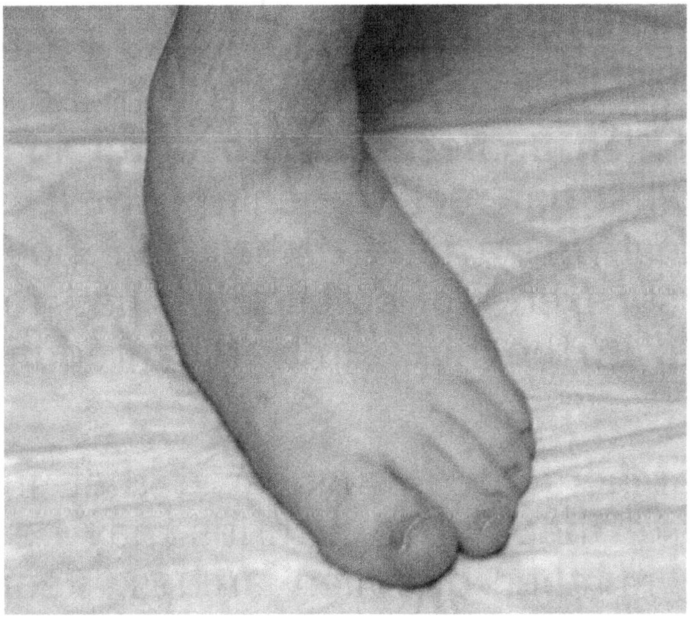

FIGURE 5.7 A foot with posterior tibial tendonitis exhibiting the forefoot abduction or sweeping toward the outside of the forefoot. Notice how the inner structures of the foot are under tension while the structures on the outside appear to be crushing.

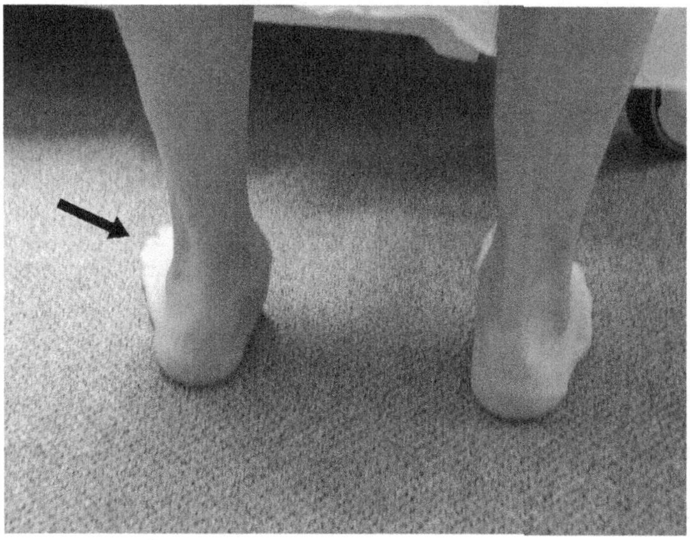

FIGURE 5.8 "Too many toes" sign. Notice how the foot on the left bows to the inside, exposing the lateral toes (arrow) along the outer border of the leg more than on the right.

Posterior tibial tendonitis or fallen arches is a common degenerative tendonitis. Although posterior tibial tendonitis can be seen in people with normal arches, frequently fallen arches seem to occur in people who have somewhat flat feet to begin with. It is likely that the persistent extra effort that the posterior tibial tendon must exert to stabilize a flat foot with its looser joints in the heel and arch gradually wears it out.

Many researchers have suggested that inflammatory conditions like rheumatoid arthritis may be responsible for a large number of fallen arches. People afflicted with rheumatoid arthritis commonly have severely flattened arches along with a number of foot deformities. There are a large number of yet unidentified forms of joint and connective tissue inflammatory conditions that most likely affect people and these conditions may be responsible for many cases of fallen arches.

Clinically, conditions associated with forefoot overload such as Achilles tendon contractures are commonly seen with posterior tibial tendonitis. It is difficult to determine whether this is a cause of posterior tibial tendon wear, but mechanically it certainly increases the pain and discomfort of fallen arches.

Posterior tibial tendon failure is frequently the initial cause of fallen arches. There are other conditions that should be looked for:

- Midfoot arthritis.
- Collapse from arthritis of the ankle.
- Stress injury in people with nerve injury (such as diabetes).
- Rupture of the plantar fascia.
- Traumatic rupture of the ligaments in the mid- and hindfoot.
- Stress fracture of the tibia can also bend the ankle leading to a flatfooted appearance.

Initial treatment of a fallen arch is usually nonsurgical. When the problem has come on suddenly, immobilization in a walking cast can decrease inflammation and help the tendon heal. This is usually continued for about six weeks. Steroid injections can also help with inflammation. However, the steroids can weaken the tendon temporarily and, too frequently, cause worsening of the problem by completely rupturing the tendon.

After the initial acute inflammation has subsided, arch supports and braces may be used to support the arch. Unfortunately, these devices do not restore the arch, but they do realign it while the device is worn. This can improve pain and walking endurance. By reducing the force and stress on the tendon, these devices can further aid healing, eventually allowing for transition to less cumbersome braces to stabilize the foot. In many instances, these devices may need to be continued indefinitely, because, once the arch has changed shape, it does not return to normal and may continue to be painful without the brace.

Treatment of this disorder follows the guidelines for a foot overload syndrome outlined in this book. Stretching the Achilles, hamstring, and improving posture and balance will lessen the force applied to the forefoot. Short courses of physical therapy may aid in decreasing inflammation and improving strength and flexibility.

Surgical treatment can be considered when the above measures do not give adequate relief or when high demand is required of the ankle. The surgical approach is individualized to the problem and the patient. However, often it requires fusion or cutting of the bones in order to realign the ankle and foot along with repair of the damaged tendons and ligaments. This can necessitate multiple incisions. Recovery from these procedures is prolonged and can require 6 to 12 weeks of weight restriction and up to a year before maximum improvement. The majority (80% or more) of people who undergo these operations note significant improvement. Complications from reconstruction of posterior tibial tendonitis specific to this operation include arthritis of surrounding joints, nonunion, over- and under-correction of the deformity. Rarely, these complications require further surgery.

MELVIN'S STORY

Melvin is a 68-year-old man who is retiring as a railroad foreman in one year. He noticed swelling and pain about eight months ago and over the past four months has a decided limp. He now feels as if his ankle is giving way. He purchased some inserts at the drugstore that initially seemed to help quite a bit, but overall he is feeling worse and worse.

Melvin has boggy swelling and tenderness along the back and inside of his ankle, behind his medial malleolus. He is unable to raise his heel off the ground and his weight onto the ball of his foot without a lot of pain. When standing, the arch is flatter than the other side, the inside of the ankle bows toward the midline, and the heel juts laterally. He is unable to invert his foot against force.

Standing x-rays show instability and abnormally large degrees of sliding of the hindfoot joints relative to one another. The end of the fibula bone on the outside of the ankle is in contact with the heel bone, causing erosion of the fibular tip.

Melvin has fairly severe posterior tibial tendonitis that has allowed his tendon to lengthen and weaken. Over time, the ligaments of his arch have stretched out and the foot has developed a flattening of the arch.

Melvin was initially placed in a walking cast for six weeks. After this, his swelling was improved and his ability to invert the foot increased slightly. However, when he stood up, he continued to have the fallen arch posture. He was begun on a therapy program and placed in a short-articulated ankle foot orthosis. He has been released from therapy and his pain continues to improve six months later. In addition, he has returned to work in a light-duty status. He requires a slightly larger shoe size to accommodate his brace. He fills the extra room on the other side with an extra liner in the shoe. Although the flattened arch deformity never returns to normal, often the swelling, inflammation, and acute pain of posterior tibial tendonitis can resolve so that normal activity with mild pain can resume.

FOOT MASSES

Key points:

- The vast majority of foot masses are not malignant or cancerous.
- Usually, the masses can be observed until symptoms necessitate removal.
- Excision of ganglion cysts, common gel filled masses arising from the joints and tendons are associated with a 10% to 20% recurrence rate.
- Excision of plantar fibromas, connective tissue masses that form usually along the plantar fascia in the arch, often fails to alleviate the pain and can result in recurrence.

Foot masses are any lump or bump on the foot. Feet have a lot of lumps and bumps, some of them are serious, most of them are not. Some foot masses are painful and some interfere with wearing shoes and often need to be removed. Nearly all new foot masses need to be evaluated by a physician. Although the vast majority of masses are not serious, cancer can occur in the foot very rarely. Often cancers of the foot can be effectively treated if caught early. To give you a sense of how rare this is, in the past 10 years, as a foot specialist, I have diagnosed two cancers of the foot and six noncancerous tumors of hundreds of patients with masses.

Ganglion Cysts

By far the most common foot mass is the ganglion cyst. Ganglion cysts are noncancerous masses that can appear suddenly around joints or tendon sheaths. Common locations for ganglion cysts are the lateral portion of the ankle and along the lateral part of the midfoot, although they can be seen nearly anywhere on the foot. The cyst cavity usually is connected to a joint or tendon sheath. The cyst is filled with a straw-yellow-colored, jelly-like substance that contains proteins and large sugar molecules found in joint fluid. Basically, the gel within the cyst is concentrated joint fluid, a little like maple syrup is boiled down from gallons of maple tree sap. The cysts can get larger or smaller depending on the fluid production of the joint. It is usually larger with increased activity.

No one completely understands why ganglion cysts form. They originate from defects in the joint capsule. Some people seem to be more prone to them.

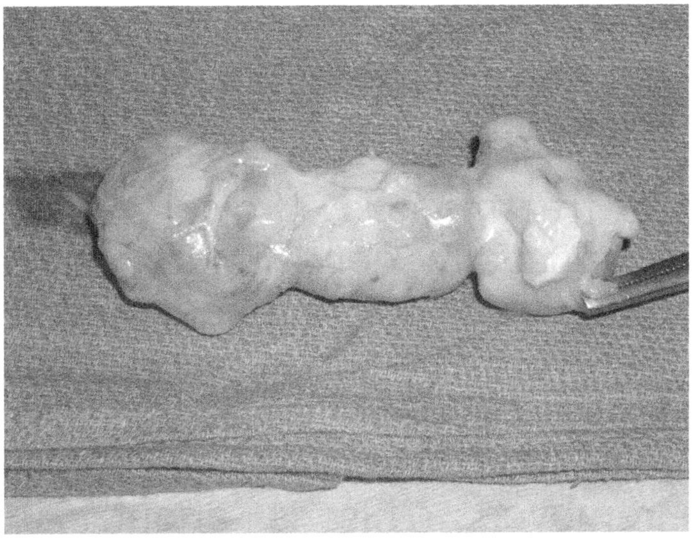

FIGURE 5.9 Ganglion cyst specimen from the midfoot. The cyst is composed of a filmy capsule containing a thick gelatin-like clear fluid.

There are several ways to treat them. One is to ignore them and, on occasion, the cysts will go away. If they are causing difficulty with shoe wear or causing pain, which they occasionally do, they can be more aggressively treated. However, they can be observed indefinitely with no ill effects.

One common form of treatment is aspiration and injection. This is usually done in the office. After cleaning and perhaps numbing the skin with a local anesthetic, a large needle is placed into the cyst and the contents removed. This may be difficult if the cyst has many separate compartments, which is sometimes the case. Often the cyst is then injected with a steroid. The success rate for this procedure is about 30% to 50%. The steroid can discolor the skin or leave a depression if the steroid causes the fat in the tissue to atrophy or melt away. This is almost never dangerous, but can leave an undesirable and probably permanent mark.

A final form of treatment is surgical excision or cutting it out. This is usually done under general or local anesthesia. An incision is made and the cyst is dissected away from the surrounding tissue. The neck of the cyst should be identified as it enters the tendon sheath or joint and usually a portion of the joint capsule is removed. This is about 70% to 90% successful and is accompanied by all the potential complications of surgery.

Bursitis

Bursitis is very similar to ganglion cysts. Under the microscope, they can look identical. Bursitis, however, is usually caused by something rubbing on a bony prominence. A bursa is a space in the tissue that forms to decrease friction between tissue planes. Mechanically, the effect is much like stepping on a sandwich bag. Like a bursa, a sandwich bag has a lining that can be filled with anything. However, when it is empty and you step on it, the slick lining will will roll on itself and slide under your feet. When it is subject to repetitive rubbing and pressure, the space can fill with fluid like the ganglion cyst and the lining can become thick. This will increase the prominence of the bursa.

Common places to form these are under the metatarsal heads, especially under the big toe MTP joint. Another common area is in the back of the heel, along where the counter of the shoe contacts the foot. The most important way to treat bursitis is to decrease the pressure on the area. Some ways of doing this are to off-load the pressure on a prominent bone, or to shift the weight on the foot with an orthotic or foot wedge.

If this is unsuccessful, then all of the options available for treatment of a ganglion cyst are reasonable. However, if the pressure on the prominence is not treated, it will likely come back. In some situations, a surgical osteotomy or cutting of a bone is necessary to reduce the pressure on the bone.

Plantar Fibromatosis

Plantar fibromatosis or Ledderhosen disease is the most common cause for bumps on the bottom of the foot. Although it is not cancerous and does not become cancer, it is called *locally aggressive.* This means that it has the potential to get larger over time and can recur after surgical removal.

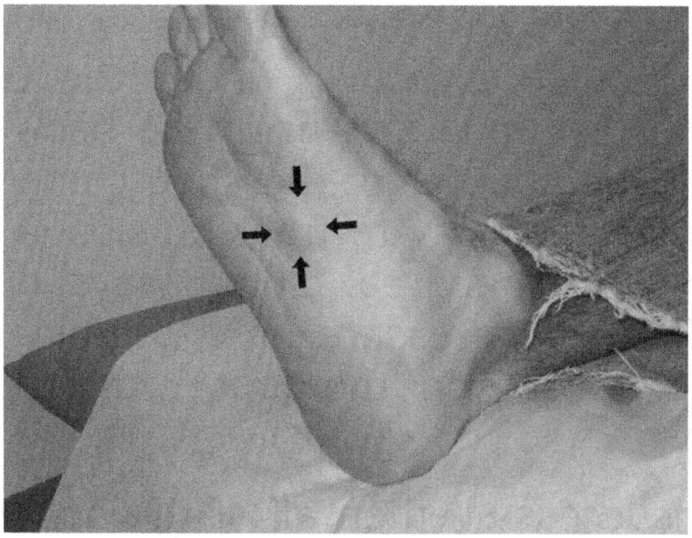

FIGURE 5.10 Plantar fibroma causing pain in the arch of the foot. These benign masses are almost always located along the plantar fascia.

No one knows for sure what causes plantar fibromatosis, but it does seem to occur in fascial tissue along the plantar fascia from the toes to the bottom of the heel. It seems to be a combination of genetics and environmental causes. An association with phenobarbital therapy, a treatment for seizures, seems evident. This abnormal tissue can occur in the palms of the hand, in the shaft of the penis, and in the soles of the feet. When a person develops it in one of these places, it is common for it to occur in other places, on the other side of the body, or in different places on the same extremity. It can occur at any age. It is more common in men and in people with diabetes.

Most commonly, people come to the doctor worried that the bumps may be cancerous, but the masses can be painful or cause problems with rubbing on shoes. If possible, they are best treated through bracing, orthotics, and stretching exercises, but, if these fail and the discomfort associated with them is considerable, surgical removal can be considered.

Simply removing the bumps results in a greater than 50% chance of recurrence. Adequate surgical treatment is possible through near complete removal of all fascial tissue. This fascial tissue extends from the heel to all of the toes. This means that the scars after this surgery are extensive. The sensory nerves to the bottom of the feet also lie underneath the fascial tissue, so they can scar or become sensitive after surgery to the plantar fascia. Finally, because large flaps of skin are raised to expose the plantar fascia and the attachments that occur between the fibromatosis and the skin, some of the skin may die after the surgery, leaving wounds that may take a while to heal or even require further surgical reconstruction.

Tendonitis and Other Pseudotumors

Tendonitis can cause masses that are often mistaken for serious disorders. The small tears that occur in the individual fibers of the tendon, without tearing the entire tendon apart, can begin a reparative or healing reaction that can become quite large, painful, and can grow quickly. The most common place for this is back of the heel at the attachment site for the Achilles tendon and is often called a *pump bump.* It can rub on the back of the heel of the shoe. The Achilles tendon can also form a similar reaction, often about two or three inches above the attachment of the tendon, more or less directly behind the ankle. Usually, a physician can make this diagnosis on clinical grounds and special diagnostic tests are not necessary unless other diagnoses are suspected.

Another common process that can mimic a tumor is a stress fracture. The healing bone that forms around a stress fracture can cause enlargement of the bone that can feel like a knob. Usually pain is intense over the knob and the whole area is swollen. These injuries should be evaluated and protected until healed. Common areas for stress fractures that mimic tumors are the metatarsals, along the fibula on the lateral portion of the ankle and along the tibia or shin.

A final mimic of tumors is bone prominence or spurring when the joints become unstable and begin to sag. This instability may be associated with arthritis (see the chapter on midfoot arthritis) or loss of sensation due to diabetes and other forms of neuropathy. When the bones shift out of place due to instability, prominences can be seen in the foot. The areas of the foot most commonly affected by this are the bottom of the midfoot and the forefoot. Sometimes, they can become so prominent that ulcers can develop.

MIDFOOT FRACTURES AND SPRAINS

Key points:

▪ Midfoot sprains are much more serious than ankle sprains.

▪ Midfoot fractures and complete sprains are sometimes missed on x-rays because the abnormalities can be subtle.

▪ Even mild midfoot sprains can take a long time to heal.

▪ Surgery is common for complete midfoot sprains. Left untreated, they can lead to arthritis and foot deformity.

Ligaments that bind the metatarsals and tarsal joints are key to the stability of the midfoot. Another key ligament is the plantar fascia, a thick band of tissue that connects the toes to the heel of the foot. This ligament is easy to feel in the arch if the toes are extended. The plantar fascia is a large ligament that tenses as pressure is placed on the front of the foot. Without it, stresses within the bones of the arch would be much less uniform and would damage these joints quickly.

Midfoot fractures and sprains are a group of injuries to the arch of the foot that vary from mild to very severe injuries. Despite using the term *sprain* for this injury, a sprain of the midfoot can lead to changes within the foot that result in permanent pain and early arthritis of these joints. The midfoot relies heavily on the ligaments to maintain stability and to keep the arch from collapsing.

On the milder side of injury is the flexion sprain of the midfoot. In this sprain, the foot is forcibly pushed toward the sole of the foot while the hindfoot does not move. An example of this injury is when the body lands on the top of the foot and the foot is forced into flexion. In this injury, the ligaments of the top of the foot joints are torn. Often small fragments of bone are popped off along with the torn ligaments. Although often very painful, these injuries will heal even while continuing to bear weight fully. These injuries usually completely resolve.

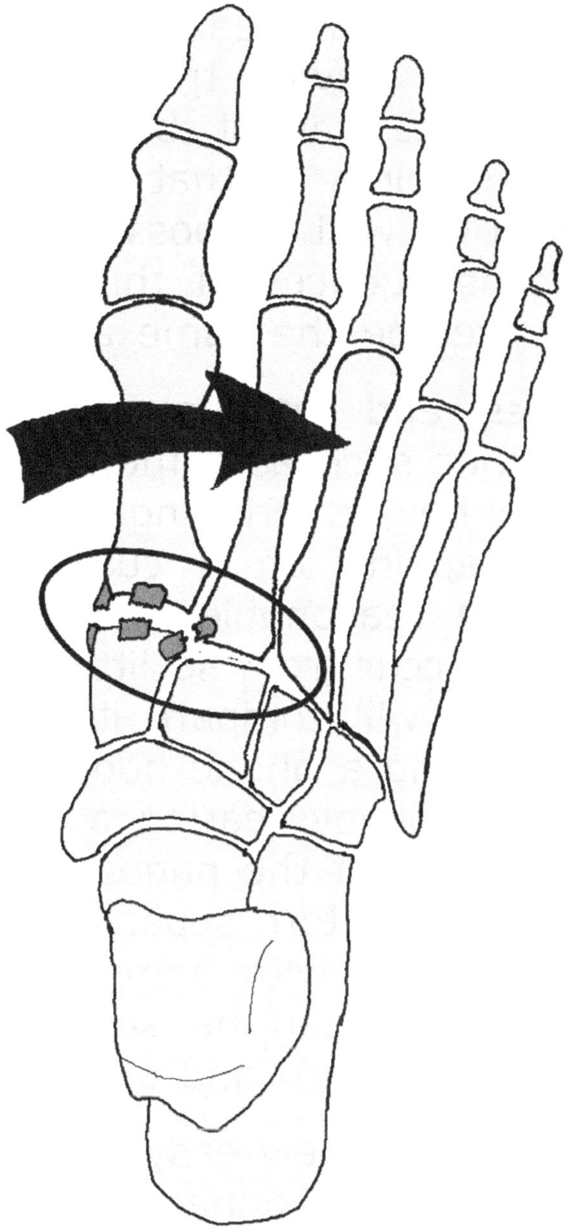

FIGURE 5.11 Illustration of the mechanism and tissue injury after a midfoot sprain.

More serious injuries involve the tearing or fracture of the bones and ligaments on both the top and bottom of the foot. Usually, the forefoot is forced to the outside or upward relative to the hindfoot. These fractures and sprains can tear the ligaments on the bottom of the foot, leaving the joints unstable and loose. These injuries cannot be treated as easily. Restoration of the joints so that the anatomy of the joints is restored as well as possible is necessary to minimize the consequences of this injury. It is rare for the foot to ever be the same after this injury.

Midfoot fractures and sprains can be caused by high-energy injuries such as a motor vehicle accident or a fall from a height. Tripping injuries such as a twisting when stepping on a curb can also cause midfoot sprains. A reasonable question is "how can so much damage occur from so little force?" In order to answer this, we will compare it to the commonly known trick of tearing a phone book. If one attempts to tear a phone book by tearing all of the pages at once, it is impossible. If the pages are fanned apart, essentially each page is torn separately and the phone book may be ripped with very little effort. The structures of the foot can be sequentially torn like this until a completely torn and unstable joint results.

These injuries are extremely easy to miss on an x-ray. The muscles and other connective tissue often pull the joints back into a near-normal position after injury. When the injury is only within the ligaments and does not involve bony injury, the x-rays can be unimpressive. However, the injuries that involve primarily the ligaments are often more serious than the ones that primarily result in fractures.

One form of midfoot fracture that occurs in people who have developed nerve damage most commonly from diabetes is fully discussed in Chapter 9. It is treated much differently than the injury seen in people with normal sensation within the feet.

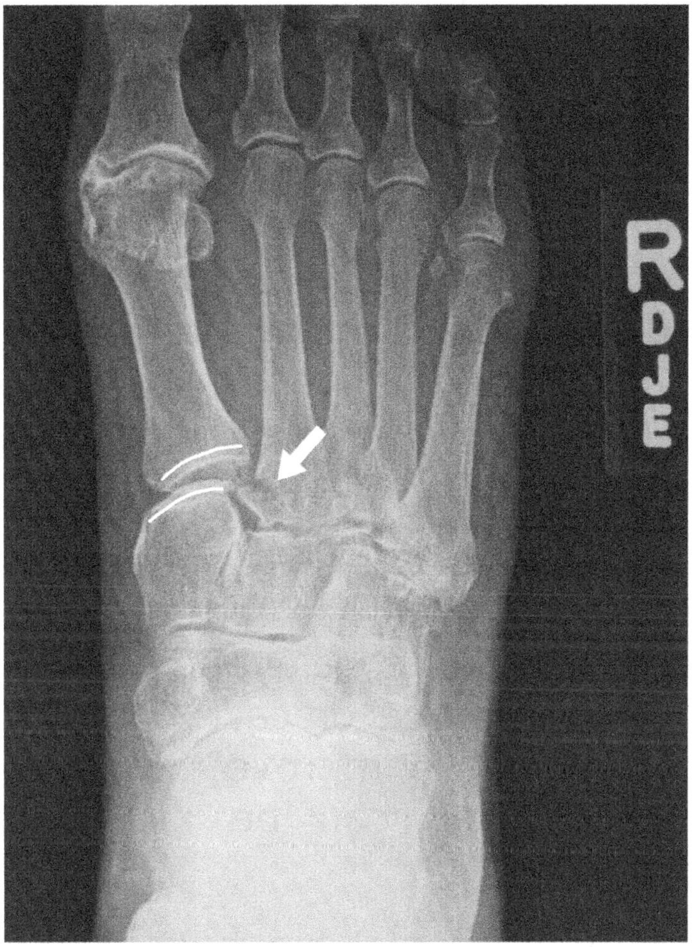

FIGURE 5.12 A fairly subtle but serious midfoot injury represented by an incongruent or poorly fitting first tarsometatarsal joint (white lines) and an avulsion fracture of the base of the second metatarsal (white arrow) reflecting a tear of a crucial midfoot ligament called the Lisfranc ligament.

What else could it be? The important issue is to ensure that these common, serious, but unfortunately often overlooked injuries are adequately treated.

Injuries to accessory bones within the midfoot.

- Bruises from direct blows such as having a car run over the foot.
- Midfoot arthritis.
- Masses most commonly ganglion.

Most importantly, a physician who routinely sees these injuries and is comfortable determining whether surgical reconstruction is necessary should evaluate the injury. This is always best done sooner rather than later.

If surgical reconstruction is not necessary, then standard treatment like that for any other sprain is recommended: rest, ice, elevation, and sometimes immobilization in a brace or cast. These injuries take considerably longer to improve than ankle sprains. Some degree of pain can be present for several months or longer.

Often, a prefabricated walking boot can help walking in the early stages of healing. These boots control the amount of stress on the front of the foot and can decrease pain. After the swelling subsides, a rocker soled shoe and an arch support may help with the remaining discomfort.

Persistent symptoms suggestive of painful arthritis are common (30%–60%)[4][5][6] even with optimal surgical reduction. When pain continues, nonoperative treatment can be instituted in a manner similar to that recommended for midfoot arthritis.

Surgical treatment involves setting the joint back into its original position and placing screws and pins across the joint to keep it aligned until the ligaments heal. Surgeons are relying on the ligaments to heal at their natural length and strength because there is no technique for reliable ligament direct repair. After the operation, weight bearing is restricted for six to twelve weeks and the screws are often removed at some point afterward. People who have sustained these injuries often continued to have pain despite the normal appearance of the radiographs.

A recent study has caused many surgeons to consider changing their approach to the treatment of ligamentous midfoot injures.[7] The approach is arthrodesis or fusion of the midfoot joint in an effort to reestablish the stability of the arch. In this procedure, the joint and the hard bone directly underneath it are removed. The bones are then pressed together and allowed to heal like a fracture would so that the two (or multiple) bones become a single bone. The study comparing people with ligamentous midfoot injuries who have been treated with the traditional fixation and those who have had their joints fused found that the people with the fusions had less pain and better function than people who had traditional fixation. Although this is a reasonable treatment, completely recommending this more aggressive technique requires agreement by other investigators and should not be based on one study.

NOTES

[1] Ester mans A, Pilot to L. Foot shape and its effect on functioning in Royal Australian Air Force recruits. Part 1: Prospective cohort study. *Mil Med.* 2005 Jul;170(7):623–628.

[2] Wenger DR, Mauldin D, Speck G, Morgan D, Limber RL. Corrective shoes and inserts as treatment for flexible flatfoot in infants and children. *J Bone Joint Surge Am.* 1989 Jul;71(6):800–810.

[3] Rao UB, Joseph B. The influence of footwear on the prevalence of flat foot: A survey of 2300 children. *J Bone Joint Surge Br.* 1992;74:525–527.

[4] Hardcastle PH, Reschauer R, Kutscha-Lissberg E, Schoffmann W. Injuries to the tarsometatarsal joint. Incidence, classification and treatment. *J Bone Joint Surg Br.* 1982;64(3):349–356.

[5] Wilppula E. Tarsometatarsal fracture-dislocation. Late results in 26 patients. *Acta Orthop Scand.* 1973;44:335–345.

[6] Kuo RS, Tejwani NC, Digiovanni CW, et al. Outcome after open reduction and internal fixation of Lisfranc joint injuries. *J Bone Joint Surg Am.* 2000 Nov;82-A(11):1609–1618.

[7] Ly TV, Coetzee JC. Treatment of primarily ligamentous Lisfranc joint injuries: Primary arthrodesis compared with open reduction and internal fixation. A prospective, randomized study. *J Bone Joint Surg Am.* 2006 Mar;88(3):514–520.

6

Hindfoot and the Heel

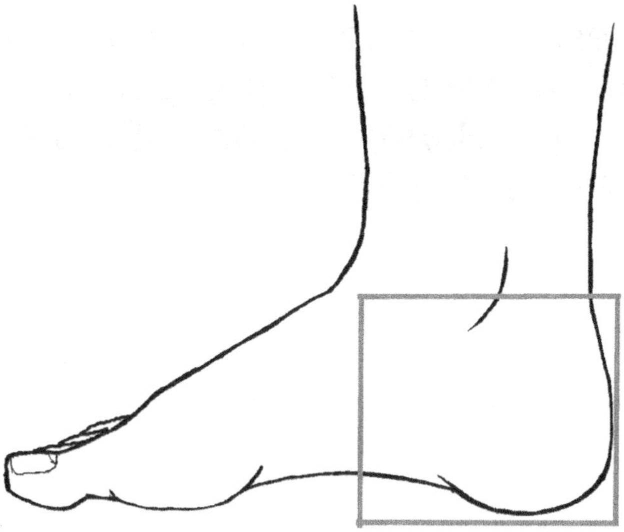

ANATOMY

The bones of the hindfoot include the heel or calcaneus bone, the talus, the navicular, and the cuboid. These bones form the subtalar joint (under the talus) between the calcaneus and talus and the talo-navicular joint between the talus and navicular and the calcaneo-cuboid joint. Together the joints give the foot the ability to turn from side to side to adjust to changes in the contour of the ground.

The plantar fascia, an important stabilizer of the midfoot, attaches to the heel at its lower prominence along with several small muscles that aid in movement of the toes and arch. A tough ligament that extends from the calcaneus to the medial and plantar aspect of the navicular also controls the talo-navicular joint. This ligament is called the spring ligament and cups and supports the head of the talus, thereby keeping the arch from sagging.

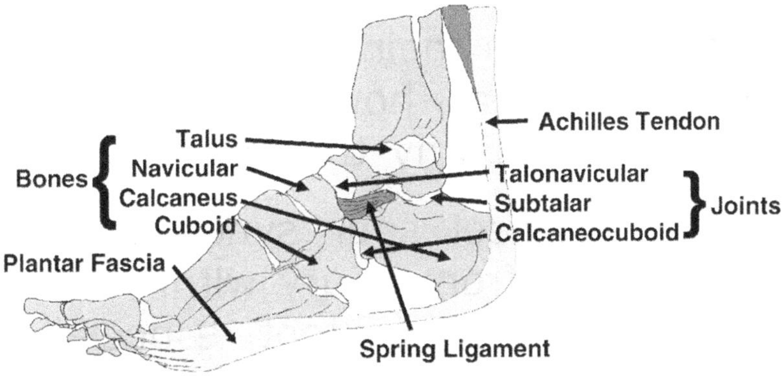

FIGURE 6.1 Anatomy of hindfoot.

PLANTAR FASCIITIS/HEEL SPURS

- Plantar fasciitis is an irritation of a ligament that extends from the base of the toes to the heel. It is most commonly painful near its attachment on the heel.

- This injury is caused by many things including age, weight, and overuse.

- Most cases of plantar fasciitis resolve without surgery.

- Expensive custom inserts are no more helpful than over-the-counter inserts.

- Many effective nonoperative treatments exist. No one treatment is successful for everyone.

Many people who suffer from plantar fasciitis say that it can be an exquisitely painful and limiting condition. It is by far the most common problem in our practice. It has been estimated that 1 in 10 people will suffer from plantar fasciitis in their lifetime. It may be higher than this. Ninety percent, however, will recover without surgery, some without any treatment whatsoever.

Plantar fasciitis or heel spur syndrome is a painful condition that arises from injury within the connective tissue on the bottom of the foot, especially the heel. The plantar fascia is a tough, stiff strip of connective tissue that covers the smaller muscles within the arch. This structure extends from the base of the toes to the front of the heel. You can feel it as a band along the inside of the arch area when you pull your toes up. The normal job of the plantar fascia is to help control the arch during walking and standing. When the toes extend at the end of a step when the weight is on the ball of the foot, the fascia tightens making the arch rigid. This allows you to push through the foot with the strong muscles of the back of the calf without the arch sagging. Many of the fibers of the plantar fascia pass around the heel and become a part of the Achilles tendon in the back of the heel.

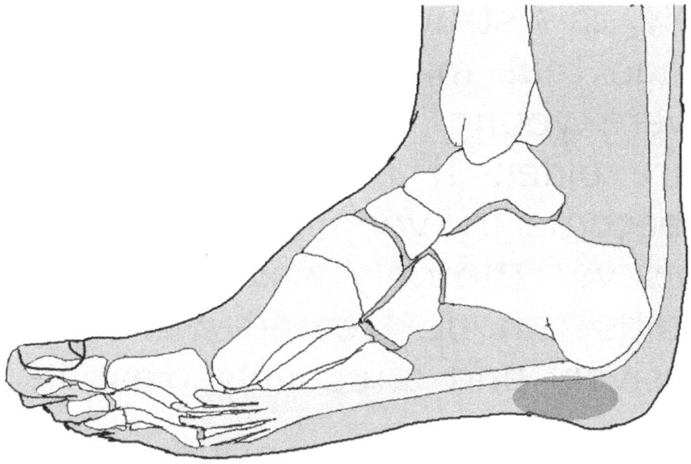

FIGURE 6.2 Localization of heel pain in plantar fasciitis.

Many things increase the stress on the plantar fascia while walking or engaging in other activities. Factors that can injure the plantar fascia include:

- Being overweight.
- Overuse.
- Athletic activity.
- Not having proper flexibility.

A sudden or powerful blow as can happen during a fall from a height can also cause an injury directly to the heel although this is less common than the repetitive overuse injury. Anything that increases the amount of tension on the plantar fascia or the amount of time that the plantar fascia is tensed will aggravate the condition. This includes posture, both of the body and the foot, shoe wear, occupation, and recreational activities. Forefoot overload may play an important role in this condition.

Unfortunately, this structure deteriorates with age and activity. Usage that may have been easy to tolerate when we were young may cause pain and irritation when we are older. It is more common for plantar fasciitis to become irreversible and potentially require surgery. However, the only way to determine whether plantar fasciitis can be treated without an operation is to aggressively and effectively treat it.

Other diagnoses need to be considered. Plantar fasciitis is localized to the bottom of the weight-bearing portion of the heel. It is often on the forward (toward the toes) and inside part of the heel pad. Occasionally, other parts of the plantar fascia can be tender, such as the outside of the heel pad or in the arch.

Other problems that may be confused with plantar fasciitis include:

- Pinched nerve behind the inside of the ankle/Tarsal Tunnel syndrome.
- Pinched nerve around the plantar fascia/Baxter's nerve.
- Arthritis of midfoot or hindfoot.
- Stress fracture of the heel/calcaneus.
- Tumors of the heel.
- Fallen arch/posterior tibial tendonitis.
- Pinched nerve in the back/sciatica.

Radiographs are commonly taken to evaluate heel pain. When the problem has not responded to initial treatment, it is important at some point to ensure that a rare tumor or uncommon stress fracture is not present.

Heel spurs are often seen in x-rays in the evaluation of heel pain. Plantar fasciitis is even sometimes referred to as *heel spur syndrome.* In fact, 50% of people with heel pain will have a plantar fascial spur of some size, but so will 15% of people without heel pain.[1] Commonly, the heel spur is blamed for the pain. However, this blame is misplaced. The problem with this assumption is that the logical response to it is that the heel spur must be removed before the pain will go away. This is not true. Even though it may feel as though a knife is piercing through the heel and it may seem logical that the heel spur is responsible for this, the spur is in reality fairly small, usually about 2mm to 5mm. The heel spur extends parallel to the floor and so does not actually gouge into the skin of the heel. The heel spur is covered by 10mm or more of fat and skin on the bottom of the heel and is usually deep to the tough plantar fascia. The swelling often felt along the bottom of the foot is enlargement of the plantar fascia, which is commonly two or three times as thick as normal in patients with plantar fasciitis.

Bone scans, MRIs, and CT scans are necessary only when the diagnosis is in question. Certainly, they often show abnormalities in plantar fasciitis, but this fact is not enough to make them useful in the evaluation of plantar fasciitis. In order to be useful, these tests have to potentially change the recommendations that are made to treat the problem or help to exclude other possible diagnoses.

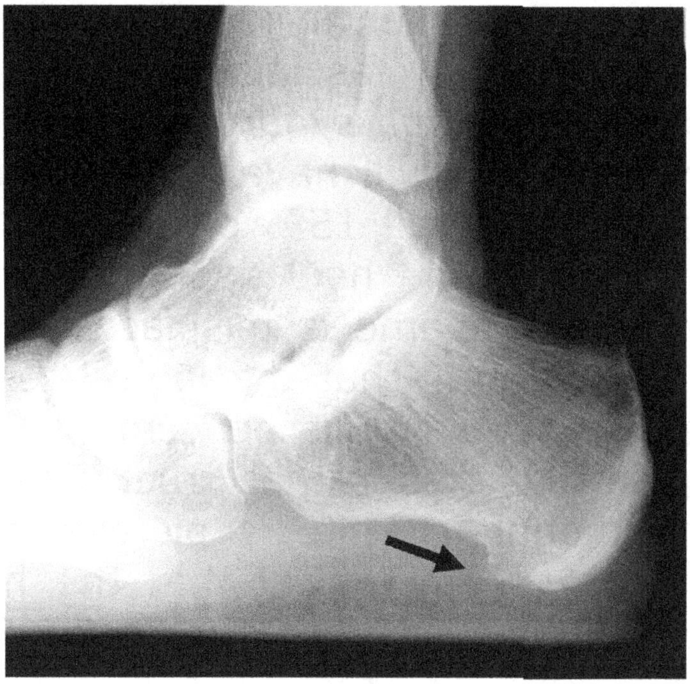

FIGURE 6.3 Typical appearance of plantar heel spur.

The first step in treatment is to decrease the excessive tension and stress on the plantar fascia. The goal is to maximize the plantar fascia's ability to heal itself by limiting its stress to a level that will allow it to heal. One long-term approach is weight loss and that certainly should be started if it is necessary. Flexibility exercises that loosen the plantar fascia, Achilles, hamstring, hip, and back are strongly recommended. The key to stretching exercises is repetition. They should be done three or more times a day. The exercises stimulate the muscles to become longer. This is an adaptive response, which takes months, so sustained effort is necessary to see results. In addition, exercises designed to improve your posture and normalize your center of gravity are helpful.

It is not advisable to begin a jogging routine while in the midst of a case of plantar fasciitis, but it may be possible to begin a low-impact exercise program such as water aerobics, stationary bike or spinning, swimming, or Pilates. Appropriate exercises should not cause sustained or severe aggravation of the pain. If there is worsening of the pain, activities should be scaled back until the pain has subsided.

Anti-inflammatory pain medications, such as ibuprofen (Motrin®) and naproxen (Aleve®), or acetaminophen (Tylenol®) can be helpful pain medications, but should not be expected to cure the problem alone. These medications are also unlikely to do much to relieve swelling.

Reducing strain on the plantar fascia with the use of heavier, stiffer shoes and arch supports can also be helpful. Heavier, stiffer shoes may be obtained by simply carefully selecting shoes at a shoe store. To gauge the stiffness of a shoe, grab the heel and toe of the shoe and try to bend it. If it bends easily through the arch and toe area, then it will be less effective at protecting the plantar fascia from stress. An excellent choice is a rocker bottom shoe.

Arch supports, orthotics, or inserts have been helpful and nearly routine intervention in the treatment of plantar fasciitis. Stress in the plantar fascia and forefoot is reduced with inserts. Custom inserts often cost $100 to $300 and are commonly prescribed by physicians. However, the cheaper, noncustom inserts are just as effective as custom inserts. Find an insert that is comfortable and relieves the pain. Silicone or gel inserts are sometimes not comfortable. The harder plastic inserts are also not often tolerated well, because they press the intensely tender heel. A firm foam insert with a moderate arch commonly has the right combination of support and comfort. Taping the foot is effective in relieving pain, but requires supplies and expertise on proper application.

Cortisone or steroid injections are commonly prescribed. Complications of this include rupture of the plantar fascia and atrophy, discoloration, or dimpling of the skin. Serum glucose measurements taken commonly in diabetes after steroid injection often become elevated for one or two days, but generally return to normal after this. Fifty to 70% of people will experience significant prolonged relief.[2] It is difficult to determine if steroid injections can cause permanent improvement. One study has documented improvement in pain one month after the injection, but little difference between people treated with steroid and people treated with placebo after that point.[3] It still can be helpful to relief early in treatment.

Supervised rehabilitation through regular evaluation by a physical therapist can assist in recuperation. A physical therapist can also make appropriate adjustments and gradual intensification of the exercise program as the sensitivity improves. This is especially helpful when the intention is to return to high-level athletic competition. Deep tissue massage and other treatments such as ultrasound and phonophoresis—the use of ultrasound to enhance the delivery of topically applied drugs—are most appropriate early in the course of the problem. Although the effectiveness of deep tissue massage techniques such as Graston has not been definitively proven, many seem to respond to it. Others find it aggravating and painful. Don't do it if it is excessively painful.

Casting the foot in a nonremovable fiberglass cast, immobilizing both the ankle and the toes can help 50% to 70% of people with resistant plantar fasciitis.[4][5] The goal is to almost completely eliminate the stress on the plantar fascia by limiting motion and muscle usage within the hindfoot. It is usually applied for three to six weeks. Casting is always inconvenient and leads to loss of muscle tone in the legs, which may also need treatment. It is also uncomfortable, so it is usually a last resort prior to surgical treatment.

Night splinting, or splinting the foot in a neutral position with a prefabricated brace while sleeping, seems to be losing some of its initial popularity. These premanufactured splints are made in several different styles with some models fitting to the front of the leg and some to the back. Results from studies evaluating these devices were encouraging, but more recently have been disappointing and some recent studies have shown that it is completely ineffective. One simple technique that is often helpful is to keep the foot in a neutral position when resting or sitting. Many people when sitting have the habit of curling their feet under their chair or resting their feet on a surface such as a stool. Often when they get up, the contracted tissue is painful as it resumes the posture necessary to walk. There is an adage in the treatment of plantar fasciitis that "the first step is the worst step." The cycle of rest and re-aggravation of the plantar fasciitis while intermittently sitting and walking is at least painful and possibly injurious to the plantar fascia. Keeping the feet on the floor with the heels closer to the chair than the knees can eliminate this problem. This seems to make getting up less painful for the first several steps.

Surgery is directed toward releasing and cutting the plantar fascia to unload the painful attachment of the ligament on the heel. Unfortunately, it also interferes with some of the critical functions of the plantar fascia. Generally, anywhere from 25% to 50% of the plantar fascia is released during surgery. This can be done either through an open procedure with an approximately 1 to 2 inch incision or endoscopically. The endoscopic procedure is done by using smaller incisions and a fiberoptic camera or scope is used to see the fascia while it is being cut. Both procedures cut an important structure in the foot. Many people do well after this procedure, but a few may actually have worse pain due to changes in the mechanics and stress within the bones and joints of the foot. It results in the slight flattening of the arch and the degree of flattening is related to the amount of the plantar fascia released. Another common complication is numbness in the heel.

Several alternatives to open surgery have been introduced, but their effectiveness has not been consistent in studies. Orthotripsy, or the application of repeated ultrasonic shockwaves to the heel, was a procedure that was introduced about ten years ago, but the effectiveness in scientific studies has been inconsistent.[6][7][8] Promising results have been seen with the use of Botulism toxin injections but this requires further study before it is used routinely.

Enthusiasm for blood products including platelet-rich plasma (PRP) has been increasing recently with several orthopedic and podiatric publications that have reviewed this treatment. Platelet-rich plasma is a product derived from blood usually taken from a vein of the person being treated. The blood is placed in a centrifuge, a machine that spins the blood sample at high speed, separating the components of the blood. One portion of the blood is injected into the plantar fascia. It was hoped that this part of the blood would contain concentrated proteins that would help the plantar fascia to heal, but recent studies have not conclusively shown a large benefiting. These treatments are expensive, even more so because most insurances do not cover them at this time. Until there are well-performed scientific trials, use of this treatment should be done sparingly and with caution.

PAUL'S STORY

Paul is a 51-year-old computer technician who has noticed pain in the left heel. He didn't injure it and his activity level has not changed, but he had put on about 20 pounds after his recent divorce. At first, he noticed the pain when he got out of bed. His heel hurt usually only until he got into the bathroom and then during his long drive into work. However, over the past month, the pain has been nearly continuous, especially when getting up from a seated position.

He has a slightly flat-appearing arch that is identical to the right foot. The heel is tender along the front and inside of the bony prominence on the plantar aspect of the calcaneus. A vague swelling was located there. His hamstrings were definitely tight—he couldn't touch his toes from a standing position without bending his knees. His x-ray was normal without a heel spur.

Paul was put on an anti-inflammatory medication to help control his pain. He was given a stretching and postural program. An over-the-counter arch support was given to him with a recommendation to use rockersoled shoes. At four weeks, he had 40% improvement. At three months, the pain went away.

We believe that with these simple interventions that the recovery from this painful condition can be accelerated much of the time.

ACHILLES TENDONITIS

- Achilles tendonitis most commonly affects the insertion of the Achilles tendon at the heel and the portion of the tendon about two to three inches above the heel.
- Achilles tendonitis can be associated with an enlargement or bump on the tendon.
- It can be effectively treated with immobilization and rehabilitation.
- Steroid injections have a significant risk of rupture.

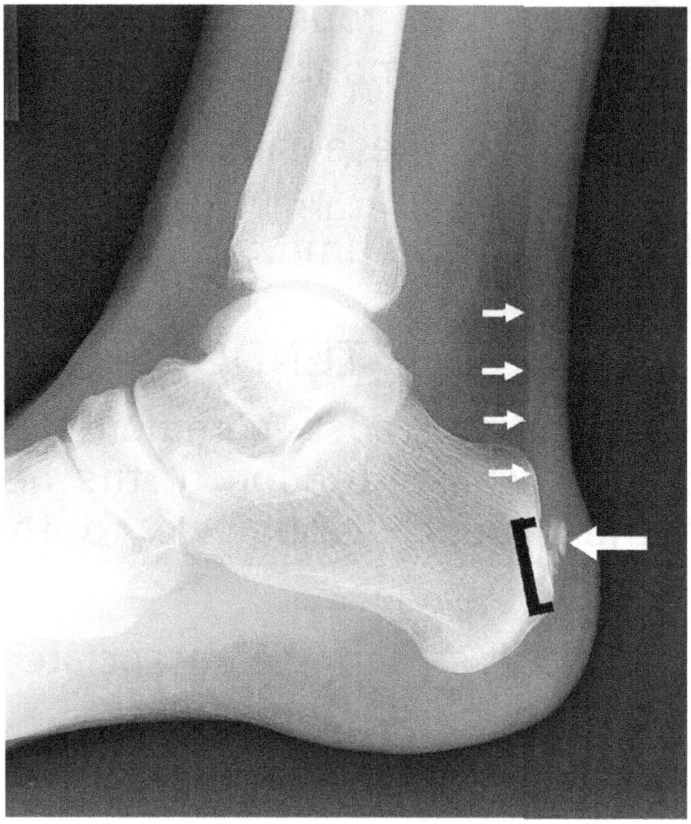

FIGURE 6.4 X-ray of an ankle with Achilles tendonitis. The Achilles tendon is faintly visible and the anterior border of the tendon is outlined (white arrows). The attachment of the Achilles tendon is about halfway down the back portion of the heel (black bracket). In this case, there is calcification within the tendon.

Tendonitis is a term used to describe a chronic overuse injury of the tendon. A tendon is dense connective tissue that connects a muscle to a bone. Certain areas on the tendon have limited blood supply. The blood supply is the fuel that powers tendon repair and metabolism. All tendons are injured slightly every time that they are used. If the injury is small enough that the body is able to repair itself completely, then no pain is sensed. However, if the injury surpasses the body's ability to heal, then the injury persists and accumulates eventually causing pain and tenderness.

As one gets older, this blood supply decreases and the tendon deteriorates even more. Sometimes, the tendon may not heal and will continue to be painful. More aggressive treatment is then needed. Attempts by the body to repair the tendon can lead to scarring, which is often noticed when the tendon becomes enlarged. Even doctors sometimes describe this as inflammation, but when it is looked at microscopically, inflammatory cells are not usually present. What is seen is scarring, blood vessel formation, and small incomplete tears of the tendon fibers.

The Achilles tendon is in the back of the leg and is responsible for plantar flexing the foot or for pointing your toes. Its most important job is slowing the forward progress of the body. The muscle attached to the Achilles tendon is most active when you go from the position of your step when the foot is flat on thc ground until the heel is lifted at the completion of the step. It is only used to push the body forward when you are running or walking quickly.

The Achilles tendon is commonly damaged in tendonitis either at its attachment to the calcaneus on the very back of the heel or about two or three inches above the insertion at about the level of the ankle. Persons with Achilles tendonitis occasionally worry that they have tumor, but cancerous tumors in this area are extremely rare while Achilles tendonitis is extremely common.

Swelling, prominence, pain, and tenderness are all signs of Achilles tendonitis. Sometimes, the pain will radiate up the calf or into the heel. The nerves that sense pain follow the course of the muscle into the tendon and are responsible for this. Rarely, a rupture can occur after tendonitis. Ruptures do occur frequently during sudden stretches of the tendon often during athletics, but Achilles tendon pain is not common prior to this. The percentage of people with Achilles tendonitis that subsequently rupture the tendon is probably much less than 5%.

Most of the time, the pain increases for the first few steps after inactivity such as when arising from sleep or after sitting. This occurs because the muscle is allowed to recoil when sitting or lying down, since the foot normally assumes a flexed position. It takes extra force to stretch the muscle out to working length. The extra force is felt at the point of the tendon damage.

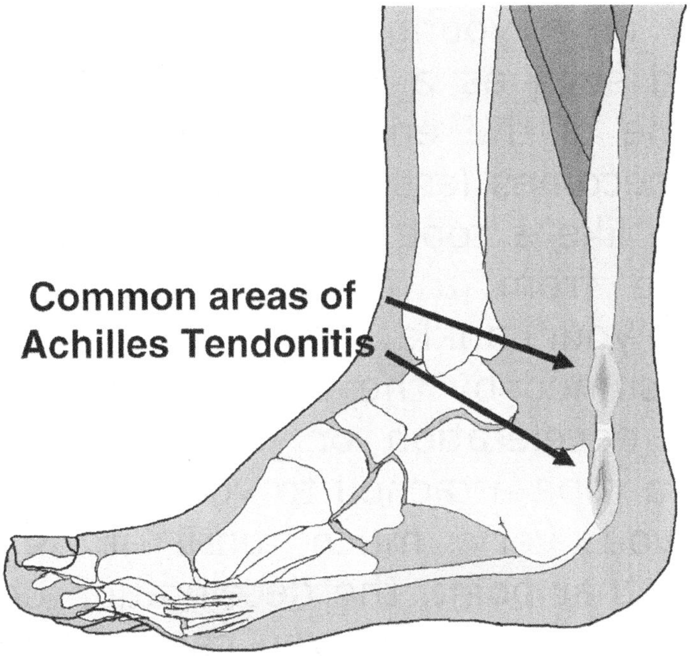

FIGURE 6.5 The two common locations for Achilles tendonitis are at the attachment of the Achilles tendon (insertional tendonitis) or two to three inches above this (noninsertional tendonitis).

As mentioned earlier, the most important cause of tendonitis is injury and scarring beyond the ability of the tendon to repair. This changes the tendon structurally. The ability of the tendon to repair itself is intimately related to blood supply and the blood supply of the tendon is poor. Blood supply is worse in the center of the tendon as it gets farther from the bony insertion at the heel and the highly vascular muscle belly. The area in between these points is called the *watershed area,* because neither the blood supply from the bone nor the muscle quite adequately supplies it. This makes it prone to injury. Age, smoking, hypertension, diabetes, and other factors can accelerate tendonitis.

The tendon of a young person is very elastic and when a load such as a step occurs, it stretches and absorbs some of the energy of the step. With time, the tendon becomes less stretchy. The tendon absorbs energy more like a rope and less like a bungee cord. If you jump from a bridge with a bungee cord attached to your ankle, the energy of that fall is gradually assumed by the bungee cord so that there is no quick deceleration or jolt. If you jump off a bridge with a rope attached to your leg, the rope does not slow you very much until it is completely extended. At that point, the deceleration occurs rapidly with the disastrous results you can probably imagine. When the tendon is inelastic, you are much more likely to injure it.

Anything that increases the stress on the Achilles tendon will increase the work that it does and increase the chance for tendonitis. Weight is certainly a factor. Any excess weight that you carry, whether it is fat or muscle, will increase the amount of stress on the Achilles. However, even more important is the way in which the weight is held. Posture has a great deal to do with this. If you carry your weight in front of your body by slumping shoulders, a slouched back, pendulous breasts, or an extra big belly, extra stress will be put on the Achilles tendon. Otherwise, the weight would cause you to fall over. In addition, all of these factors rotate your pelvis backward, making it difficult to take a full step. If the step is begun on the flat foot as opposed to the heel, then a larger portion of the step is spent with the Achilles musculature activated. This adds up over time to overuse and injury of the Achilles tendon.

People who have a tight Achilles muscle that does not allow the ankle joint to have a full range of motion, have a difficult time getting their heel on the floor when they are standing upright. These people spend a greater proportion of their step on their toes and you may even notice that they are toe walkers. Many times, the gait abnormalities can be too subtle to notice casually.

Athletic activity can increase the chance of injury. Surveys have reported that the rate of Achilles tendonitis in serious runners is approximately 5% to 7% per year. While, in general, athletic activity is good for health, the stress that it applies to the heel is significant and injuries happen. Youth protects you from these injuries, but as you get older, you must pay attention to factors such as flexibility and the type of running shoes you use more and more in order to avoid injury.

Finally, there are a number of systemic inflammatory conditions that may predispose one to Achilles tendonitis. We think of these primarily when there are multiple areas of tendonitis seen in one person. Rheumatoid arthritis, lupus, psoriatic arthritis, scleroderma, and anklylosing spondylitis are a few of the several dozen conditions that can be associated with multiple tendonitises. A rheumatologist can diagnose these conditions.

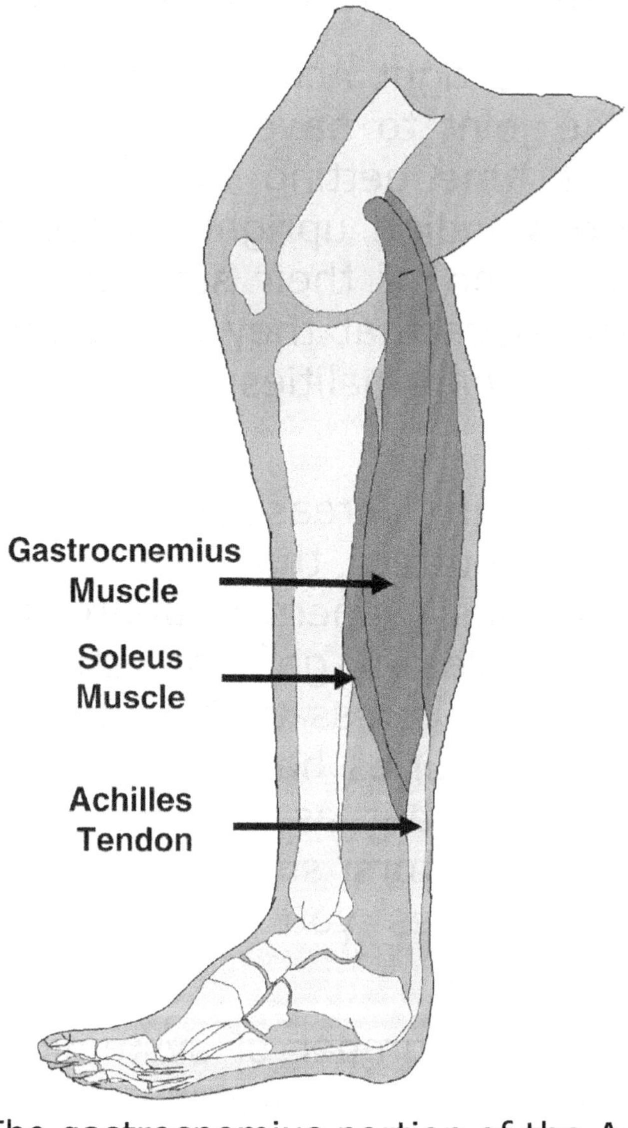

FIGURE 6.6 The gastrocnemius portion of the Achilles tendon attaches above the knee. This makes them both tighter when the knee is in full extension.

Achilles tendonitis is so common and characteristic that there are few other things that it resembles.

- Calcaneal stress fracture (uncommon, often associated with swelling, pain is along the heel).
- Tendonitis of other tendons in the back of the heel.
- Achilles tendon tear.

Like other forms of tendonitis, the goal of treatment is to make the tendon can heal as much as possible. This includes rest, improving flexibility, and reducing stress to the tendon. By doing so, we hope that the limited ability of the tendon to heal will be adequate to allow for eventual painless function. It is a long process and patience is definitely required.

Initial treatment of an acute and severely painful Achilles tendon centers on rest. Although it is usually not necessary to be at bed rest, you need to eliminate activities that aggravate the tendon. If jogging, sports, or even walking for exercise is a part of your regular routine, you should substitute other activities for them. Exercises such as water jogging or aerobics or riding on a stationary bicycle may be more appropriate early in treatment. A frank discussion with your employer may be necessary if your job requires prolonged walking or standing such as retail sales or working in a warehouse. It is always tempting to suggest vacation as a means of rest, but rarely does a severe case of Achilles tendonitis go away that fast.

In severe cases, a period of immobilization is recommended. Applying a short-leg walking cast to the leg, extending from the end of the toes to the upper shin, can drastically reduce the stress on the Achilles tendon. This cast is worn for three to six weeks. A prefabricated cast boot is not as effective. Immobilizing your leg with a short leg cast is good for immediate pain relief during this relatively short period.

Nonsteroidal anti-inflammatory medications are often helpful in relieving pain. However, often because of the name—nonsteroidal antiinflammatory—it is often expected by people that they do much more. It is not anticipated that the swelling or knots will be improved by these medications substantially. It is also not expected that it will do much to cure the underlying tendonitis. It is simply a pain medication. It should be continued only if it is effective as a pain medication, at the minimum dosage necessary to control the pain.

In less extreme cases of tendonitis, a less aggressive approach is reasonable. A prefabricated heel wedge can be inserted into the shoe to relax the Achilles musculature and to reposition the foot during gait. If there is a specific foot abnormality such as flat foot, a prefabricated arch support may be helpful.

Regular stretching exercises that concentrate on the Achilles and hamstring muscles can decrease the tension within the back of the calf, reducing the stress and work of the injured tendon. These exercises should be done regularly so that you stretch and lengthen the muscle. Exercises are outlined in Chapter 10.

A lot of research has been done to evaluate the types of strengthening exercises that help Achilles tendonitis. Several studies have shown eccentric exercises to be specifically helpful for this condition. "Eccentric exercise" means an activity in which there is an overall lengthening of the muscle in response to external resistance. In this case the tendon and associated muscles are worked at high resistance to the point of pain. An experienced therapist can teach and supervise these exercises to avoid greatly aggravating the injury.

Enlisting the help of a competent, enthusiastic physical therapist can help in many ways. The coaching and encouragement of a physical therapist can improve motivation and improve the outlook. In addition, specific adjustments can be made to the rehabilitation routine in order to minimize any aggravation that the exercises may be causing. Ultrasound, phonophoresis, and contrast baths are often added to treatment, but there isn't a lot of evidence to prove their long-term effectiveness. Anecdotally, it is our feeling that they give temporary relief that still may be of benefit on the road to rehabilitation.

A brace is helpful in some cases of Achilles tendonitis. It works by limiting ankle motion and to some extent by applying counter pressure to the tension within the Achilles tendon. Many braces also reduce the motion of the foot and thus the work that the Achilles is required to do. All braces to some extent sacrifice freedom of motion, and fit within the shoe for increased stability and protection of the damaged structure. On the lighter end of this spectrum, an elastic ankle sleeve is light and minimally cumbersome, but not very supportive. On the heavier end, an AFO (ankle-foot-orthosis) is a rigid usually plastic shell that restricts motion considerably. This brace is sometimes uncomfortable especially if it does not fit properly. It can be difficult to fit in shoes unless they are very loose, and it is more expensive, especially if it's custom. The right brace is the one that gives the most relief with the fewest disadvantages. To some extent, your physician or therapist may be able to guide you. Some trial and error may be necessary, too.

Steroid injection in the treatment of Achilles tendonitis is controversial. Our recommendation is to avoid it. More than half of the ruptures of the insertion of the Achilles tendon that we have seen in practice have occurred after steroid injection. These medications inhibit the metabolism of the tissue. The use of steroid injections is discouraged around weight-bearing tendons such as the Achilles tendon because of this significant incidence of rupture.

Surgery is directed toward removal of the damaged tendon, any calcaneal bone pressing on the tendon and repair of the Achilles tendon. This includes removing any spurring within the tendon. Occasionally, in situations where the tendon damage is severe, the flexor tendon to the big toe can be used to reinforce the tendon repair. This sacrifices some amount of toe strength, but is usually well tolerated. After the surgery, the leg is restricted in weight bearing for up to four weeks. Good results are found in 70% to 80% of cases but may take up to one year to fully recover from the surgery. Complications include rupture of the repair, wound healing problems, and continued local pain.

AMANDA'S STORY

Amanda is a 63-year-old retired teacher who had heel pain for nine months. Her pain increased gradually, making her daily walks with her Yorkie difficult. The pain was worse in the morning when arising and after sitting. She noticed a lump on the back of her heel. This knot is so tender that she couldn't stand having it touched by the heel of her shoe and she started wearing clogs. The x-rays showed prominence of the top of the calcaneus and calcification within the tendon.

The shoes that Amanda has purchased are completely appropriate for her, as they do not press on the tender knot and have a slight heel. A stretching program was begun under the guidance of a physical therapist and Amanda's tendonitis improved rapidly in the first month. The improvement over the next three months was less rapid, but the pain was completely gone at six months.

ACHILLES TENDON RUPTURE

- Achilles rupture is a common athletic injury that is frequently overlooked.
- People often describe the rupture as feeling as if they were kicked in the back of the heel. Usually a palpable defect in the tendon is clearly evident.
- Operative and nonoperative methods are effective in treatment. It is unknown which method is superior. The activity goals are important in making this decision.

The Achilles tendon is directly behind the ankle. It attaches the large muscles in the back of the calf to the heel. The Achilles tendon actually attaches to the heel or calcaneus bone about midway down the back portion of the bone. The large muscles that attach to the Achilles tendon are the medial and lateral gastrocnemius and the soleus muscles. The primary job of these muscles is to draw the entire foot toward the floor. This muscle action is used to press on the gas pedal of a car or to stand on tiptoes. More importantly, it slows the body's progress forward so that you don't fall forward when you walk or stand and gives you a spring or thrust at the end of your step.

A rupture occurs when the fibers of the tendon fail and tear away from each other. The sensation from the actual rupture is usually misinterpreted as "getting kicked in the back of the leg." It usually occurs while jumping and happens a lot in basketball.

After the rupture, walking may be possible, but usually is painful to some degree. There may be a sensation of instability and inability to push off the foot at the end of the step. It is often mistaken for an ankle sprain. Bruising is common along the heel and a palpable gap is often felt along the course of the normally uniform tendon. Usually the area is painful.

The circulation of the Achilles tendon enters the tendon from the insertion on the bone and from the muscle. The circulation gradually decreases the farther away you are from these points on the tendon. The midportion of the tendon, which is about six to eight centimeters above the heel, has less blood supply than the portions at the ends and, as a result, this decreases its potential to heal itself.

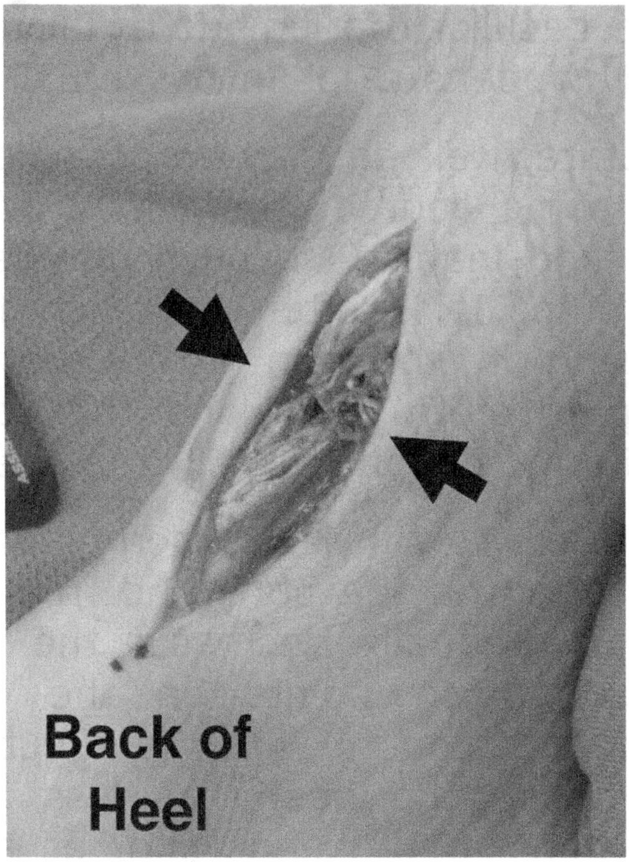

FIGURE 6.7 Picture of ruptured Achilles tendon. The edges of the tendon are ragged and irregular, which aids in the healing of this tendon.

The Achilles tendon can be subjected to forces that are many times your body weight during vigorous activity. Activities such as coming down on the foot after a jump are particularly stressful to the tendon. Scarring and partial injury may cause a weak spot within the midportion of the tendon. However, it is rare to have pain or symptoms in the tendon prior to injury.

Certainly many medical conditions predispose people to these injuries. Diabetes can lead to arterial damage and commonly contributes to all forms of tendonitis including the Achilles tendonitis. Inflammatory diseases such as rheumatoid arthritis can cause tendon rupture, as can many of the drugs used to treat these diseases, including steroids and other drugs that suppress the immune system. Quinolone antibiotic usage such as ciprofloxacin has been associated with a number of cases of tendon rupture. Finally, steroid injections have been reported many times to be associated with Achilles rupture.

Achilles rupture can be fairly well diagnosed by the location of the tenderness and the loss of power from the muscle. The tenderness, depending on the location of the tear, can range from the top of the heel bone or up to two or three inches into the calf. Usually, a gap or palpable dip is felt at the location of the tear and may be up to an inch in length. Often the foot itself will assume an unusual posture when the foot is in the resting position. In rest, the foot is in a more extended posture than normal. This makes the bottom of the heel seem more prominent. The reason for this unusual posture is that the Achilles is no longer opposing the muscles that extend the ankle.

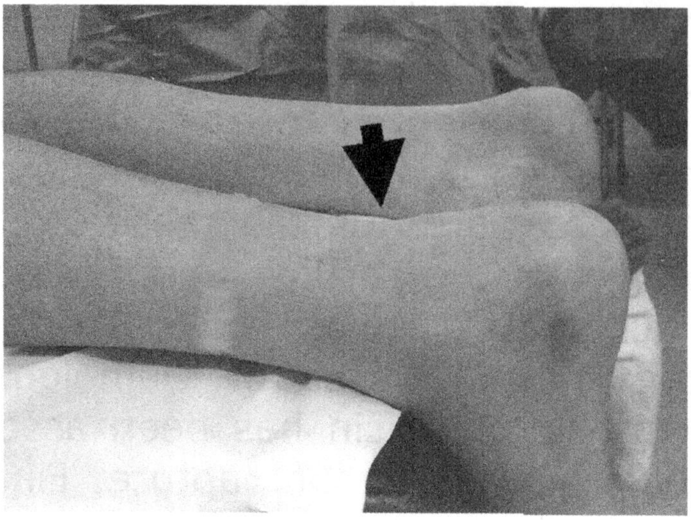

FIGURE 6.8 A leg with ruptured Achilles tendon. The stump of the residual tendon and indentation of the tendon are obvious when compared to the uninjured side.

Other problems that may be confused with Achilles tendon rupture include:

- Achilles tendonitis
- Ankle sprain
- Peroneal tendonitis
- Posterior tibial tendonitis or tendonitis of the flexor to the big toe
- Calcaneal or ankle fracture
- Muscular tear of the gastrocnemius muscle

The diagnosis of Achilles tendon rupture can be made on a clinical basis alone. That being said, radiographs are almost always taken to rule out other issues problems such as fractures of the ankle and calcaneus.

The tendon itself and its rupture are not distinctly visible on most radiographs. Other radiographic tests such as CT and bone scan are not helpful. MRI is certainly capable of imaging an Achilles tendon rupture, but in general is not necessary. However, the diagnosis is usually quite clear by physical examination. Ultrasonic evaluation can also diagnose it, but is not usually needed.

There are few questions in orthopedics that are quite as controversial as the decision to treat Achilles tendonitis surgically or nonsurgically. One thing that is not controversial is that some form of treatment is necessary to reestablish the function of the Achilles tendon. If Achilles tendon rupture is not treated, then the tendon generally heals in a lengthened position. The lengthened tendon is weakened and the gait becomes abnormal and often unstable.

Standard nonoperative treatment involves casting or bracing for six to eight weeks. The ankle is placed in a flexed position to allow the torn edges of the tendon to come into contact. The hope is that the torn edges of the tendon will heal at their normal length. This reestablishes the tension within the musculature and the strength. Regaining strength through nonoperative treatment can, however, be prolonged and occasionally some degree of weakness may remain.

Surgery is often selected especially in younger and more athletic people, in whom the sometimes modest loss of strength is not well tolerated. Here, the choice of the surgical technique is also controversial.

Some surgeons who value the reliability of the technique promote open management of the rupture with formal sewing of the tendon ends. Using this technique, the heavy suture is braided into the stumps of the torn tendon and sewn together. The incision using this technique may be several inches long. Techniques that repair the tendon through smaller incisions have been recently developed. There is no consensus on which technique is better yet.

With all forms of treatment, light activity is generally possible and early motion after surgery seems to help prevent adhesions between the skin and underlying healing tendon. Some form of bracing after surgery is required for at least four weeks. You can return to sports in three to six months.

One of biggest problems in the treatment of Achilles rupture is that it often is misdiagnosed. In some studies, up to 25% to 35% of people with Achilles tendon rupture have a delay in diagnosis of greater than one week. This can make it more difficult to treat this problem without surgery because the adhesions that develop very early within the torn edges of the tendon can keep the tendon edges from apposing properly.

Operative treatment, both percutaneous and open, can result in wound-healing problems. There is little soft tissue between the Achilles tendon and the skin.

The blood supply to this area is commonly decreased especially in the elderly, in people with diabetes, and in smokers. This limited blood supply makes healing after surgery difficult and may even lead to wounds with frankly dead edges. The Achilles tendon, like most tendons, is enclosed in a filmy sheath that allows it to slide between the skin and the underlying tissue without friction. However, the space within this sheath is also a place where infection can start. The tendon, as a structure without a good blood supply, does not heal well and sometimes the tendon can die if it is allowed to dry out or become infected. Skin healing problems and infections happen about 10% of the time and routinely require months to close.

A sensory nerve passes over the Achilles tendon in the area where it is commonly approached operatively. When it is damaged, there can be numbness in the outside of the foot and an exquisitely painful area can develop. This is especially a danger in limited incision approaches when the nerve may not be protected directly and needles and sutures placed blindly through the skin may injure it.

On the other hand, in some large studies of treatment of Achilles tendon rupture, the satisfaction rate is not as high as with surgery. Decreases in push-off strength are sometimes noted and the rate at which the tendon ruptures again can be as high as 20%.

This is one area where large substantial objective studies should be done. Figuring out who would benefit from open, percutaneous, and closed treatment of Achilles ruptures is one of the glaring gaps in medical knowledge.

LEON'S STORY

Leon is a 36-year-old salesperson for a local farm implement dealership. He is an avid athlete and basketball player. When going up for a rebound, he came down on another player's shoe and felt a pop. He thought initially that he had been kicked by a fellow player. He was helped off the floor and could still walk, but his ankle felt like it was "dead" when he tried to walk.

He was seen at the emergency room and diagnosed with an Achilles tendon tear. X-rays were normal. He was then referred for orthopedic evaluation.

The risks and benefits of both operative and nonoperative treatment for the Achilles rupture were explained to Leon. On the one hand, not operating on Leon would have fewer wound complications. On the other hand, the rerupture rate is higher.

Leon decided to have it operatively repaired. His surgery was done as an outpatient and he was placed in a walking cast within a few days. His ankle was protected with a walking boot for two months out from the surgery. He gradually increased his activity and was able to return to competitive sports in five months.

HEEL FRACTURES/CALCANEAL FRACTURES

- Calcaneal fractures usually occur after falls from a height or motor vehicle accident.
- They are sometimes easy to overlook on x-rays.
- The tissue swelling that is normal after this severe injury can make the skin prone to healing complications after surgery.
- Stiffness, arthritis, and some degree of pain are common even after optimal treatment.

The calcaneus is a peculiar bone. It is the largest of the tarsals, the bones of the mid- and back portion of the foot. The joint beneath the ankle, between the calcaneus and the talus called the subtalar joint, is responsible for adjusting to uneven surfaces such as sodden ground or rocks by shifting to the inside or outside as the need arises. It is the link between the strong muscles of the calf and the thrust through the forefoot needed to jump or run. The stresses applied to it are generated by direct contact with the heel when weight is on the heel such as in the beginning of a step, and by the force of the Achilles tendon and the counterforce from the forefoot at the end of the step. The bone has the consistency of balsa wood and can be dented fairly easily by a blunt tool such as a hammer.

Researchers continue to argue about the best treatment for calcaneus fractures. H.L. McLaughlin in 1959 described fixing calcaneus fracture to be similar to "nailing custard pie to a wall" because the fragments are so damaged and fragile that it is difficult to get them properly aligned and stabilized. The general current consensus among surgeons is that if repairable joint damage is present, then surgery is necessary.

Although studies do suggest that precise realignment of the bone and its joint give the best possibility for adequate function, the complication rate for these fractures is high and the complications can be disastrous. The skin envelope is thin and usually highly damaged after the fracture. Often a prolonged period between injury and surgery is necessary to allow for recovery of the skin from the initial trauma. Although some might disagree, most fractures can be treated without surgery.

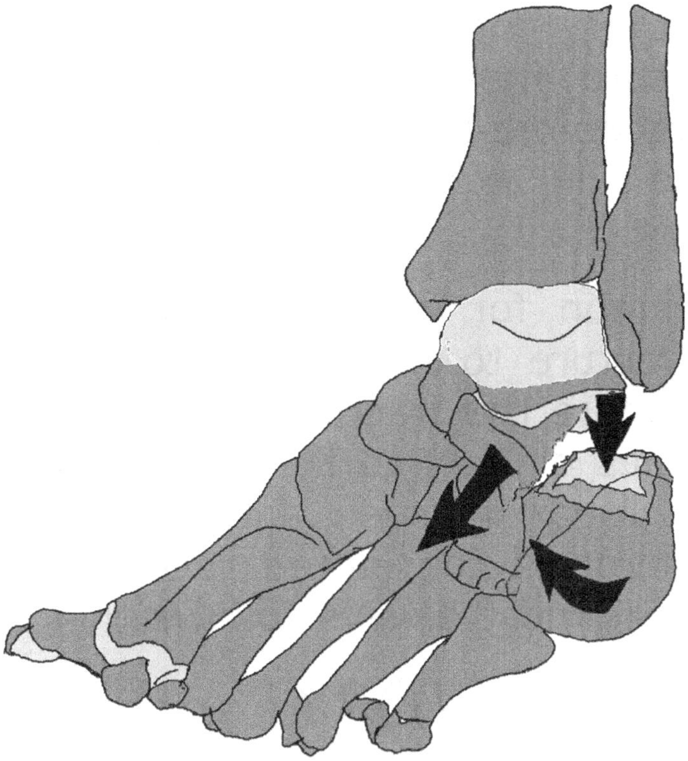

FIGURE 6.9 A typical calcaneus fracture as viewed from the back. The talus shears a portion of the inside of the calcaneus from a high-energy impact. The remainder of the joint surface crushes into the body of the calcaneus. The body of the calcaneus itself rotates.

The tongue fracture is the one exception. This fracture is essentially a tearing of the attachment of the Achilles tendon off the calcaneus by cracking it off through the calcaneus. Often the movement of the fracture fragment can stretch and compress the skin over it, damaging the circulation. Necrotic patches of skin can follow, complicating treatment of the fracture that must be realigned.

New techniques and improved hardware have allowed for surgery that requires smaller, less dangerous incisions. It is important for your doctor to be absolutely sure that this joint can be adequately reconstructed before attempting it. If the surgeon does not have the skill, experience, or, mostly, the patience, go elsewhere.

It is uncommon for a person who has suffered a calcaneus fracture to have a foot that functions the way it did before the fracture. The heel is often wide and sometimes difficult to fit into a shoe. Stiffness in the joint is routinely seen and maintaining 50% of the joint motion is considered successful. Arthritis to some degree almost always follows this injury.

JONATHAN'S STORY

Jonathan is a 27-year-old roofer. He is unmarried and didn't complete high school. He is fairly happy with his job even though it is physically demanding.

The morning of the accident, it was particularly hot. Perhaps it was the heat, perhaps it was the lack of water, but around 10 a.m., he noticed that he felt a little dizzy. He didn't think much about it until he was wiping sweat from his eyes and suddenly began to feel like the horizon was swimming around his head. He slid on his side to the gutter when the gutter caught his shirt tilting him upright and slowing his decent temporarily until the shirt tore. He plummeted 10 feet to the grass. Although he did not lose consciousness, for the next hour he was in a dream-like state. It was only in the emergency room that he realized how much his left heel hurt.

The emergency room physicians started intravenous fluids and examined Jonathan's swollen heel. X-rays were taken and he was admitted for pain control. After consultation, a CT was taken to better clarify the injury.

Jonathan was young and a nonsmoker. Both of these factors are associated with a decreased risk of complication. Surgery was suggested.

Jonathan's recovery was prolonged and difficult. Fortunately, his skin healed uneventfully, but he continued to have pain and swelling for months. He required narcotic pain medications for 10 weeks and began to walk about three months after surgery. He was not fully functional for four months and had a limp for a full seven months. Just when it seemed like it would never go away, it finally subsided. Unfortunately, his motion and pain in his foot did not allow him to return to be a roofer and he had recurrent dreams about his fall. When we last saw him, he was planning to return to vocational school to become an auto mechanic.

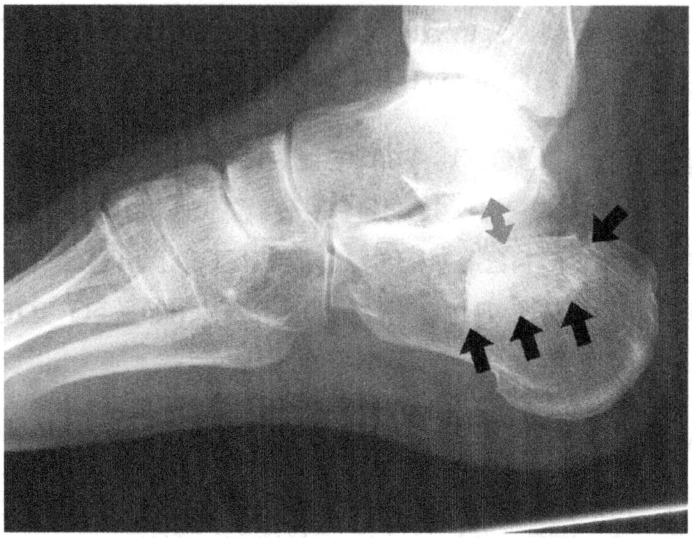

FIGURE 6.10 Jonathan's calcaneus fracture. A portion of the calcaneus (arrows) that consists of much of the subtalar joint has been punched into the body of the bone.

TARSAL TUNNEL SYNDROME

- Tarsal tunnel syndrome is a compression of the posterior tibial nerve as it travels from the back and inside of the ankle into the arch.

- Usually, numbness or tingling is sensed on the bottom of the foot with normal sensation of the top of the foot. The sensation of the heel may or may not be affected.

- The nerve may be irritated by tight musculotendinous or ligamentous structures. Masses such as ganglions have also been reported to cause tarsal tunnel syndrome.

- The outcome after surgical treatment of tarsal tunnel syndrome is often less than excellent.

▪ Surgery should only be considered for severe symptoms.

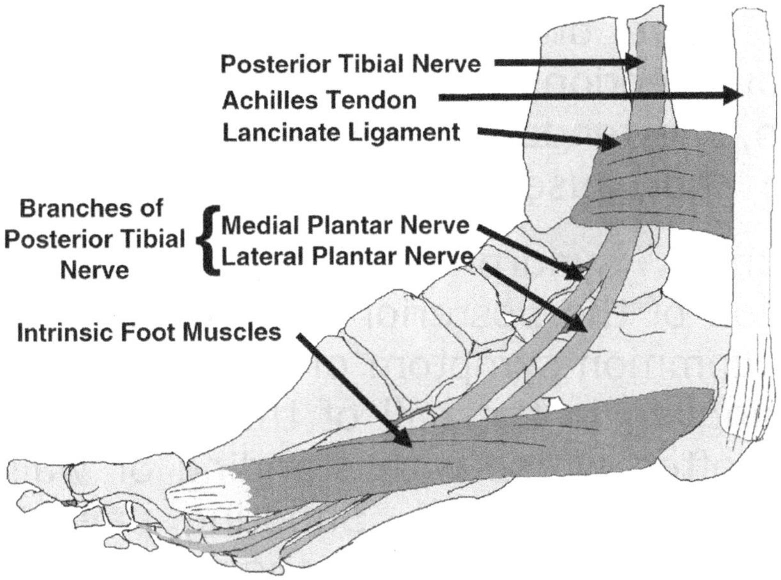

FIGURE 6.11 The posterior tibial nerve and its path through the ankle into the arch. Bands of connective tissue within the foot musculature and ligaments behind the ankle can compress it.

Like in other parts of the body, the nerves of the foot serve important functions. Nerves allow us to feel what is touching our skin and help us control our muscles. The nerve is a pathway to and from our tissue and communicates constantly with other nerves. These pathways must remain open and unconstrained along their entire course to be useful. The blood vessels must also be able to that nourish them adequately.

Compression of the major nerves of the foot is an occasional problem and usually occurs as the nerves pass through several anatomical structures that are there to protect our nerves. As they pass through these spaces, they are prone to strangulation. Tension from a bowed ankle or flattened arch can increase this. The nerve often passes through these spaces with various tendons and if the tendons are enlarged or swollen, the tendons can choke the circulation from the nerve and cause a tingling sensation.

Tarsal tunnel syndrome (TTS) is an injury or compression of the posterior tibial nerve at the ankle. The most common symptom of tarsal tunnel syndrome (TTS) is tingling in the ball of the foot and arch. The tingling is often worse with standing or walking for a prolonged period of time. Shooting pains can often accompany these sensations especially when pressure is applied to the skin overlying the nerve.

Nerve damage from diabetes or other systemic causes is the most common problem that closely resembles tarsal tunnel, so a physician needs to exclude those before she diagnoses you with TTS. It is fairly common for TTS to accompany other problems such as ankle swelling and inflammation, masses around the ankle such as ganglion cysts, arthritis, or fallen arches.

Firm flat shoes with an arch support seem to help. Elevating the inside of the edge of the heel and arch with the arch support will take some tension off the nerve and often the symptoms will disappear. Stretching exercises help, but no definitive studies have demonstrated predictable improvement.

Most cases of tarsal tunnel syndrome resolve with stretching, and new shoes, but surgery on the nerve is sometimes necessary. This does not mean that it is uniformly successful. Satisfaction from this type of surgery is notoriously poor. Scar sensitivity, numbness of the heel and forefoot, and persistent pain are common complications.

SHARON'S STORY

Sharon is a 34-year-old woman who works as an executive for a local business. She noticed tingling on the ball of the foot when she is on it for more than an hour. The problem seems to bother her primarily when she is in pumps. When the tingling begins, any pressure on the inside of the foot causes shooting pain. The pain is otherwise difficult to predict.

Sharon's foot exam was fairly normal. When the nerve was tapped along the arch area, a "lightning-like" sensation was noticed extending to the arch and big toe. Sustained pressure on the foot in this area caused the tingling sensation in the arch.

Sharon's treatment involved reducing irritation of the tendons and muscles that lie next to the posterior tibial tendon. She was asked to wear flatter shoes and over-the-counter arch supports. Her pain and tingling gradually improved and eventually stopped three months later.

NOTES

[1] Tanz SS. Heel pain. *Clin Orthop.* 1963;28:169–178.

[2] Buchbinder R. Clinical practice. Plantar fasciitis. *N Engl J Med.* 2004 May 20;350(21):2159–2166.

[3] Crawford F, Atkins D, Young P, Edwards J. Steroid injection for heel pain: Evidence of short-term effectiveness. A randomized controlled trial. *Rheumatology (Oxford).* 1999 Oct;38(10):974–977.

[4] Gill LH, Kiebzak GM. Outcome of nonsurgical treatment for plantar fasciitis. *Foot Ankle Int.* 1996 Sep;17(9):527–532.

[5] Tisdel CL, Harper MC. Chronic plantar heel pain: Treatment with a short leg walking cast. *Foot Ankle Int.* 1996 Jan;17(1):41–42.

[6] Alvarez R. Preliminary results on the safety and efficacy of the OssaTron for treatment of plantar fasciitis. *Foot Ankle Int.* 2002 Mar;23(3):197–203.

[7] Haake M, Buch M, Schoellner C, et al. Extracorporeal shock wave therapy for plantar fasciitis: Randomised controlled multicentre trial. *BMJ.* 2003 Jul 12;327(7406):75.

[8] Buchbinder R, Ptasznik R, Gordon J, Buchanan J, Prabaharan V, Forbes A Ultrasound-guided

extracorporeal shock wave therapy for plantar fasciitis: A randomized controlled trial. *JAMA.* 2002 Sep 18;288(11):1364–1372.

7

The Ankle

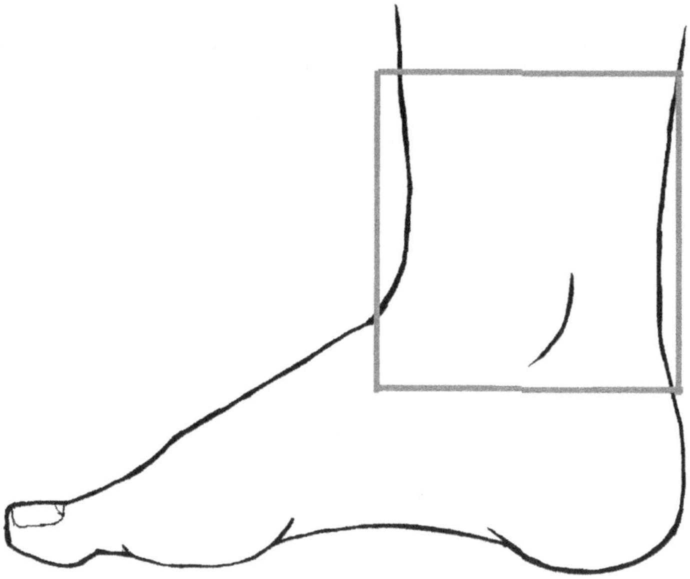

ANATOMY

The ankle joint is a hinge joint that extends, so the toes go to the sky, and it flexes, so that the toes go toward the floor. It is composed of three bones. The tibia and fibula join together to create the roof, and the inside and outside walls of the ankle. The talus is a spool-like surface over which the tibia and fibula rotate. The tibia and fibula are joined together at the syndesmosis, a joint that is tightly bound together by strong ligaments. The motion between the tibia and fibula is small but gives the unit just enough flexibility to adapt to the assortment of things that we ask the ankle joint to do. Ligaments of the inside and outside of the ankle control the motion so that the surfaces of the hinge joint hold together properly and securely. The ligaments of the ankle act like the pin in a door hinge. The ligaments insert on the tibia and fibula near the center of rotation of the ankle joint so that the ligaments do not tighten or loosen with motion. The ligaments then fan onto the talus and other parts of the foot. The ligament on the inside of the ankle is the deltoid ligament. The ligaments on the outside of the ankle are the anterior talofibular, and calcaneofibular ligaments.

The ankle is a very durable joint. Unless you sustain an injury that disturbs the joint or its ligaments, arthritis or wear of the ankle is extremely rare. However, injuries as small as an ankle sprain can wear the joint quickly.

A number of important tendons pass to the back and inside of the foot along with the posterior tibial artery and nerve. The posterior tibial tendon supports the arch and turns the ankle to the inside. The flexor tendons to the toes lie behind the posterior tibial tendon. The back and outside of the ankle—behind the fibula—is where the peroneal tendons turn the foot toward the outside travel. They are restrained within a groove in the back of the fibula by a ligament called the superior peroneal retinaculum.

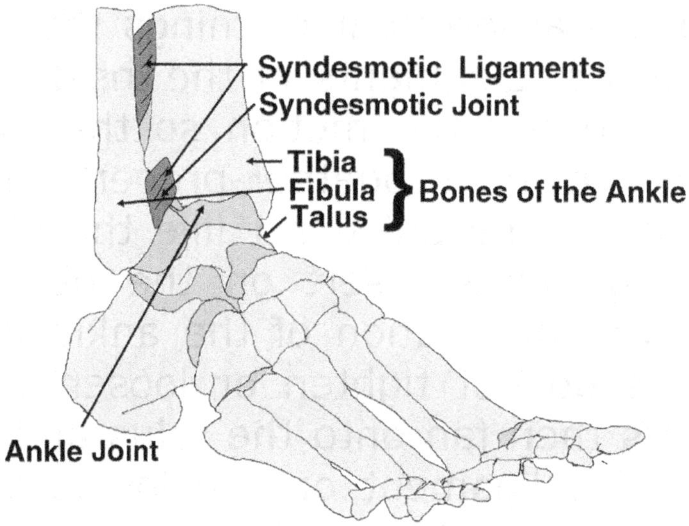

FIGURE 7.1 The major bones and joints of the ankle.

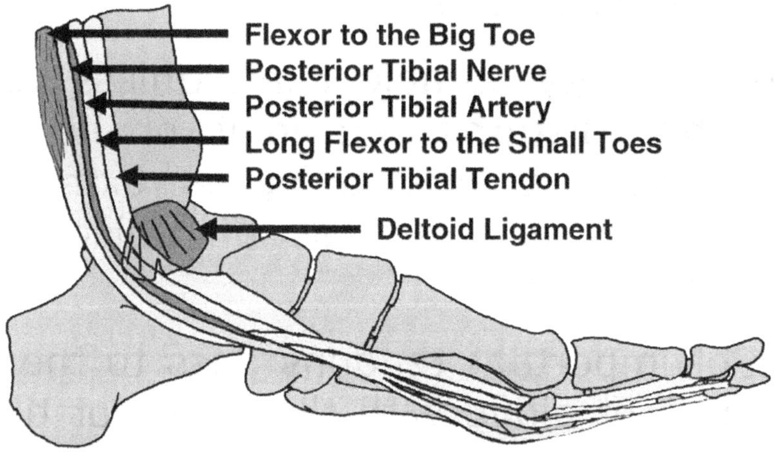

FIGURE 7.2 Major ligaments, tendons, and other structures on the inside of the foot.

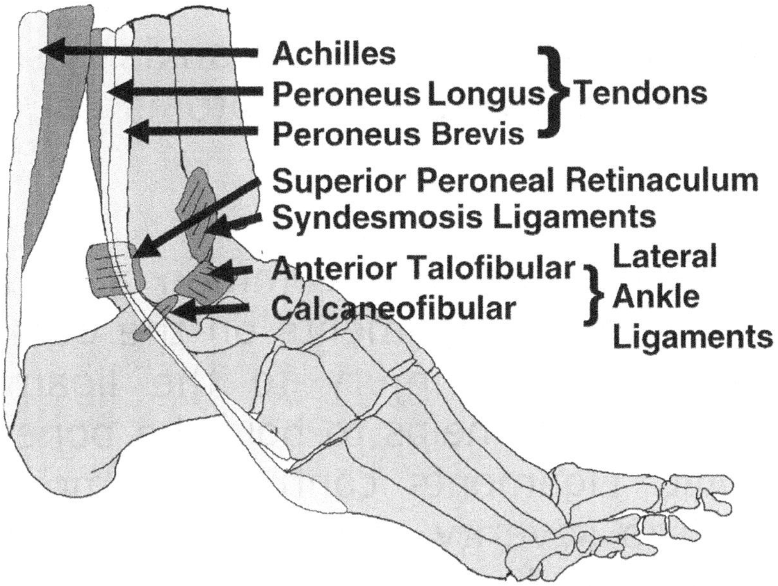

FIGURE 7.3 Major tendons and ligaments of the outside of the ankle.

ANKLE SPRAINS

- An ankle sprain is an injury of the ligaments, connective tissues that support the ankle and guide its motion. The most common ankle sprain involves the ligaments on the outside of the ankle when the ankle is forced to rotate toward the inside.

- Ankle sprains are common injuries, but sometimes lead to chronic pain and instability. It is common to take a long time to recover from an ankle sprain.

- Initial treatment includes rest, bracing to avoid re-injury, and rehabilitation to regain muscular control of the ankle.

- Repair or reconstruction of the ankle is sometimes necessary for persistent symptoms of pain or instability.

Ankle sprains are the most common athletic injuries and usually affect the ligaments on the outside of the ankle. A sprain is an injury to the ligaments, the connective tissue that helps to hold the bones together within a joint. Ligaments control the motion of the ankle joint. The severity of the injury can vary from only stretching the ligament to a complete rupture.

It is normal to experience pain, weakness, swelling, and bruising around the ankle after an ankle sprain. It can be as painful as a fracture and can be very difficult to walk on. There is usually a lot of bruising, which occurs due to bleeding underneath the skin. The bleeding usually continues around the torn ligaments on the outside of the ankle until the vessels spasm closed and clot. The blood can appear to spread by leaking into other parts of the foot and into the calf muscle. Usually the blood will move with gravity. You will see bruising along the back of the calf, along the inside and outside of the heel, and along top of the forefoot over the ball of the foot.

A typical ankle sprain occurs when the muscles and ligaments are not able to counteract a shift of the force of body weight to the outer portion of the ankle. Sudden changes in the direction of body motion such as while running during a soccer game may cause the shift in the direction of force of the body weight across the ankle from the center to the outside edge of the ankle. This is much like leaning too far over on a stool while you are sitting on it, which can cause it to topple. You topple when your body weight shifts from the center of the stool to beyond the edge of the stool. As the ankle begins to roll and invert, the ankle collapses and the lateral ligaments rupture. If an x-ray of the ankle were taken at the exact time of the injury, it is likely that it would show the ankle joint to be almost completely dislocated or disconnected. Since the body weight is still transferred to the ground through the ankle, excessive force is applied to the edges and corners of the joints in its severely disjointed position. This can cause bruises of the bone under the joint surface and can even fracture the bone.

A second type of ankle sprain, the "high ankle sprain," is an injury of the ligaments that bind the tibia and fibula, the syndesmosis. This type of ankle sprain accounts for about 25% of ankle sprains in athletic injuries. The pain in the high ankle sprain is a little higher on the leg than the typical ankle sprain, usually about three centimeters above the tip of the fibula. Sprains in this area take considerably longer to heal than a lateral ankle sprain.

Sprains are slow healing. If the torn edges of the ligament do not heal at the correct length, then the ligament will remain loose. As a result, ankle sprains can become recurrent. Persistent instability due to stretched-out and nonfunctioning ligaments after an ankle sprain occur in approximately 30% of ankle sprains.

Certain abnormalities can make ankle sprains more likely. If your heel is shaped so that it tilts toward the inside of the foot, it's much easier to direct the force from the weight of the body to the outside of the leg. Ankle sprains are common in people with abnormal ankle alignment.

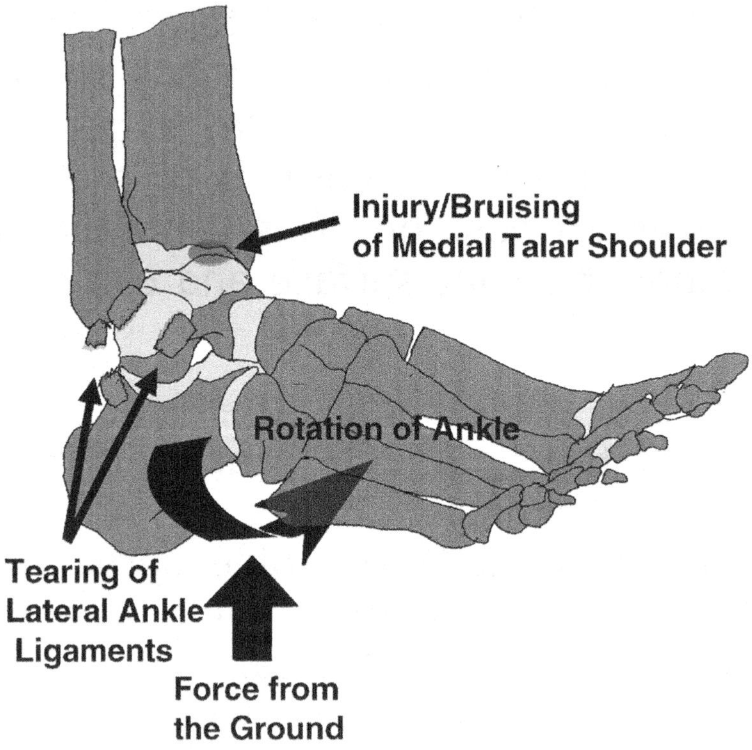

FIGURE 7.4 Ligaments on the outside of the ankle usually tear during an ankle sprain. In addition, the bone of the talus can become bruised from the force of the foot placed directly on the foot.

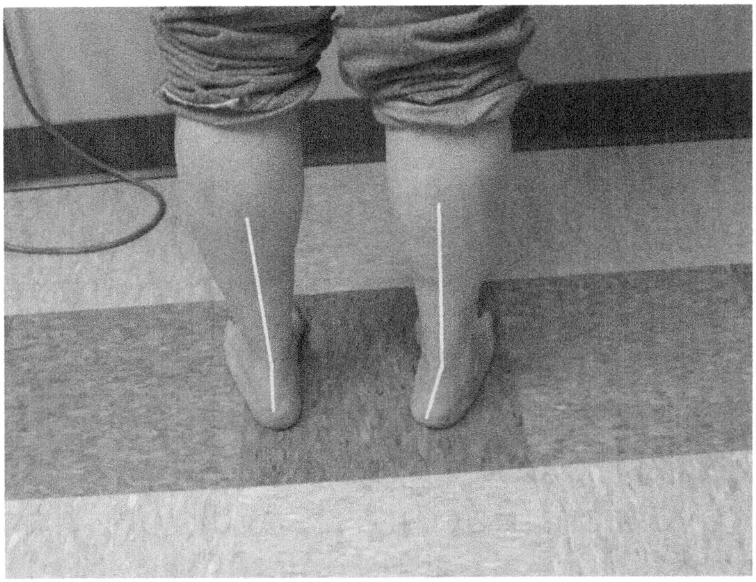

FIGURE 7.5 The right heel is inverted, an abnormal position. Weight applied to this ankle will tend to invert the foot more, making it prone to sprains.

Although an ankle sprain is a serious injury, it usually can heal without a lot of medical attention. Other more serious traumatic injuries are easy to confuse with ankle sprains. It is important to get a physician to look at an ankle sprain to make sure it is not a more dangerous injury. A thorough physical examination, in addition to proper x-rays, is usually necessary. A few of the injuries include:

- Ankle fracture.
- Osteochondral injury of the talus (chipping of the joint).
- Fracture of the base of the fifth metatarsal.
- Lateral process fractures of the talus.

- Fracture of the body of the talus.
- Achilles tendon rupture.

Peroneal tendon tears or peroneal tendon dislocation/tear of the superior peroneal retinaculum that holds the peroneal tendon within its groove.

Although it is possible to chip off pieces of the joint or bones into the ankle joint during a sprain, most small fractures along the periphery of the ankle represent avulsion fractures. Avulsion fractures are small chips of bone that break off in the process of tearing the ligaments. These fragments are usually less than one centimeter in size. Although they are bony injuries and are fractures, these injuries are usually not treated differently than the sprains. Despite the appearance on x-rays, these fragments are not loose. The bone fragments are firmly attached to the ligaments that are torn and have no potential to drift within the body.

Initial treatment of even severe ankle sprains is not surgery. Rest, ice, elevation, immobilization, compression, and pain medication are traditional methods of treatment.

Resting an injured body part, whether an ankle or other area of the body, is certainly logical. The injured ankle is painful to walk on or move. However, there is no evidence that complete rest actually improves the recuperation after ankle sprain. Certainly, it makes sense to reduce daily activity to avoid aggravating the pain, but rest need not be extensive and in most situations weight bearing can be started immediately.

Ice is also a mainstay of treatment. Why? Cooling ankle tissue may decrease the blood perfusion and slow the metabolism of the cells within the tissue. It is unclear whether this is desirable. Studies on the use of cold therapy or cryotherapy on ankle sprains are few and for the most part are poorly done, but some studies have evaluated this question using effective cooling devices on the shoulder and knee after surgery. They fail to show that the deep tissue temperature changes much after hours of icing.[1]

Ice does have the ability to improve pain, however. There are many different types of nerves that come from the skin, sending signals to the brain. Pain, temperature, light touch, pressure, and vibration senses all have separate nerves. Within the spine and brain, these nerves interconnect. They talk to one another. Stimulation of another sensory nerve, such as a temperature nerve through ice or a pressure nerve through rubbing, inhibits the transmission of the pain signals to the brain where we become aware of them. This interferes with the perception of pain, but does little to the ankle itself. Ice is a completely reasonable method of treating an ankle sprain or other injury as long as the benefit of it is understood. The benefits are a small effect on swelling and bleeding within the tissue immediately after the injury and a significant effect on the perceived pain. There is likely to be very little benefit on the ultimate result or the speed of healing.

Elevation is also commonly used in the treatment of an ankle sprain. It is probably the one effective way of decreasing swelling. However, is it important to control swelling? Despite the fact that swelling is extremely common complaint in musculoskeletal injuries, it is poorly studied. It can be observed in people with prolonged swelling from lymphatic and venous diseases, injuries such as cuts and sores do not heal well in chronically and severely swollen extremities. In these cases, the skin also begins to develop a leathery, scarred texture. This is different from the moderate and brief period of swelling experienced with most ankle sprains. It is not clear that meticulous control of swelling is beneficial. Certainly, swelling decreases motion, but modest degrees of swelling do not likely have much effect on recovery from an ankle sprain. The throbbing pain that often accompanies any injury for the first days to a week or two is very responsive to elevation, however.

Compression is helpful in controlling severe swelling. In most ankle sprains, the swelling is modest and located over the area of injury or on the top of the foot. Elastic bandages such as Ace wraps are a common dressing used in the treatment of ankle sprains, but are not effective at controlling swelling or in stabilizing the injury. The most effective and even compression can be obtained from an elastic sleeve or low compression support hose or sock.

Of all of the points above, immobilization has been studied the most extensively. Most of the scientific information indicates that when it comes to immobilization, less is more.[2] It is beneficial to protect the ankle from re-injury, but you don't want to go overboard. The consensus of most of the evidence suggests that people who are casted and completely immobilized take longer to return to sporting activity, have more residual instability, and more pain than the people who were treated with a less restrictive brace or none at all.

Nonsteroidal anti-inflammatory (NSAIDs) medications such as ibuprofen (Motrin® or Advil®) or naproxen (Naprosyn® or Aleve®) are helpful pain medicines. It is unfortunate that this class of medication come with the description *anti-inflammatory.* It gives the impression that these medications are capable of reducing swelling or accelerating recovery, neither of which has been conclusively proven. The pain-relieving effect may be delivered by topical application of NSAIDs in people who have side effects such as upset stomach with oral NSAIDs

As the most common athletic injury and a significant cause of prolonged pain, there's a lot of interest in preventing sprained ankles. There seems to be good evidence that sports braces and taping techniques are helpful in the prevention of ankle injuries, decreasing in the incidence of ankle sprain by 70%.[3] This improvement in the incidence of ankle sprain is sometimes balanced by the brace's cost, and impact on the athlete's performance and comfort, as well as the possible negative effects of the brace on the movements of other joints. One type of brace or taping technique is not clearly superior to another. Shoes that are specially designed to prevent ankle sprains have recently been introduced into the market by a new shoe company, Ektio. Several aspects of the design of these shoes may be effective at preventing ankle sprains and reducing re-injury. Although they appear to be well constructed for this purpose, their effectiveness at preventing and treating ankle sprains has not been established yet except anecdotally.

A reasoned and balanced approach to ankle sprains is recommended. There is sometimes a tendency to overtreat many disorders that tend to resolve without treatment such as ankle sprains. It is helpful when selecting tools to use to treat ankle sprains to focus on the goals of treatment. The goals are to control the pain, increase the function of the ankle, and prevent re-injury. Pain medication, ice, and braces are helpful in this regard. It is important to realize that these treatments do not necessarily lead to a faster and more successful outcome. They provide a measure of safety and decrease the pain experienced getting there.

Prolonged problems after an ankle sprain are extremely common. In one study, 96 cadets in the United States Naval Academy with ankle sprains were followed for six months. At the conclusion of the study, 40% of the cadets continued to have residual symptoms.[4] The symptoms did not seem to correlate with ankle instability. Syndesmosis sprains tended to do even worse. Many persistent chronic ankle pains will not have a specific treatable or repairable problem.

Surgery for ankle sprains is suggested only if you are unable to trust the ankle or you keep on spraining it. Generally, surgery involves repair of the ligaments. If the ligaments are so damaged as to make repair impossible, then reconstruction using nearby tendons can be considered, but adds significantly to the recovery and extensiveness of this surgery. It is done as an outpatient. A period of immobilization and protection after surgery is very commonly advised. Complications include continued instability, nerve damage, ankle pain, and wound problems.

ANKLE ARTHRITIS

- Ankle arthritis is a wearing of the joint cartilage in the ankle joint.

- Ankle arthritis is usually caused by an injury such as a fracture or a disease such as rheumatoid arthritis. Osteoarthritis in the absence of trauma or another disease is much less common in the ankle than it is in the knee or hip.

- Nonoperative treatment of ankle arthritis revolves around immobilization the ankle in a comfortable position for walking, weight reduction, and pain control through medications.
- Elimination of the joint through fusion is the traditional surgery. Although replacement surgery for the ankle is improving, this procedure is much less reliable and more complicated than in joint replacement in the hip or knee.

Primary arthritis of a joint is wearing out of a joint through nontraumatic means in absence of another reason. People with primary arthritis usually have genetic traits that affect the mechanical flexibility of the bone, causing premature damage to the joint by jarring it with normal activity. Mechanical abnormalities such as stiffness of the underlying bone cause premature wear of the cartilage. This form of arthritis is common in the knee and hip, but it is actually uncommon in the ankle.

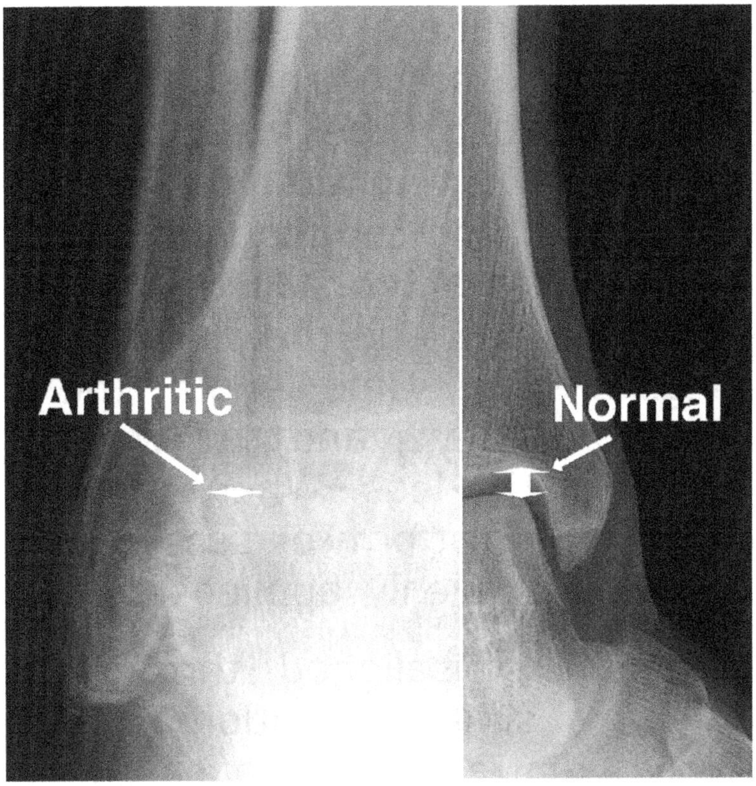

FIGURE 7.6 Primary joint arthritis. The joint is uniformly destroyed and the alignment of the joint is otherwise normal. An x-ray of a normal ankle is superimposed to the right to contrast the extent of the narrowing of the joint due to arthritic destruction.

Most ankle arthritis occurs because of another underlying condition. Many cases of ankle arthritis are caused from inflammatory arthritises. The most common cause of ankle arthritis is trauma. This initiates gradual deterioration of the joint. If fragments of an ankle fracture are not restored perfectly, the deterioration of the joint can happen in months or years instead of decades. The ankle joint surfaces normally mate nearly exactly. When damaged, the joint does not tolerate irregularity well.

Changes in the alignment of the foot can radically alter the forces across the ankle. If the balance of the ankle is disturbed, the wear within the joint accelerates. The ankle and foot can be compared to a three-legged chair. The corresponding foot structures to these three legs are the ball of the first toe, the lesser toes and the heel and the platform is the ankle. When the legs are the same length, the platform or seat of the chair is level and the weight is equally applied to each of the legs. When one leg is shorter than the others, the platform or seat wobbles or leans and the weight is unevenly applied to the legs.

When the foot is misaligned through fracture or ligament injury, a similar situation can arise. If the foot becomes flattened because the arch is unstable—such as occurs during an ineffectively treated midfoot fracture or dislocation—the ligaments beneath this joint no longer are tight enough to stabilize the joint in its correct position. As a result the big toe extends. In effect, the big toe elevates off the ground. In order to maintain the three primary "legs" of the foot on the floor, the foot must evert and the arch sag even more. This strains the ligaments of the inside of the ankle and applies more compression force to the outside of the ankle, causing shear, wear and eventually arthritis.

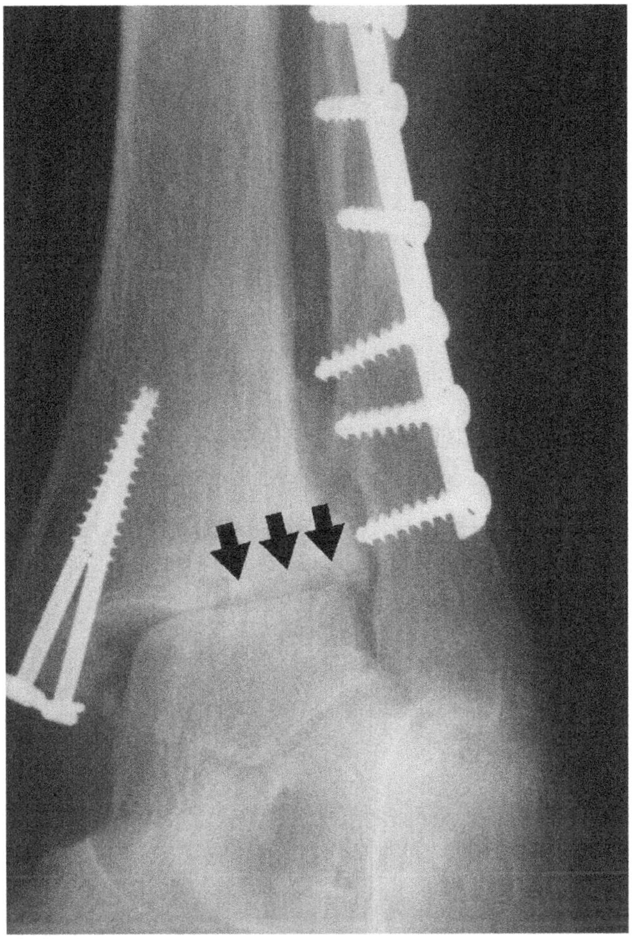

FIGURE 7.7 Rapid deterioration and malalignment of an ankle joint after failure of the fixation of a fracture, and unrecognized or untreated syndesmosis injury. The outside portion of the tibial joint surface has eroded severely as a result (black arrows).

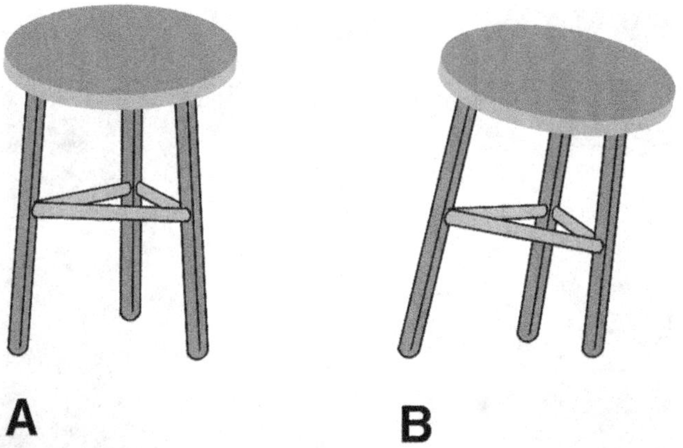

FIGURE 7.8 When the supports of the stool are equal in length (A), the seat of the stool is level and it is easy to sit on (representing a flat level ankle). When one leg becomes shorter or unstable (B), the stool becomes unlevel and thus difficult to sit on. In addition, if you were able to balance on it, your weight would be unequally distributed on the legs.

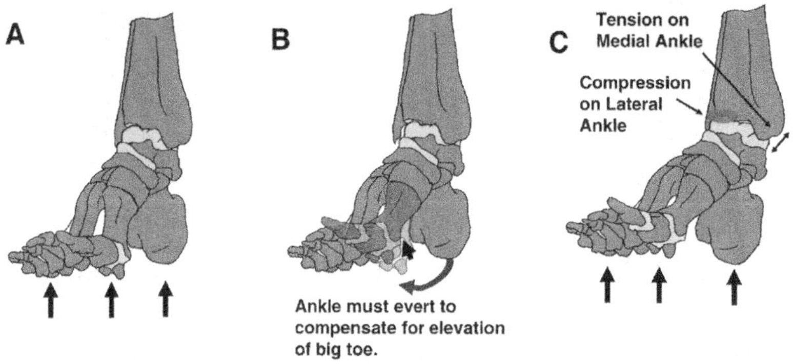

FIGURE 7.9 When the heel, the first and the fifth metatarsal head contact the ground with equal pressure, the ankle is stable. B. When the arch sags such as when the midfoot is injured and unstable, the first metatarsal elevates or extends away from the floor (small arrow). The ankle must evert or rotate to the outside of the foot for the big toe to maintain contact with the floor. C. This rotated position strains the medial ankle ligaments and crushes the outside of the ankle joint as in figure 7.10.

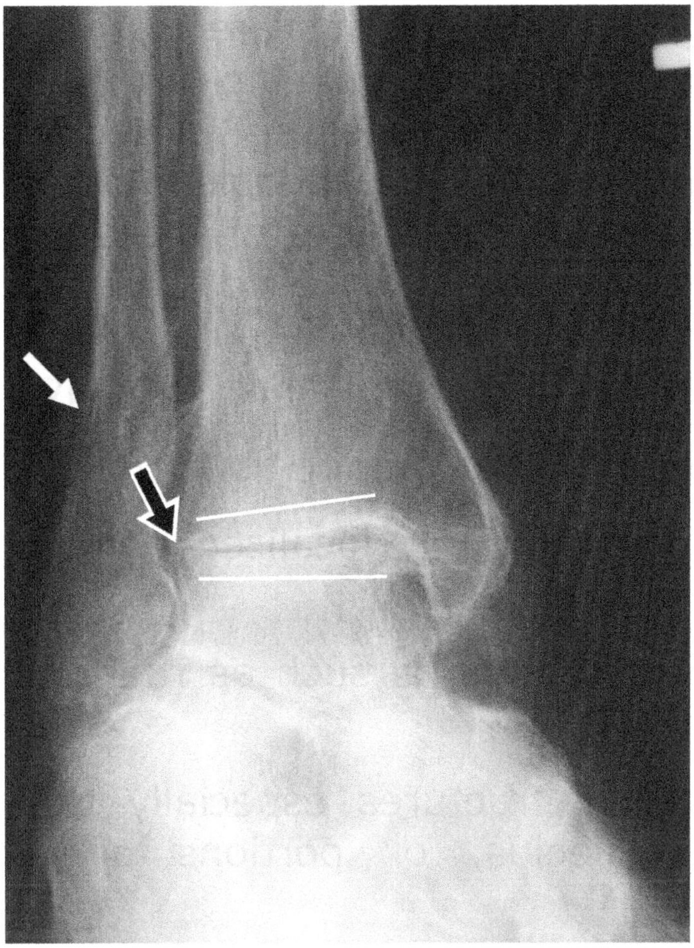

FIGURE 7.10 Valgus or eversion type of ankle arthritis. This type of ankle arthritis could be caused by a fallen arch, untreated syndesmosis injury, or an old unstable midfoot fracture.

Arthritis in the ankle is caused more frequently by trauma than deterioration, so the people suffering from ankle arthritis tend to be younger and more active than the people with knee and hip arthritis. This is important when considering treatment for ankle arthritis. An average person with knee arthritis is about 64 years old. The average age of a person with ankle arthritis is 58 years old and a greater proportion of people with ankle arthritis are in their thirties and forties than with knee and hip arthritis. Long-term planning is even more necessary in deciding treatment for ankle arthritis because people with ankle arthritis are likely to live long lives after the surgery.

Other causes of ankle pain:

- Avascular necrosis (the talus bone dying).
- Tendonitis of the posterior tibial or Achilles tendon.
- Osteochondral injury (localized bone and cartilage injury with the joint).
- Inflammatory arthritis such as rheumatoid arthritis and gout.
- Nonunions of fractures especially the lateral and medial malleolus, or portions of the talus or calcaneus.
- Osteoarthritis of adjacent joints such as the subtalar or talonavicular.
- Irritation of accessory bones such as the os naviculare and os trigonum.

Treatment of ankle arthritis is initially done without surgery. Antiinflammatory medication such as naproxen (Aleve®), ibuprofen (Motrin®), celecoxib (Celebrex®), and other medications such as acetaminophen (Tylenol®) can effectively decrease the pain, but obviously do not cure the arthritis. Steroid injections into the ankle joint can occasionally be done and can eliminate episodes of intense pain, but also do not cure the arthritis. Injections and oral medications of natural joint components such as glucosamine and chondroitan sulfate are shown to give temporary relief and have few side effects. You can find oral glucoamine/chondroitan sulfate at your drug store without a prescription. Strong evidence that these medications prevent or repair arthritis is not available. Use of these medications should be discontinued unless considerable pain improvement is experienced within one month.

Stretching exercises of the ankle are futile and can aggravate the pain. Ankle arthritis becomes more symptomatic when the ankle is being used at its limits of motion. Ensuring that other joints, ligaments, and tendons within the legs are as flexible as possible can help reduce the motion that is necessary in the ankle for fairly normal walking. Hamstring, back, and hip exercises are recommended, but take some time to make a difference.

Often in severe ankle arthritis, mobility is lost. Using an elevated heel can help to accommodate this. This is done either through selecting a shoe that has an elevated heel relative to the thickness of the sole in the forefoot or by using a heel pad inside of the shoe. Up to a half inch of elevation is usually possible using a heel pad. Much more than this is likely to push the heel of the foot out of the shoe and compromise the fit of the shoe. Rocker-soled shoes are not usually helpful in the treatment of ankle arthritis, because they may increase ankle motion with walking, which is likely to aggravate ankle arthritis.

Braces are an important way of treating ankle arthritis. Like the brace treatment of nearly all ankle and foot problems, there are a number of options that can be chosen. Each has its advantages and disadvantages. Usually the trade-off is weight and difficulty with placing it into a shoe for stability and effectiveness. For mild cases, an elastic sleeve or sports ankle brace such as a lace-up brace may be enough. A more aggressive brace would be a fixed or short-articulated AFO or molded Arizona brace. The goal of brace treatment is to control pain through the restriction of ankle motion. Braces are unlikely to stop the progression of arthritis. Although the brace will not work without wearing it, it does not need to be used all of the time as long as activity without the brace doesn't aggravate your ankle pain.

Surgery of ankle arthritis can be considered when all else fails. Occasionally, removal of spurs or loose bone fragments can give relief, but is usually not successful except in very specific circumstances. It is difficult with current techniques to directly repair the cartilage damage in advanced ankle arthritis. Surgery for ankle arthritis involves a substantial intervention and recovery. The choices are ankle fusion or ankle replacement.

Ankle fusion involves removing the joint cartilage and tough bone beneath it, called the *subchondral* bone.

The raw bone surfaces are then pushed together to allow them to heal with bone crossing the joint. Screws and other devices are often used to hold the bones still, helping the new healing bone to cross the joint. The ankle can no longer move after this, but the other joints in the foot can often move allowing a near normal gait. This can be done through an open incision or by using smaller incision and a fiber optic camera called an arthroscope. An arthroscope is an instrument about the caliber of a pencil that is placed into the joint through one-half inch incisions to clearly visualize the joint. These procedures generally require an overnight stay in the hospital and the ankle is immobilized in a nonweight-bearing cast for 6 to 10 weeks.

Ankle replacement is removal of the joint surfaces and placing a plastic and metal device into the defect left after removing the joint. Most people are familiar with similar procedures done on the knee and hip. However, the technique of ankle replacement did not enjoy the initial success of hip and knee replacement. In fact, for many years it was not done in the United States because of poor results and complications. With further research and improvements in design, the current ankle replacements seem promising.

When choosing between these techniques, a frank consideration of the risks and benefits of each should be carefully weighed (Table 7.1). Ankle fusion has the disadvantage of permanently eliminating your ability to move your ankle. When ankle motion is eliminated, the stress on the surrounding joints in the middle of the foot is increased, leading to further deterioration and arthritis of these joints eventually. However, once the ankle is fused, it will remain fused and the ankle at least should not require reoperation. Ankle fusion also has an approximately 10% lack-of-healing rate. This prolongs recovery and often requires reoperation.

Ankle replacement retains ankle motion and, therefore, gait is more normal and stress to other joints is decreased. However, infection and wound breakdown after ankle replacement are disastrous complications. The technique for implanting the ankle replacement is more demanding and intra-operative complications are more frequent than with replacement of the hip and knee. These complications may require further medical care including surgery to repair. Most reports seem to indicate that ankle replacements may function for 10 years or more in 80% of cases. If you have an expected lifetime of decades, you will probably have this surgery more than once.

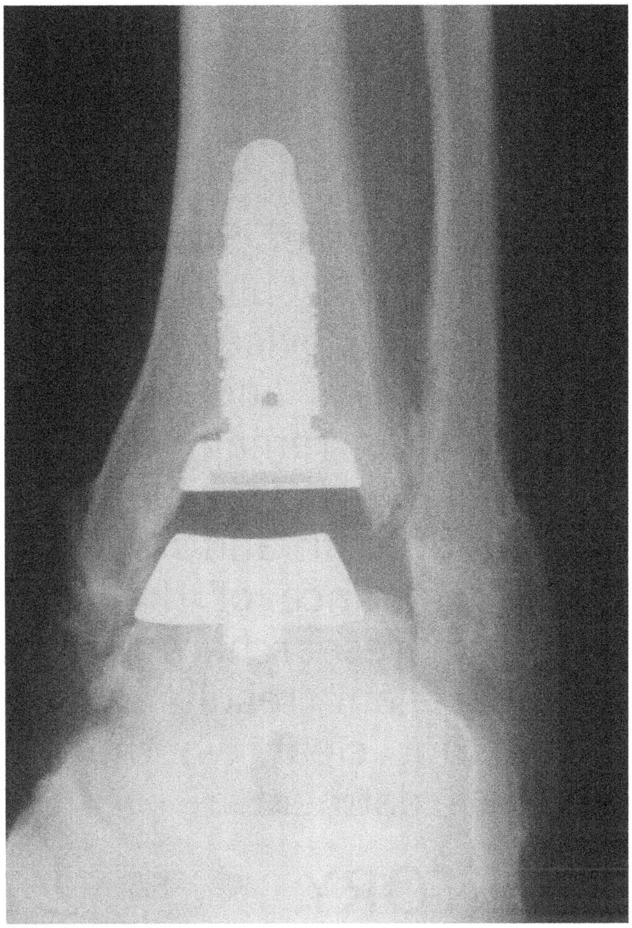

FIGURE 7.11 An example of a currently available ankle replacement.

TABLE 7.1 Factors that favor ankle replacement versus ankle fusion

Ankle Replacement	Ankle Fusion
Age > 65yrs	Age < 55yrs
Multiple Areas of Foot Arthritis	Prior Infection
Wt < 100kg	Overweight (> 100kg)
	Severe Malalignment
	Neuropathy/Diabetes
	Scarring
	Peripheral Artery Disease

Ankle Replacement	Ankle Fusion
	Active, High-Demand Occupation

Unfortunately, reversing ankle arthritis once it has occurred is not yet possible. Some researchers have begun to test devices that pull the ankle apart called external fixators. These devices attach to the bones of the ankle through wires and pins that go through the skin. These devices remain on for a period of months and ambulation is possible during this time. Improvements in ankle pain and movement, and even the radiographic appearance of the ankle have been noted. However, other researchers have not been able to replicate the excellent results that were initially reported and it is not clear whether this technique represents a future treatment.

LEONARD'S STORY

Leonard is a 71-year-old man who had recently retired from working in an auto parts store. Leonard recalled multiple ankle injuries over his life starting with a sprain that occurred during football in high school. Over the years his tendency to sprain his ankle became gradually less, but over the past two years, he had noted increasing pain especially on uneven ground, like when he mowed his lawn.

Leonard's ankle was enlarged when compared to his other ankle and prominent along the outside with the heel angling toward the midline. His range of motion was restricted with reduced ability to bring his toe up. His ankle had only mild instability when the outside ligaments were stressed.

Radiographs show tilting of the talus in relation to the tibia and fibula. The talus appears to be rotated within the joint with the medial shoulder of the talus digging into the tibial roof. The cartilage is worn from the position of the joint.

When discussing the treatment options, Leonard was against surgery unless "there was no other way." His primary concern was the prolonged restricted weight bearing and fear of complications as he is on a blood thinner for mini-strokes. Leonard was placed in a hinged ankle brace to keep the ankle from twisting out of place and a small lift was placed in the device to compensate for his restricted motion. He was instructed to take an over-the-counter anti-inflammatory medication for pain.

Abnormal and premature wear in the ankle can be caused by direct damage to the joint from trauma, or wear due to faulty balance around the joint. Leonard's abnormal foot alignment along with his ligament injury and instability lead to a gradual wear of his joint. Leonard may eventually require an operation to definitively treat his ankle arthritis, but as long as his pain can be controlled in other ways while pursuing an active lifestyle, it may be delayed indefinitely.

Over-the-counter anti-inflammatory medications are just as effective as the varieties available by prescription and are sometimes less expensive. Although few of the symptoms of osteoarthritis are caused by the body's inflammatory system, anti-inflammatory medications can still effectively mute the pain. There will still be swelling or warmth associated with osteoarthritis.

All anti-inflammatory medications have side effects—including an increased risk of cardiac death—and routine use should be discussed with your doctor.

ANKLE FRACTURES

- Ankle fractures are injuries to the bones and ligaments that do not significantly involve the weight-bearing roof of the ankle. They can occur in high-energy accidents such as motor vehicle accidents, but more commonly are caused by ordinary falls and stumbling.
- If the remaining ligaments and bones around the ankle can maintain the alignment of the ankle, the ankle fracture is stable.
- Stable ankle fractures are usually treated without surgery and often ambulation can begin immediately with proper protective immobilization.

- If the injury of the bones and ligaments allows the joint to come out of alignment, the ankle fracture is unstable.
- Unstable fractures sometimes require surgery to regain alignment of the joint and fracture fragments, although in certain instances these may be treated nonoperatively with close follow-up.

The thought of a fracture or break of a bone (this is the same thing) of the foot or ankle provokes a lot of concern and fear. Of course, even within the few days that often pass between the injury and a medical appointment in our clinic, the injured person has begun to experience the loss of independence and the pain that often accompanies the injury. Many cannot understand how a simple and mundane activity such as taking out the trash or crossing over a curb, a chore they do every day could have led to such a situation. Isn't the ankle stronger than that?

Ankle fractures are unfortunately common injuries. Typically, they occur from falls and twisting injuries, but there are few mechanisms of force that affect the ankle that cannot produce an ankle fracture. The severity varies.

Avulsion fractures are small chips of bone that detach when the ligaments are torn around a joint. These are on the mild side of the spectrum of ankle fractures because they are really ankle sprains that include a very small bony injury. Often, people wonder whether these fragments can drift around their bodies, but the fragments are attached to the injured and torn ends of the ligaments and cannot migrate. The principles outlined above in the Ankle Sprain section can be applied to these injuries.

On the other end of the spectrum are severe unstable injuries that can involve multiple bones and ligaments. Some even tear through the skin. These "open" injuries have increased damage to the soft tissues around the ankle and introduce contamination into the fracture site. Treatment of these injuries always involves some kind of surgery.

The bruising pattern after an ankle fracture can be awful, but the explanation of the distribution of the bleeding within the tissue is very simple. A broken bone tears blood vessels within the bone and in the soft tissue around the bone. The bleeding that follows often initially is seen as a lump or "goose egg." However, after the first few hours, the bleeding stops as the vessel's spasm closed and clotting occurs from the activation of platelets, small cells within your blood stream that release the proteins that begin a complex clotting cascade. There are more than 20 separate proteins within your blood that regulate and participate in the simple act of clotting. The blood meanwhile begins to seep along tissue planes, down along muscles and collect within these tissue planes. Gravity often guides this seepage. Common areas for the blood to collect are in the back of the calf if one is lying down and along the heel and top of the second, third, and fourth metatarsophalangeal joint, just on top of the ball of the foot.

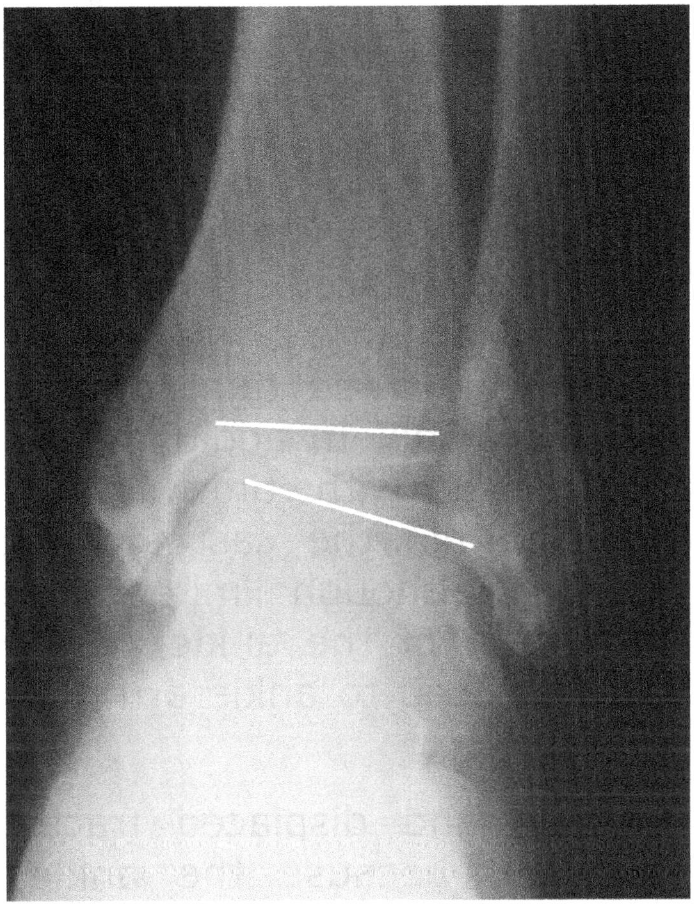

FIGURE 7.12 Leonard's ankle x-ray. The joint has begun to tilt (lines) due to ligament damage and abnormal wear.

The stability of the ankle determines the appropriate treatment. Ankle stability is the ability to maintain proper joint alignment after damage to ligaments and bones. When the damage to the ligaments and bones is severe, small amounts of pressure can slide the ankle out of its tight-fitting bony confines. The ankle joint can be visualized as a ring of structures consisting of the talus, the tibia and fibula, and the ligaments that connect them on the inside, the deltoid ligament, on the outside, the lateral ankle ligaments, and between the tibia and fibula, the syndesmosis. An interruption in the ring at one point does not compromise stability. A break in two points can allow the ring to slide out of place.

Sometimes an unstable ankle can be pushed into proper position and placed in a cast. However, maintaining perfect alignment within a cast can be difficult. A cast is never so tight that the foot and ankle do not move at all. In addition, as the swelling in the leg decreases with time and healing, the amount of room within the cast increases and the motion of the foot, although limited, also increases. A small displacement of the ankle from its perfectly aligned position can lead to ankle arthritis, sometimes quickly.

In highly unstable and displaced fractures surgery cannot be avoided, because the ankle cannot be reliably expected to heal in perfect alignment. Stability is regained through fixation and reconstruction of torn ligaments and fractures. This is especially true for the syndesmosis, the joint between the tibia and fibula. The syndesmosis controls not only the width of the joint, but also the rotation of the talus in the ankle joint. If an injury of this structure is present and not properly addressed, a bad result is nearly guaranteed.

Recuperation after ankle injury involves a significant degree of loss of independence. The inability to drive is probably one of the most inconvenient aspects of this. So, when is it safe to drive after an ankle fracture? Researchers have looked into this question and have found that reaction time is delayed in people who have recently had a fracture even one that is not treated with an operation for three to six weeks. A good rule of thumb is that you should be able to walk comfortably with a minimal limp before returning to driving. Otherwise, the delay in reaction time may mean hesitation when braking in a driving emergency. It is never safe to drive with your left foot and it is never safe to operate the pedals with a walking boot or cast.

The use of anti-inflammatory pain medications such as ibuprofen and naprosyn during fracture healing has come under some scrutiny recently. Although these medications are often effective for pain, the side effects include stomach upset, increased bleeding, and potentially serious ulcer formation. Research has indicated that anti-inflammatory pain medications may actually delay bone healing. This effect may be of little importance in some fractures that heal quickly, but there is a chance that it increases the time that it takes to heal a fracture or the possibility of fracture healing failure called *nonunion.* Typically, if nonunion develops, surgery may be necessary. It is probably safest to avoid nonsteroidal anti-inflammatories until further research clarifies the risk. Acetaminophen

(Tylenol®) is not in the "anti-inflammatory" class and may be used alternatively either alone or with a narcotic pain medication.

Swelling is often a considerable concern after a fracture. Swelling is a normal part of recovering from an ankle fracture that can persist to some degree for a long time. It is not at all unusual to have mild to moderate swelling for three to six months and enough swelling to limit certain shoe wear for 6 to 12 weeks. Although this is usually not dangerous, the foot may turn colors if it is not elevated during this period.

Physical therapy is sometimes not necessary after a fracture. When the limitation of function has been brief and mild, the ankle is able to return to normal function without a great deal of help. Stiffness and swelling may make it difficult to correctly position the leg during walking after fracture, increasing the possibility of re-injury. Positioning the ankle may take extra effort. If the ankle is not positioned properly when walking, then it is easy to step on the side of it potentially causing a twisting or falling re-injury. Loss of strength, balance, and stiffness is also common. These are things that physical therapy can help with a great deal. Physical therapy is not going to alleviate pain.

It is extremely common to be unable to return to full activity after a severe ankle fracture. Modern surgical techniques have developed ways to restore the anatomy of a fracture and to restore the majority of function such as walking, but there are a number of instances with athletes where they will be unable to go back to their pre-injury playing level. There are many structures besides bones that are injured during an ankle fracture. Many of these structures scar and become less compliant than prior to the injury. One of the most common complaints is of pain after getting up from a seated position or after getting up out of bed. This undoubtedly is due to loss of compliance of the soft tissue after the injury and the increased strain that is necessary to stretch these structures to a working length after relaxation.

A frequent concern from patients is the potential problem with the metal used in repairing the fracture and airport security. A recent study[5] looked at metallic implants and their detectability by airport scanners. Archway scanners generally in use by airports usually do not detect stainless steel implants weighing less than 145 grams. An implant of this size is unusual in even the most extensive foot and ankle reconstruction. Titanium implants are detectable at considerably lower weights. Wand-type scanners are much more sensitive and can detect implants weighing as little as twelve grams. Usually, airport security pays no attention to the cards that are sometimes given to people to identify their implants. These cards would easy to reproduce by anyone with a laptop computer and a laminator. The newer backscatter and millimeter wave airport scanners do not penetrate far beneath the skin and, therefore, are unlikely to detect orthopedic implants.

AMY'S STORY

Amy is a busy mother of three who worked at the postal office sorting packages. She was walking the family dog who suddenly bolted when he saw a rabbit across the street one snowy night. Amy who is barely 130 pounds at five foot four inches was texting on her phone at the time and was immediately and unexpected pulled to her left side. An audible snap and a jolt of pain in her right ankle indicated to her that she was in trouble. She phoned her husband and he immediately took her to the hospital emergency room.

The ER physician who saw her announced that the ankle was broken and that she should see a specialist. "You may need an operation for that," he announced. Amy began to sob as they had plans to go to Florida in two weeks.

In Amy's case, her fibula broke at the level of her ankle joint. Amy was seen in the orthopedic clinic the next day. She was in a wheelchair, and her face plainly showed that she was anxious and in pain. Her husband was in the room looking worried as well. Amy's leg was several shades of deep red and blue. The bruising was located along her heel, back of her leg, and along the tops of her toes. Her ankle was swollen and painful with any motion. Her tenderness was mainly over the fractured bone with mild tenderness over the inside of her ankle near her medial malleolus. When her heel was gently pushed to the outside, it did not move and this maneuver hurt only a little.

Although Amy's ankle was tender and would be for some time, it was not unstable and therefore surgery was not necessary. This came as a huge relief to her. In fact, even though the ankle was clearly too painful for walking now, it would not be long before she could begin to put pressure and walk on it. She was given crutches and fitted with a removable walking boot—a Velcro®, metal, and rubber device that would control and limit the motion of the ankle while she began to bear weight on it. This would both eliminate the painful motion of the ankle while walking and protect the ankle from further aggravating stress and potential injury. Her vacation was saved although she would have to curtail long walks on the beach.

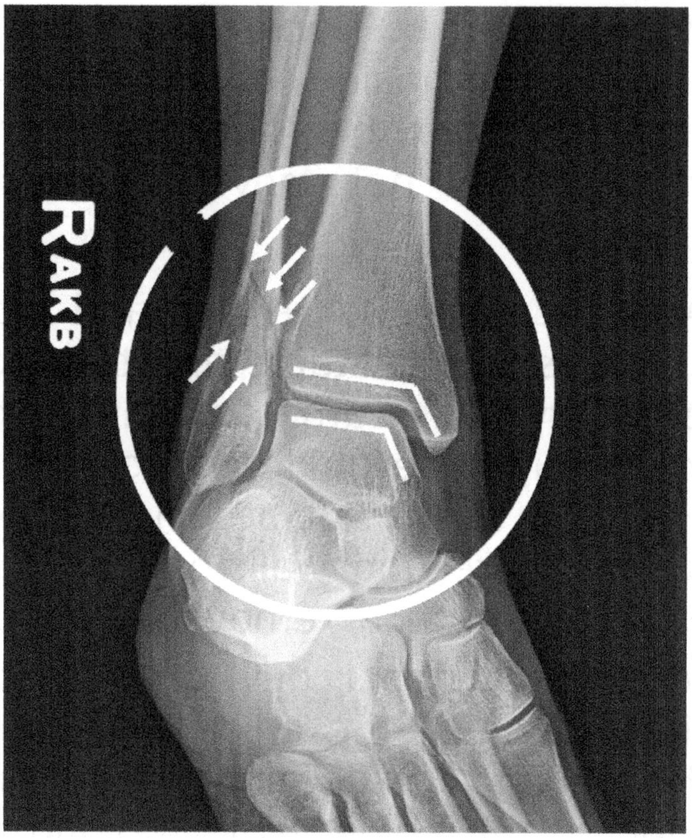

FIGURE 7.13 A. Brandon's fracture includes both a fracture of the shaft of the fibula and a tear of the medial supporting ligaments. The joint was unstable and incongruent represented by the double break in the circle. B. An illustration of the fibular fracture and ligament tear on the inside of the ankle, leading to an unstable ankle injury.

BRANDON'S STORY

Brandon's injury was quite different. He was a 34-year-old lawyer who was an avid soccer player. He was hit from the outside of the knee while playing soccer and fell to the ground in agony. There was absolutely no way that he could put weight on his leg and was carried off the field by his teammates and was driven to the emergency room. Orthopedic consultation was obtained after x-rays showed an ankle fracture dislocation.

This is a tear of the medial joint ligaments and a fracture of the fibula above the level of the ankle joint. Variants of this fracture can fracture the fibula so high that it may not be seen on standard ankle x-rays, but should be apparent from the pain near the outside of the knee. This variant called a *Maisonneuve fracture* can show no fracture or other abnormality on ankle radiographs. Brandon's x-rays show abnormally increased space between the medial talus and the medial malleolus, which indicates that the ankle joint surfaces are not longer in proper position. This alignment is critical for good function.

Brandon was told about the risks, potential complications, and benefits of surgical stabilization of his ankle. Remarkably, even through Brandon was an enthusiastic athlete, he was also a one-half-pack per day smoker. This is always a complicating factor in recovery.

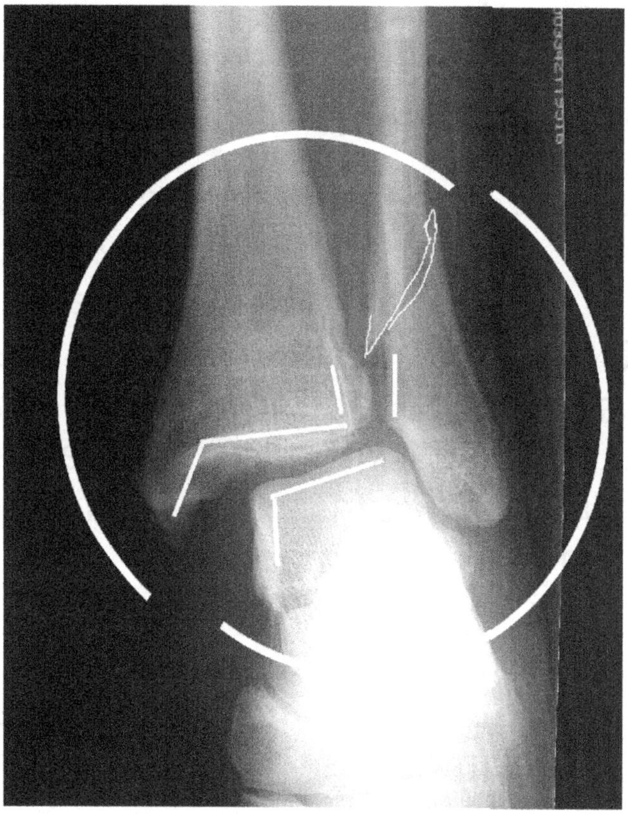

FIGURE 7.14 A Postoperative images showing the lateral plate with screws. The joint surfaces are aligned congruently.

Brandon's surgery went great. The operation took slightly less than an hour. The fixation involved placement of a plate and screws on the fibula. The ligament tear was not repaired.

When Brandon was seen two days after the procedure, he still was in considerable pain and it hurt to even move his ankle slightly. His wound looked good and had stopped bleeding. He was placed in a cast. In two weeks, his cast was removed and the sutures in his wound were removed. He was placed in a cast boot, but was not allowed to bear weight on it until six weeks after the injury. He was able to shower, and return to his law practice after a week on crutches.

At six weeks, he was allowed to progressively begin to bear weight and at 10 weeks, he was weaned from the boot into a tennis shoe.

He began to work out and progressively returned to nonimpact aerobic activity. However, he was unable to return to impact exercises such as running or soccer. He had a CAT scan done. It showed only healed fractures without other evidence of injury. Brandon eventually was able to return to recreational jogging although he gave up soccer. Two years after the injury, he was seen for knee pain and he said that he rarely thought about his ankle now, but it took over a year to it to recover completely.

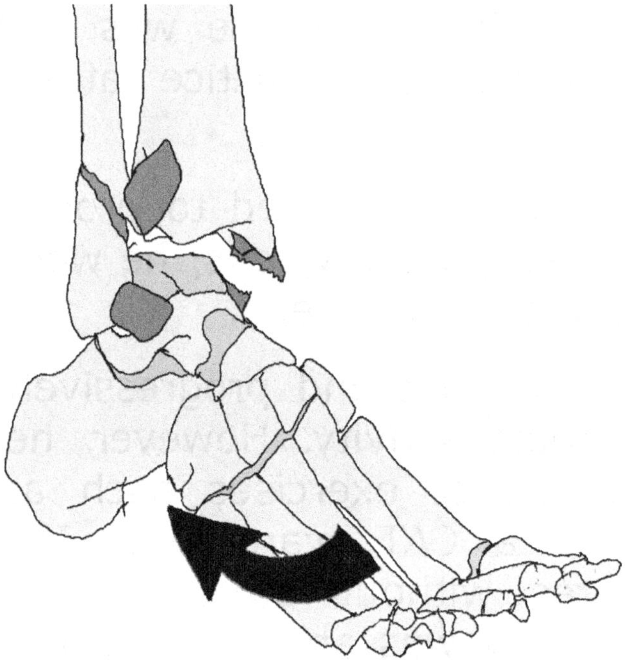

FIGURE 7.14 B Amy's fracture is a fairly typical fibular ankle fracture showing the apparent presence of two fracture lines arises from the ability to see both the front and back crack in an x-ray. Importantly for Amy, the ankle joint surfaces between the tibia and talus are congruent. The injury is stable as represented by the ring with a single break within it.

"CHIP FRACTURES"—OSTEOCHONDRAL DEFECTS OF THE TALUS

• Osteochondral defects or injuries of the talus can cause ankle pain.

• Fifty percent of these injuries are hidden on x-rays.

• There are several ways that osteochondral talar defects can form. Trauma is certainly a frequent cause.

An osteochondral defect (OCD) is an injury of the joint surface usually of the talus. It is a somewhat rare problem. The cause of it is far from completely understood and there are probably multiple causes. Although osteochondral damage can occur in any joint, the ankle seems to be most commonly affected. The talus is surrounded in the ankle by opposing joint surfaces on the top, inside and outside. This makes the joint very stable, but severe ankle sprains and fractures that can temporarily dislocate the joint will cause these surfaces to hit one another in unusual ways, which can lead to bruising and chipping of the joint. When the joint surface is bruised, the healing can result in a painful cyst or crater-like lesion. This type of osteochondral injury can be found on the inside shoulder of the talus. Finally, vascular injuries can cut off the blood supply to portions of the joint and cause it to fragment. These lesions can form in young children and adults.

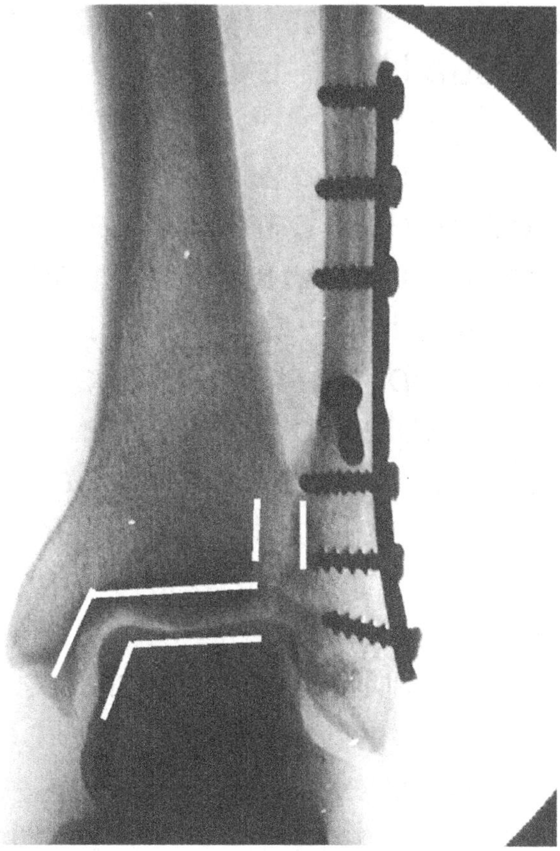

FIGURE 7.15 Medial talar OCD in an adolescent boy.

OCDs may be variable in size, location, and degree of joint damage. The cartilage surface over the OCD may be normal and smooth. At other times, the fragment can be large and separated from the remainder of the joint. Still other times it may contain only scar and fragmented cartilage.

It is treated initially by immobilization and weight restriction. Chronic osteochondral injuries can be initially treated with physical therapy, analgesics such as Motrin®, and occasionally through injections of steroid medications and weight bearing immobilization in a devise such as a fracture brace. Although often worthwhile, these treatments sometimes don't work.

Surgery of these injuries is a balance between the severity of the reconstruction and the degree with which the joint can be reconstituted. None of the techniques will leave the joint completely normal. When the fragment is large, the joint can be opened, and the fragment replaced and stabilized with pins or screws. If it's small, the fragment can be removed. The defect left is cleaned back to living bone and allowed to fill with blood clot. The blood clot can regenerate into fibrocartilage, an immature disorganized form of cartilage, which often decreases pain but is not as resilient as normal articular cartilage.

More complete reconstruction of the articular cartilage is necessary in some situations where the techniques above are unsuccessful in relieving the pain. This is done through an open surgical procedure. In order to get to the problem area a cut in the tibia or fibula bone is often necessary. One technique involves harvesting a portion of the knee articular cartilage and bone and replacing the damaged portion of the talar joint with it. Another involves the growing cartilage in a laboratory and implanting it into the defect. Recovery after this procedure is often prolonged and weight bearing on the ankle must be delayed until the graft and bony cuts heal. This procedure gets good results in 80% to 90%. Some insurances fail to cover this procedure, however, citing it as investigational.

MICHAEL'S STORY

Michael, an athletic physical therapy student, had an ankle fracture four years ago. He fractured it after making a lay-up during a weekly basketball game. He came down on his opponent's foot twisting his leg. He heard a distinct pop, felt significant pain, and was helped by his friends to a hospital. X-rays revealed a nondisplaced fracture or "cracked" distal fibula.

He was treated by a physician without surgery for a stable ankle fracture. He gradually recovered but noticed that the injury, while improved, really never completely went away. Over the past two years, he noted sudden fleeting pains in the ankle with small injuries and missteps, which caused sharp pains on the inside of his ankle that usually improved quickly. Because of this, he gave up basketball. Then he twisted his ankle while walking down the stairs at his home, causing sudden pain that did not go away and his ankle started clicking. Radiographs showed a dark area in the medial aspect of the talar shoulder on one view, an osteochondral injury.

Michael was placed in a cast boot. His pain decreased over the next two months as he was weaned out of the boot. He gradually returned to full activity at four months but still occasionally has momentary pains with twisting injuries. He chose not to have surgery.

PERONEAL TENDINITIS

- The peroneal tendons lie behind the fibula bone on the outside of the ankle. They run along the outside of the foot to attach in the midfoot.
- Dislocation of the peroneal tendons around the fibula can occur after ankle sprains. Usually, this problem does not resolve unless the supporting ligaments are repaired.
- Deterioration of the tendons can occur and cause swelling along the course of the tendons. This deterioration is sometimes associated with abnormal alignment of the heel and forefoot.

The peroneal muscle and tendons begin in the outer portion of the calf and pass behind the fibula, the bone along the outside of the ankle. The back portion of the fibula at the level of the ankle has a groove in which the peroneal tendon slides. The tendon is contained in this groove by a ligament called the *superior peroneal retinaculum.* The tendons then proceed along the outside of the calcaneus. The peroneus longus tendon wraps around the cuboid bone to attach in the arch and the peroneus brevis tendon attaches onto the base of the fifth metatarsal.

These tendons are important stabilizers of the ankle. Although the lateral ankle ligaments hold the ankle when it "rolls," the peroneal tendons can actually pull the ankle back into proper position.

Sometimes, when the ankle is sprained, the ligaments that restrain the peroneal tendons within the groove behind the fibula can also be injured. It is common for this to be missed when the ankle is examined early after the sprain. The pain of the examination and the significant swelling that usually accompany the ankle sprain can make it difficult to see the subtle signs that the peroneal tendons are dislocated or unstable. If during the recuperation, when you start walking again you hear a popping sound, it may be a sign that the peroneal tendons are popping out of place.

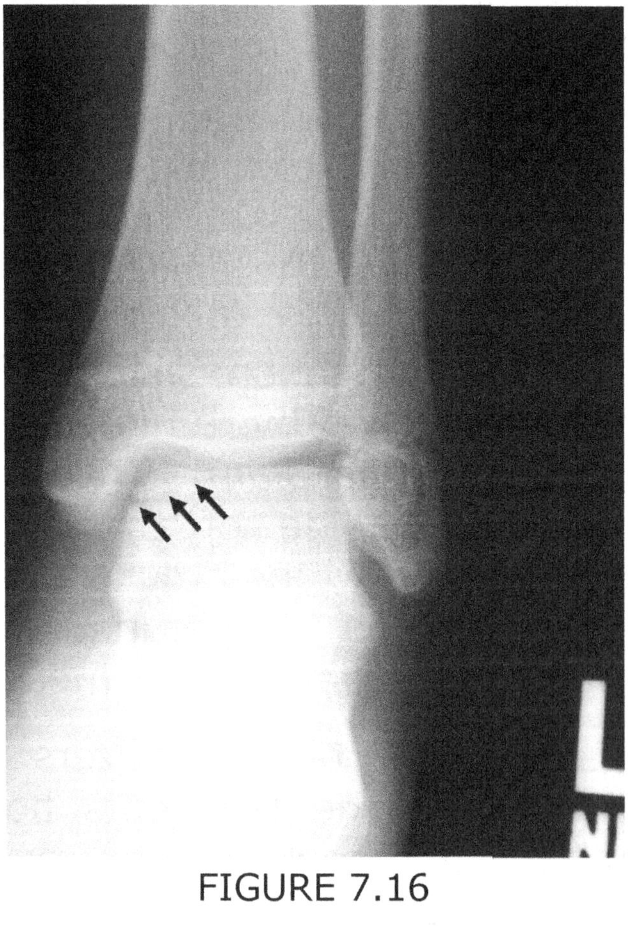

FIGURE 7.16

Once the ligament has been torn, the unstable tendon and damaged ligament rarely heal. Surgery is usually necessary and involves repair of the injured ligament.

Tendonitis of these tendons is also sometimes encountered. Peroneal tendonitis is commonly seen on radiographic tests such as MRIs, but swelling and pain in the back of the ankle can point to painful deterioration of this structure. Often it is associated with abnormal alignment of the ankle. If the ankle is in a significantly abnormal position, the peroneal tendons need to be more active to stabilize the ankle to avoid ankle sprains.

Treatment of peroneal tendonitis usually begins with reducing stress on them through braces or nonuse. Nonsteroidal anti-inflammatory medications such as ibuprofen and naprosyn can reduce pain, but often do little to improve the swelling that accompanies this condition. If several months of these treatments fail to improve the pain, surgery may be necessary.

NOTES

[1] Levy AS, Kelly B, Lintner S, Speer K. Penetration of cryotherapy in treatment after shoulder arthroscopy. *Arthroscopy.* 1997 Aug;13(4):461–464.

[2] Jones MH, Amendola AS. Acute treatment of inversion ankle sprains: Immobilization versus

functional treatment. *Clin Orthop Relat Res.* 2007 Feb;455:169–172.

[3] Dizon JM, Reyes JJ. A systematic review on the effectiveness of external ankle supports in the prevention of inversion ankle sprains among elite and recreational players. *J Sci Med Sport.* 2010 May;13(3):309–17.

[4] Gerber JP, Williams GN, Scoville CR, Arciero RA, Taylor DC. Persistent disability associated with ankle sprains: A prospective examination of an athletic population. *Foot Ankle Int.* 1998 Oct;19(10):653–660.

[5] Bluman EM, Tankson C, Myerson MS, Jeng CL. Detection of orthopaedic foot and ankle implants by security screening devices. *Foot Ankle Int.* 2006 Dec;27(12):1096–1102.

8

The Skin

Celia Ristow and Ginat Mirowski M.D.

- The skin is a complex structure that functions to safeguard our body.
- The skin acts as a barrier; it keeps water in the body and dirt and disease out.
- The skin stores fat for energy and works to control the body temperature.

The skin is composed of three layers. In the epidermis, the most superficial layer, the keratinocytes or skin cells divide and grow and migrate upward toward the surface of the skin, flattening as they are pushed to the surface by the dividing cells beneath them. It is the body's outer protective barrier against the environment. Melanocytes are the pigment-producing cells within the epidermis that absorb ultraviolet light and impart color to the skin. Skin color is determined not by the number of these cells but by the amount and type of pigment within the cells themselves. The dermis is the supportive middle layer. A network of small blood vessels, small lymphatic vessels, and nerves runs through the dermis.

The deepest portion of the skin consists of fat and moderate-size vessels that insulate the body and store energy. This fat also helps to absorb and diffuse pressure and trauma.

The thickness of the skin varies depending on its location and function in the body. The top of the foot is covered by normal-looking skin, while the sole is much thicker. Special structures within the skin include hair, nails, and sweat glands. No hair grows on the soles of the foot, but sweat glands are plentiful. Sweat is sterile and odorless; it's the bacteria on the skin that grow in the sweat that produce the odor-causing chemicals.

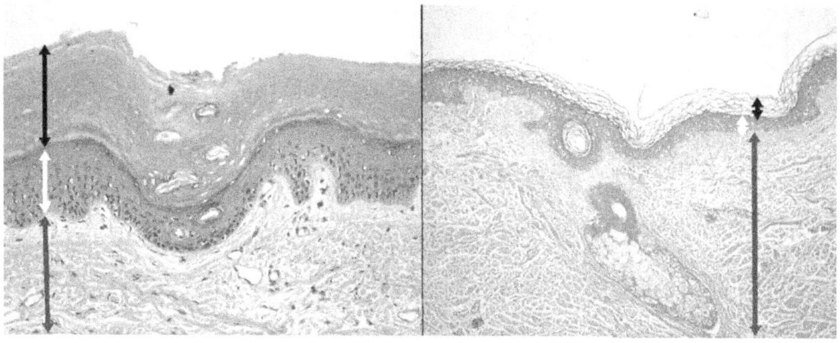

FIGURE 8.1 Microscopic picture of the skin of the sole of foot (left) in comparison to that of the back (right). The dermis (white arrow) and epidermis (black arrow) on the sole of the foot is much thicker than that of the back.

SKIN HEALING

When the top layer alone is damaged, it heals without scarring although there may be some temporary, or rarely, permanent changes in color. When the injury is deeper and the dermis is damaged, the process of healing produces scar. Scarring is permanent because it causes a change in the architecture of the skin. Some individuals tend to form very thick scars called *keloids.* In other people, scars can result in thinning of the skin.

Blisters form when rubbing causes a separation between the dermis and epidermis of the skin. The most common cause of blisters on the feet is ill-fitting shoes, but swelling from trauma or other forms of inflammation can also cause them.

If your skin is kept moist for a prolonged period of time, the keratin within the epidermal layer swells and becomes white and soft. You can see this on your toes and fingers after immersion in water such as after a long bath or swim. Prolonged moisture softens keratin layer so that it peels off, leaving thin, irritated skin.

ATHLETE'S FOOT (TINEA PEDIS)

- Athlete's foot is a fungal infection of the feet.
- It is facilitated by prolonged contact with moisture or contaminated shoe wear.
- The problem is initially treated with topical anti-fungal creams.
- More resistant cases may require oral anti-fungal medications.

Athlete's foot causes a rash that appears as flaking, redness, or "scaly" skin involving the soles of the feet, especially between the toes. Your foot itches and burns. As it gets worse, the skin weeps and sweats. It may be difficult to keep your toes dry. The fungus may cause the web spaces to crack. Bacterial infections may develop when cracking occurs. A bad smell can be the sign of a bacterial infection.

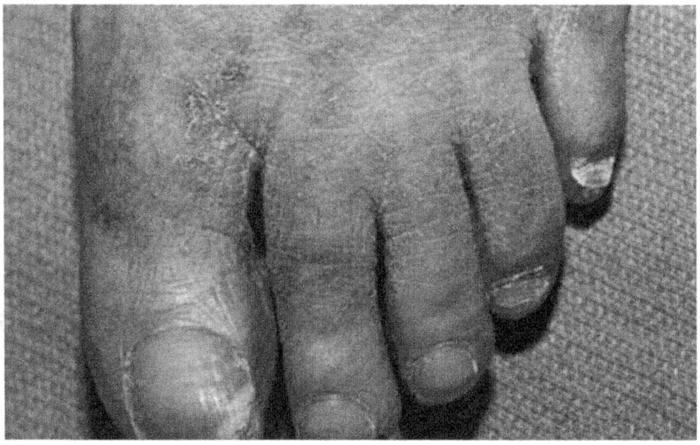

FIGURE 8.2 Cracked skin on the foot in Athlete's foot.

Athlete's foot is caused by a fungal infection. Fungus thrives in warm, moist areas. As the name suggests, athletes are especially prone to contracting the fungus, because their feet are often in wet or sweaty shoes that are not allowed to dry completely in between workouts. Walking barefoot in locker rooms, communal showers, and swimming pools can also cause Athlete's foot. Allergic rashes, psoriasis, or eczema may cause similar appearing rashes.

You can take steps to help prevent this common fungus. Keep your feet clean and dry, as it helps to reduce the presence of fungus and the opportunities for it to grow.

Other ways to prevent and treat Athlete's foot:

- Make sure you dry your feet well after bathing or swimming, using a towel to wipe between the toes.
- Wear sandals or well-ventilated shoes as much as possible.
- Avoid walking barefoot in public showers.
- Use shower shoes to avoid contact with communal floors.
- Use two pairs of shoes that can be alternated, so that sweaty sneakers have a chance to dry completely.
- Wear clean socks and change them at least daily.

Once you have Athlete's foot you will need medication and specific skin care. Try a topical over-the-counter antifungal cream or spray. However, if the condition worsens, you should see a doctor who can prescribe a stronger topical or oral medication.

PLANTAR WARTS (VERRUCA PLANTARIS)

- Plantar warts are caused by a virus, a strain of the human papilloma virus (HPV).
- The virus is highly contagious and usually spread by contact.

- Most warts will go away on their own, but it may take months to years.
- Warts can be painful.
- It is important to treat warts in a way that is both effective and minimizes scarring.

Plantar warts are common skin problems on the bottom of the foot and around the nail folds. Warts often appear on weight-bearing areas such as the ball by foot. Plantar warts are benign skin growths caused by an infection by HPV, which enters the body through small breaks in the skin. When your skin is infected by HPV, it begins to grow more rapidly than normal, resulting in lumps. The virus can spread into the surrounding skin causing a cluster of warts. Unlike warts on the hands, plantar warts appear as thick, hard bumps that can be yellow, gray, or white in color. Small dark specks in the center are often mistaken for "roots" of the wart, but are actually small blood vessels feeding the rapidly growing tissue within the wart. These blood vessels are visible from the surface. The warts can be painful when standing or walking, much as a pebble would be if it were lodged in one's shoe.

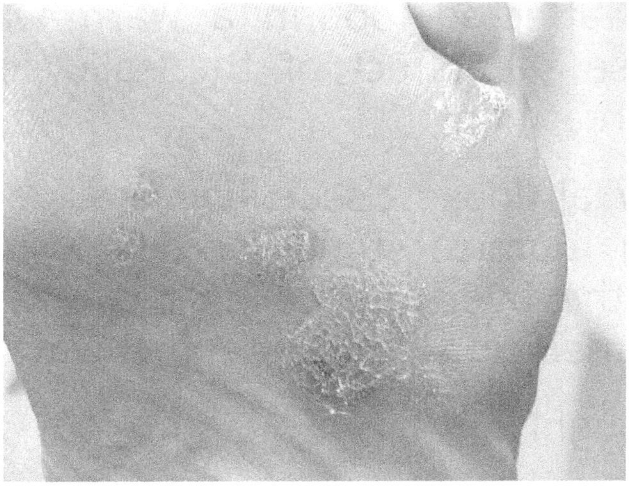

FIGURE 8.3 Multiple warts on the weight-bearing surface of the foot.

If you have a plantar wart and you cut it, small points of bleeding would be seen within the lesion. Corns have a firm smooth rounded surface when pared.

Most warts will eventually go away without treatment. Unfortunately, this may take months to years and, in the mean time, they may spread to other parts of the skin or to other people, so it is best to treat them.

Most nonprescription wart medications can work, but may be too weak to be effective. Salicylic acid is available as a liquid, gel, ointment, or impregnated into a pad. Some OTC brand names include Dr. Scholl's Wart Remover®, Compound W®, Freezone®, and Wart-Off®. Be careful when applying! Other advice:

- Soak the affected foot in a warm-water footbath to increase the effect of the salicylic acid before starting treatment.
- Rub away all loose tissue using a small nailbrush, washcloth, pumice stone, or emery board. File as much of the overlying callus tissue as possible to help the medicine penetrate the wart properly.
- Dry thoroughly.
- Remember to closely follow the directions on the individual product to limit the painful side effect of the acid on healthy skin tissue.
- Treat the lesion nightly. Clean in the morning. Reapply for up to two months before giving up.

Another treatment is to use duct tape. Although this treatment seems effective, it is unknown how it works. You apply duct tape on the wart anywhere from seven days to two months. After each week, look to see how much of the wart remains. You may gently file the top of the wart by rubbing with a pumice stone or nail file to remove off any excess skin.

A fast-drying solution of 17% salicylic acid and 17% lactic acid (for example, Duofilm® or DermaTech Wart Treatment®) is another effective treatment. This solution should be applied after showering and permitted to air-dry. Cover it with waterproof tape until the next shower or bath. Once a week pare or file any excess skin to further enhance the treatment.

If these treatments do not work and the warts are painful, or the warts continue to grow or multiply, it is best to seek treatment from your doctor.

Children are likely to tolerate only the less painful treatments, but this may mean a slower response. Cantharidine, a painless blistering solution that comes from the blister beetle, is applied in the office. The treated area is covered by a dressing that should be removed in four to eight hours. The area should be washed and dried. If stinging or burning occurs, wash it sooner. Soon the skin will swell and become red. A blister is likely to form. The blister may be bloody and appear blue or it may be clear. To relieve the pressure of the blister, a clean pin can be used to pierce the blister roof. Every effort should be made to leave the blister roof intact to cover the affected area. This will minimize the possibility of infection.

Other treatment includes:

- Cryotherapy or freezing warts with liquid nitrogen. At a temperature of −90°C, liquid nitrogen causes the death of the both infected and normal tissues. The HPV itself is not killed. The longer the liquid nitrogen is applied to the skin, the larger and deeper the skin will freeze. To kill the infected skin, two passes with liquid nitrogen is generally needed. At the junction of the live and dead cells a blister forms. When the blister roof is removed, many of the infected cells are removed and thus the viral burden is reduced. Despite being imprecise, liquid nitrogen therapy is a highly successful treatment regimen. If used properly, the risk of scarring is small.

- Efudex (5-fluorouracil) is a chemotherapeutic agent that destroys growing skin cells and is sometimes used topically to treat warts.
- CO_2 laser treatment is a very effective and quick procedure compared to other approaches. It is performed in the physician's office or in the operating room. It is expensive and may result in some scarring.
- Surgical desiccation is a more destructive method of treatment. The area must be anesthetized by injecting a local anesthetic. Then, the physician uses an electrical or ultrasonic device to destroy the wart, the remainder of which is removed with a curette. This technique commonly causes scar formation.

CALLUSES AND CORNS

- A callus is a thickening of the skin that has formed in response to a concentration of pressure. Usually calluses are not painful.
- Corns are focal calluses on the feet, usually one to six millimeters in diameter, that have grown into the skin. They are painful because the hard skin core displaces the normal tissue away from a bony prominence.

- Treatment involves paring the hard corn on the bottom of the foot down intermittently. Other methods of pressure relief depend on the location of the lesion.
- Surgical treatment is occasionally necessary and relief is possible through removal of the bony prominence.

When your skin experiences pressure excessively or for long periods of time, the skin cells start to reproduce faster. This causes the skin to thicken. It gives rise to the calluses that we see on our hands when we work harder than we are accustomed. Usually these calluses are not painful. Calluses on your feet are also usually not painful although they tend to occur in areas where pressure is concentrated.

Calluses that would normally peel off when they get thick in other parts of the body, such as the hands, will grow into the skin in the feet. This callus tissue will displace the other important tissues on the bottom of the foot, such as the protective fat, until the callus is nearly rubbing directly on the underlying bones and ligaments. This is called a *corn.*

Corns usually occur when a relatively small edge or portion of the bone presses against another bone, the shoe, or the floor, trapping the skin in between. The skin growth is much more localized and the pressures much greater leading to growth into the foot. A shift in the position of the bones or thinning of the skin such as can occur with aging can expose the previously well-protected bone edge to pressure, resulting in a corn.

Corns come in two varieties, soft and hard. A soft corn forms in moist areas such as between the toes, where the bones pinch the skin in between them. The most common area for a soft corn is deep in the web space between the fourth and fifth toes, although they can occur in between any toes.

Hard corns form in dry environments where the bone and a point of pressure outside of the foot (like the floor or the shoe) pinch the skin. Common places for hard corns are on the sides of the toes especially along the top and outside of the fifth toe, at the tips of the toes and sides of the toenails and under the balls of your foot. Hard corns are usually one to six millimeters in diameter.

Corns can be quite painful, especially when the corn grows deep into the skin. It can feel like a rock is taped to the skin. Ulcers, resulting from corns, can cause deep infections that occasionally lead to abscesses and even to amputation. Differentiating corns and calluses from other dermatological conditions is mostly a matter of experience. Warts are often confused with corns. As opposed to a corn that is caused by pressure, a wart is a viral infection. Warts are not particularly localized to areas of high pressure although they may occur there. Warts are usually less painful than corns. Actual cancers and other tumors are rare, but a dermatologist should evaluate unusual growths.

The most important part of treating corns is to reduce the pressure near and around the corn. Paring down or trimming the lesion with a scalpel or planer will lessen the pressure on the skin. It's a little like removing a rock from your shoe. The effect on the pain is usually remarkable. Often the initial paring cannot remove the entire lesion. Over the days following the paring, the lesion will move toward the surface, allowing more of the corn to be removed. A pumice stone or Pedi-egg® can also be used to remove it, but more time is necessary to completely treat it. Patience and repeated paring can eliminate the lesion over time, but regular maintenance is usually necessary. A wart-removal product containing salicylic acid can help soften the lesion, making it easier to pare.

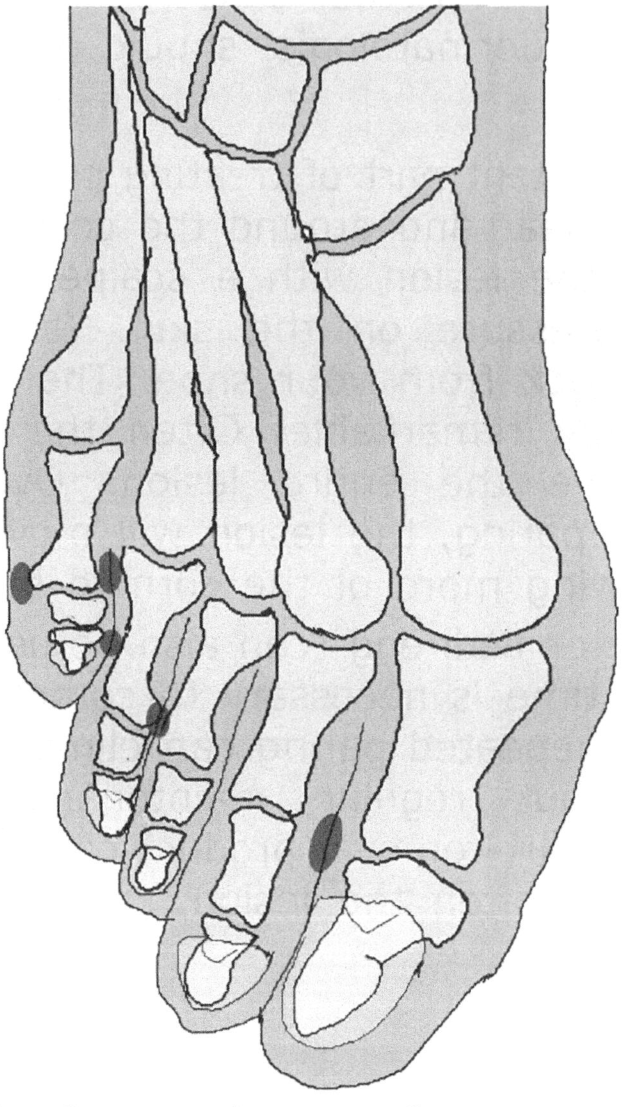

FIGURE 8.4 Common locations for interdigital corns.

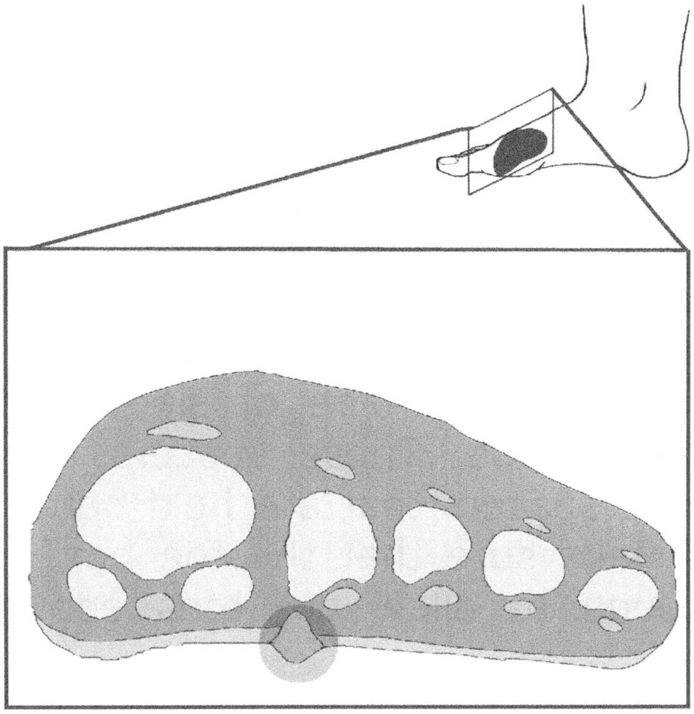

FIGURE 8.5 Cross-section of the ball of the foot showing the anatomy and a common site for a plantar hard corn.

Growth of a corn can also be slowed or stopped by removing the pressure from the area. Adhesive felt doughnuts used around the lesion can help disperse pressure. Custom inserts can be molded to increase the pressure adjacent to the callus or corn especially around the metatarsal heads in the ball of the foot. A depression can be removed from the insert below the lesion to decrease the pressure. However, custom inserts can be expensive and few insurances cover them. Corns along the outside of the foot and over the top of toe deformities can be improved by choosing shoes with a soft upper or by stretching the shoes in the area of the corn to reduce pressure from the shoes. This can be done at a shoe repair store or a pedorthotist shop.

Soft corns between the toes can be removed using toe spacers. Spreading the toes can keep the bones that are pressing against one another apart. There is an assortment of spacers made from silicone, or foam rubber that can be wedged between the toes. Some spacers come in the shape of sleeves that can be places around a toe. These spacers may shift less than the loose spacers that are held between the toes by friction. Make sure that the toe box of your shoe is wide enough to allow the toes enough room to spread.

In some cases, especially with soft corns, the inflammation around the corn can become so intense that an ulcer or infection occurs. Antibiotics may be necessary along with a medical cleaning of the wound. In resistant cases, the prominent parts of the bones can be surgically removed usually with predictable success.

MAX'S STORY

Max had developed increasing discomfort over the past two months. He worked as an engineer for a pharmaceutical company. He had pain and swelling in between his fourth and fifth toes that kept increasing. There was redness along the top of the skin of the fourth web and soft moist skin growth in the web along the inside of the fifth toe.

Using a small scalpel in the office a doctor removed Max's corn. This has to be done carefully, by a professional, as the skin around the corn may inadvertently be entered and begin to bleed. Max got a spacer to wear between the fourth and fifth toe. Max was told to clean the area of any loose skin after showers.

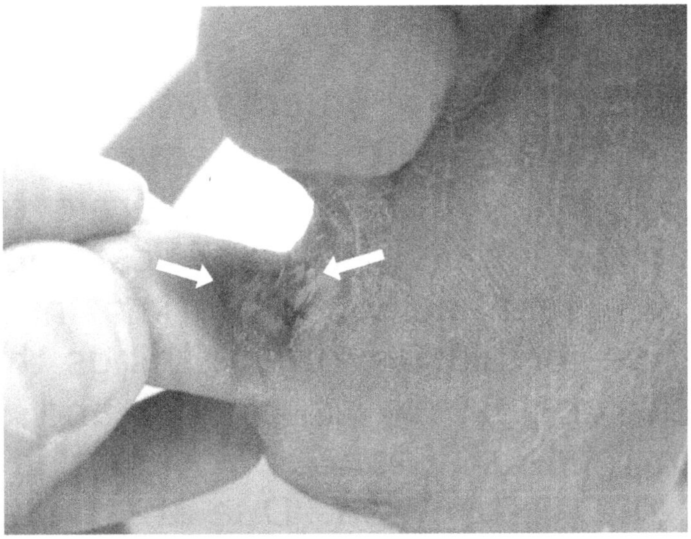

FIGURE 8.6 A corn in the fourth web space. These calluses can cause considerable pain and are not obvious unless carefully examined.

CONTACT DERMATITIS OR ALLERGIC SKIN RASH

- Contact dermatitis is an inflammatory reaction that occurs when the skin comes in contact with a substance to which it is sensitive.

- Sensitivity may be caused by an allergic or an irritant reaction.

- The reaction may appear suddenly or occur very slowly.
- Typically, sudden reactions appear as blisters while slow reaction appears scaly. Both reactions are itchy.
- The appearance and location help the doctor to identify likely causes.

Contact dermatitis is an inflammation of the skin. It is caused by contact with a chemical irritant or an allergen, anything you may be allergic to. It varies from person to person. However, common allergens that affect the feet include materials in shoes, such as rubber, glue, or plastic, or are things that are used to clean clothing such as soaps and detergents. Contact with these substances in sensitive people can result in a red, itchy rash. Due to the thickness of the soles, the rash on your foot is usually on the top. The rash may blister and look burned.

A doctor can help identify the causes and possible treatments. The pattern of a rash can often give important clues to narrow the cause of contact dermatitis. A geometric pattern (such as the lines of a flip-flop or the square of a sneaker tongue) or sparing of the web spaces of the toes suggests that the irritant may be a shoe wear material.

To try to make a more informed diagnosis and recommendation, a dermatologist can perform a patch test. A patch test is a test that places samples of 20 or more different common allergens on the skin. The allergens are removed and the skin evaluated at 48 and 72 hours. When a positive result is obtained identification of the specific substance is possible. Other conditions that may be confused with contact dermatitis include fungal rashes such as Athlete's foot or autoimmune rashes such as psoriasis.

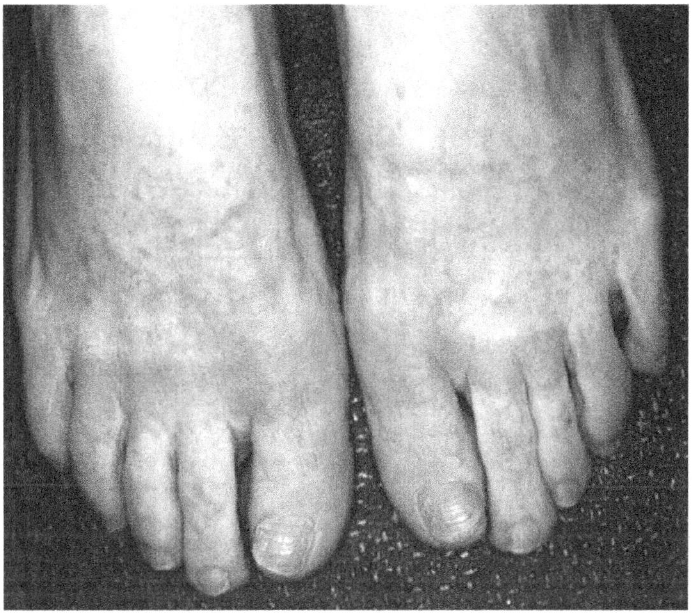

FIGURE 8.7 Contact dermatitis. Note the geographic pattern with sparing of the web spaces.

The most important point is to avoid contact with the irritant. For some people, this means wearing special types of shoes or socks that are constructed with materials that do not contain common irritants. Occasionally, anti-inflammatory creams or medications are necessary to reduce the symptoms.

FISSURING

Fissures are cracks in the skin of the foot, caused by dry or overly moist skin, a fungal infection, or uneven distribution of weight across the foot. The cracks can become deep if they are untreated and begin to bleed and become painful. This can eventually become infected.

Prevention or at-home treatment of small fissures involves regulating the moisture levels of your feet; dry skin causes cracks in thick callused skin, while moist skin can be a breeding ground for bacteria or fungi that can also produce fissures. The healthiest foot is neither too moist nor too dry. Overly dry skin can be helped by moisturizing daily, especially after showering, concentrating on the most dry portions of the foot (typically the heel). Avoid using a pumice stone or walking barefoot. If your feet are sweaty and moist, dry them thoroughly after showering and do not apply moisturizers. Cotton in socks and shoes helps moisture evaporate easier than synthetic materials do.

If fissures in your feet persist or enlarge, it is important to seek medical attention. A doctor can prescribe appropriate medications including topical steroids and antibiotics, make recommendations regarding moisturizer, special socks, callus removal (calluses, or thick skin, exacerbate the problem of fissuring), or even suggest an adhesive that holds cracks together, helping them to heal as well as providing a protective barrier that seals in moisture and seals out dry air. Also, a consistent moisturizing and exfoliating routine can prevent fissuring to start.

SKIN PROBLEMS IN DIABETES

People afflicted with diabetes must take special care of and be especially vigilant about caring for their feet. Diabetes affects both the circulatory and nervous system, making the skin susceptible to injury. Wounds or ulcers are common in people with diabetes. When you have diabetes, poorly fitting shoes or the breakdown of a callus can cause ulcers. Ulcers can become infected, creating an even more serious condition, sepsis. Even if they are painless, ulcers should be brought to medical attention immediately. Circulatory problems can increase the risk for poor healing.

Ways to Keep Feet Healthy

- Develop a habit of performing a visual inspection of the feet every morning or before getting into bed every night.
- Check for changes in color.
- Look for breaks in the skin or other abnormalities.
- Early identification and treating a problem can help before it becomes serious.

- Keep the skin of the feet moist by applying lotion after bathing (avoiding the webs between the toes and applying a thick cream to your feet just before bedtime. Make this a ritual to be performed in conjunction with the skin check).
- Sleep in socks to seal in the moisture.
- Talk to your doctor about what steps you can and should take to ensure that you have adequate blood flow to your feet.
- Talk to your doctor if you sense something out of the ordinary—even if it doesn't seem like a big deal.

PSORIASIS

- Psoriasis is an extremely common condition that can affect the feet as well as other parts of the body.
- Psoriasis commonly causes inflammation of joints.
- Psoriasis causes the skin to grow very quickly, forming a characteristic whitish or silvery scale.
- One third of people with psoriasis have family members who also have the condition.

Psoriasis is an itchy inflammatory skin condition that affects people of all ages. The rash starts out gradually but it rarely disappears completely. The cause of this condition is unknown but it may be initiated by infection, trauma, or stress. Drugs such as lithium and beta-blockers can aggravate psoriasis.

Psoriasis most commonly involves your scalp, elbows, hands, feet, and lower back. Although the appearance of psoriasis is usually characteristic of the disease, only a biopsy can differentiate psoriasis from similar skin conditions.

Use moisturizers or emollients for psoriasis. They create a barrier to prevent water loss from evaporation. Lukewarm baths followed by an appropriate emollient improve skin hydration. Thicker, greasier emollients are more effective than creams or lotions. Cleansers should be limited to mild bar soaps (i.e., Dove® or Basis®) or soapless cleansers (i.e., Cetaphil® or Aquanil®). Bubble baths and body gels should be avoided.

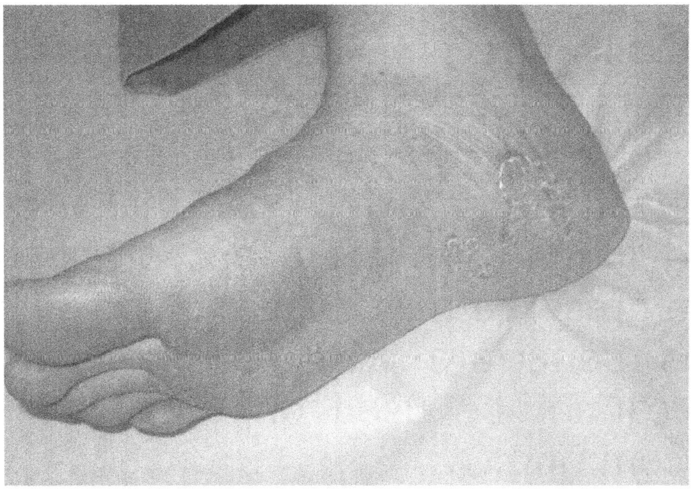

FIGURE 8.8 Psoriasis on the heel.

Skin in people affected by psoriasis is prone to irritation. Exposure to irritating substances, infectious agents, and/or environmental or emotional factors results in the worsening of itching and the psoriasis rash. Some people believe that sweating and overheating may aggravate psoriasis. Wearing natural fabrics such as cotton or silk is recommended. Scented detergents, fabric softeners, and other scented products should be avoided. Vacuuming living areas frequently, removing or cleaning carpets regularly, and eliminating pets may prevent exposure to dust mites, which is suspected to aggravate psoriasis. Psychotherapy, including behavior modification and stress reduction, can also help reduce the itching of psoriasis.

Topical corticosteroids are used in psoriasis treatment. Steroids reduce inflammation. They are available in many varieties (ointments, creams, lotions, and gels) appropriate for the specific body site. Ointments penetrate more effectively and are more potent than creams or lotions. However, greasy ointments may block the sweat glands, which can make itching worse. Creams and lotions are more acceptable on the skin but contain preservatives that can be allergenic. Gel preparations penetrate well and help to dry moist areas, but cannot be used on open skin or cuts as burning is common.

Long-term treatment with all corticosteroids can result in stretch marks and thinning of the skin. Intermittent usage and using the least potent steroid that effectively controls the psoriasis is the best way to minimize these side effects.

Medications that are derived from vitamin D, such as calcipotriene (Dovonex®) and calcitriol (Rocaltrol®), help slow the growth of skin and are highly effective for mild to moderate psoriasis. Anthralin (Drithocreme®) helps to normalize DNA activity of skin in patients with psoriasis. Side effects include skin irritation and staining of skin, clothing, and beddings. Tazarotene (Tazorac®) is a vitamin A derivative that also normalizes skin cell reproduction and decreases inflammation. Salicylic acid promotes sloughing of excess cells, and results in reduction of scale and smoother skin. Coal tar is messy but very effective in treating psoriasis. It reduces scale itching and inflammation, but how it works is still unknown.

Exposure of the skin to ultraviolet light reduces inflammation and itching. Treatments are given two to three times per week. The most common side effects are redness and pain at exposed sites, similar to sunburn. Both melanoma and nonmelanoma skin cancers may develop with long-term treatment.

Particularly difficult psoriasis or flares of otherwise well-controlled disease may require oral medications for management. Oral corticosteroids also control itching and inflammation. However, discontinuation often leads to a flare of the symptoms. Chronic use is not recommended due to serious adverse effects such as cutaneous and systemic infections, glaucoma, cataracts, osteoporosis, and bone and joint damage.

Retinoids are chemicals that are related to vitamin A that can control psoriasis. Cyclosporine (Neoral®, Gengraf®, Sandimmune®) suppresses immune cells activity. The side effects of cyclosporine include hypertension, anemia, as well as kidney or liver damage. Laboratory tests should be closely monitored when taking this medication. Other medications that suppress the immune system include recombinant gamma interferon (Actimmune®), etanercept (Infliximab®), and efalizumab (Raptiva®), methotrexate (Trexall®, Rheumatrex®), azathioprine (Imuran®), and mycophenolate mofetil (CellCept®). These medications also have serious side effects that need to be closely monitored.

SKIN CANCER

Skin cancer can be found on the feet as well as parts that get even more exposure to the sun such as your face and hands. There are three types of common skin cancer—malignant melanoma, squamous cell carcinoma, and basal cell carcinoma. With the introduction of the AIDS virus we started seeing more prevelant Kaposi's sarcoma as well.

Malignant Melanoma

Melanomas are skin cancers that arise from melanocytes, the pigment cells within the skin. Although melanomas may commonly originate from birthmarks or moles, they can occur anywhere such as under the nails, and on the sole of the foot.

Skin lesions that bleed, itch, grow, or ulcerate are suspicious for melanoma, but these are late signs. For pigmented lesions, a useful mnemonic to remember the warning signs of melanoma is ABCDE (asymmetry, border, color, diameter, and evolving). Warning signs of melanoma include:

- **A** symmetry, where one half of the mole is unlike the other half.
- **B** order irregularity, where the border appears scalloped, blurry, or poorly defined.
- **C** olor variation from one area to another, where one lesion will contain multiple shades of tan, brown, black, and sometimes even white, red, or blue.
- **D** iameter greater than 6mm (the size of a pencil eraser). However, size is the least predictive of these screening guidelines, since skin cancers may initially be very small in size, so see your doctor as soon as possible to evaluate a suspicious lesion.

- **E** volving, a mole or skin lesion that looks different from the rest or is changing in size, shape, or color.

The major risk factor for malignant melanoma is exposure to the sun, which emits harmful ultraviolet (UV) rays. These UV waves are a form of radiation that, with enough exposure, can cause mutations within cells that lead to cancer. However, on the feet, the melanoma risk is identical in light- and darkly complected individuals and so UV exposure may not be as significant a cause on the foot as in other parts of the body.

Melanoma is diagnosed by skin biopsy and subsequent microscopic evaluation by a pathologist. Early stage melanoma can be treated with high success rates. Thus, early detection of the melanoma is critical.

Treatment of early stage, nonmetastasized melanoma is done by surgical excision. However, if not detected early, a malignant melanoma can grow and spread locally and metastasize to internal organs, such as the brain and bones. Once the tumor has spread (metastasized), the success rate of treatment is much lower.

Squamous Cell Carcinoma

Actinic keratoses, a premalignant lesion, can be a precursor to squamous cell carcinoma. Actinic keratoses are more commonly found on men than women and are usually found on sun-exposed areas of the body including the legs. Actinic keratoses appear as red, scaly, and lumpy. They are rare on the feet. Approximately 5% of actinic keratoses progress to squamous cell carcinomas, so actinic keratoses should be treated.

Although squamous cell carcinomas usually develop on sun-exposed areas, it is possible to develop squamous cell carcinomas on areas that are not exposed to the sun. This is particularly true around when tumors arise around the toenails. Other sites that have a higher risk of squamous cell carcinoma include long-standing leg ulcers, radiation therapy sites, and prior burn sites.

Basal Cell Carcinoma

Like other skin cancers, basal cell carcinomas predominantly occur on sun-exposed areas. Basal cell carcinoma may appear to be nodules or ulcers. Although basal cell carcinoma may be locally invasive and destructive to surrounding tissue, the basal cell cancer rarely spreads to other areas. Common locations for basal cell carcinoma include the skin of the head and neck, including the eyes, the ears, and the nose, and other sun-exposed skin. The legs are only rarely affected, but should be suspected in nonhealing ulcers. A biopsy is needed for diagnosis. Treatment of basal cell cancers is usually surgical.

Some types of very superficial skin cancers can be treated using topical chemotherapeutic medicines.

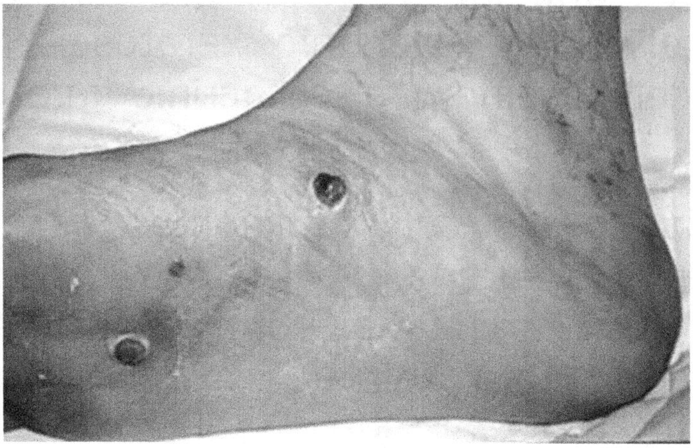

FIGURE 8.9 Multiple Kaposi's sarcoma on the plantar aspect of the foot.

Kaposi's Sarcoma

Kaposi's sarcoma is a neoplasm that was extremely uncommon in the United States before the onset of the AIDS epidemic. It is the most common malignancy in patients who are HIV positive. Prior to the introduction of effective medications for AIDS, it occurred in nearly 15% of patients with AIDS.

Kaposi's sarcoma commonly affects the soles, top of the feet, and around the toenails. It is brown, bluish, purple, or red. The cancers are flat lesions that may become nodular, ulcerate, and bleed over time. A biopsy will definitively identify it.

Although Kaposi's sarcoma may not seem immediately serious because it is initially confined to the bottoms of the feet, it may be aggressive. Spreading to the lungs and other internal organs can cause death. Chemotherapy is the most effective method of treatment. Treating the underlying immune deficiency disease is also critically important.

TOENAILS

Toenails are important parts of the tips of the toes that protect them from trauma. The nail consists of four different anatomic parts—the nail itself (nail plate), the nail bed or sterile matrix, the root or germinal matrix, and the nail fold. The nail plate is firmly attached to the nail bed. Nails are essentially modified hairs and are composed of compact, horny material that originates from the germinal matrix or root of the nail. Nails grow continuously throughout life and are not shed unless they are injured because of mechanical trauma. Individual nails grow at different rates with toenails growing at a significantly slower rate than fingernails.

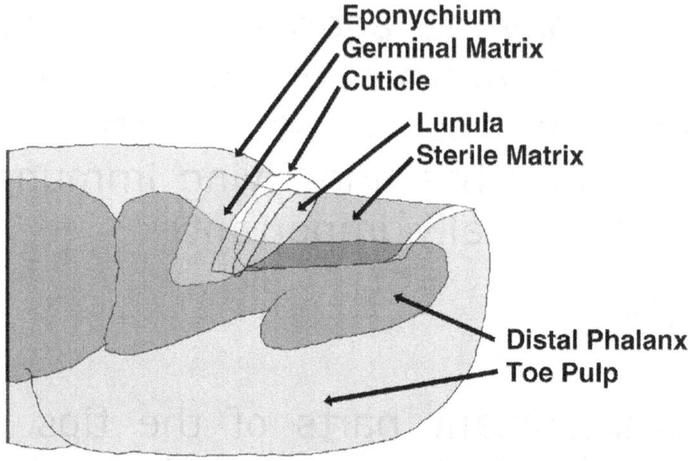

FIGURE 8.10 Parts of a toenail.

INGROWN TOENAILS

An ingrown toenail is an infection that develops when the toenail begins to grow into the skin surrounding it.

- Tenderness, swelling, and drainage occur around the outer or inner end of the nail.

- This can be caused by improper toenail care, but the shape of the nail can predispose the nail to problems.

- Treatment centers around relieving pressure on the skin. Often the nail must be anesthetized to ensure adequate removal.

Ingrown toenails can cause a nagging and unrelenting pain around the nail. An ingrown toenail causes swelling and redness of the nail fold. As time progresses, the skin around the nail can begin to drain and ulcerate. Usually, it is impossible or extremely painful to see the corner of the toenail.

An ingrown toenail occurs when the edge of the toenail begins to dig into the nail fold. As the skin begins to swell around the prominent nail, the nail digs into the skin more, causing more inflammation and infection. This vicious cycle results in rapidly progressive pain.

Many factors can predispose the development of an ingrown toenail. If the nail is abnormally wide or curved or the nail fold is particularly deep, it is more likely that an ingrown toenail will occur. Most of these risk factors are present from childhood. An ingrown toenail can even happen in infancy.

Sometimes, a shoe presses against the corner of the nail or another toe presses against the nail fold and can cause an ingrown toenail. It commonly develops as a result of improper nail care. Frequently, in the process of trimming the nail, the nail is not cut to the edge. If the nail is ripped in the process of removing the end, a fragment will be left attached to the nail and this will begin the inflammation.

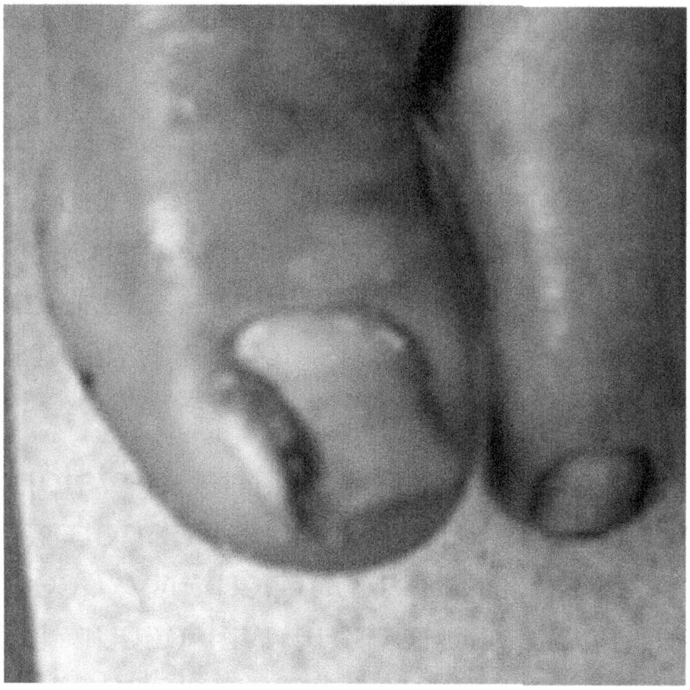

FIGURE 8.11 Inflammation and wound formation in an ingrown toenail. The inside edge of the nail is impacted into the surrounding skin.

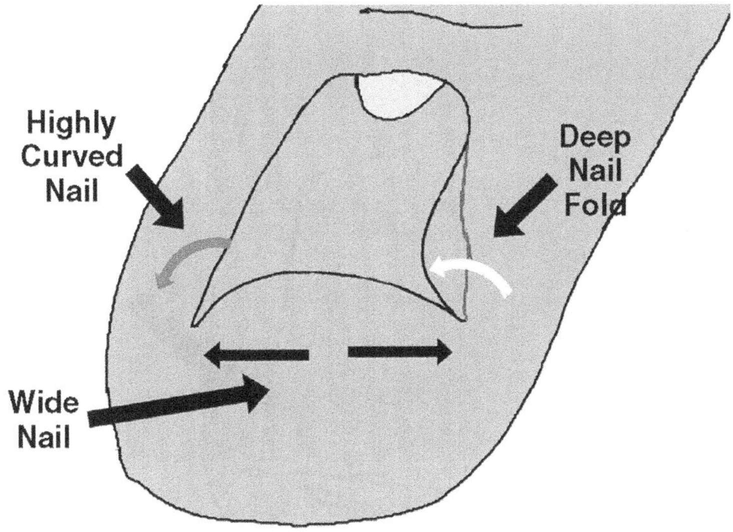

FIGURE 8.12 Factors predisposing a toenail to infection include wide toenail width, a deep fleshy nail fold, and a highly curved toenail.

Prevention revolves around proper nail care. When trimming the toenail, do not cut what you can't see. Ensure that the nail trimmer cuts past the edge of the nail. Gently round the corners of the nail, ensuring that the cuts do not end near the edge of the nail but past the edge.

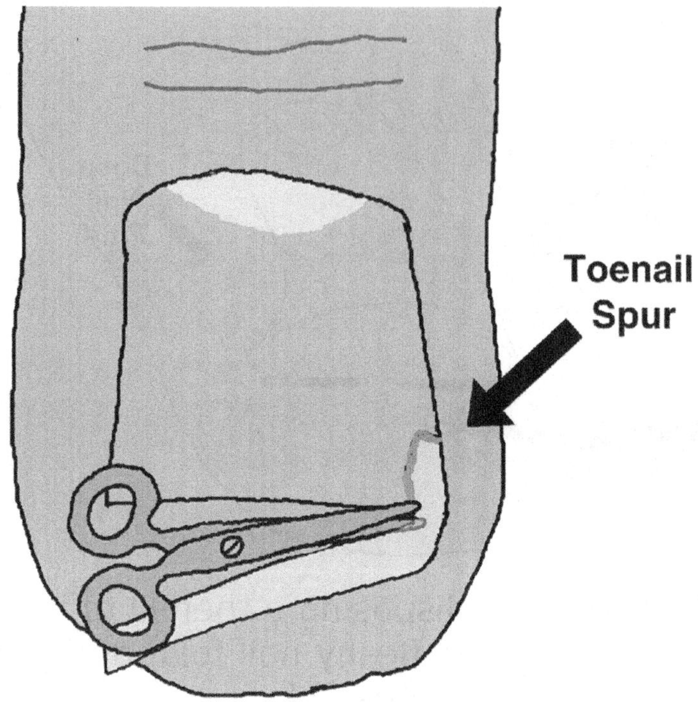

FIGURE 8.13 The inciting event in the development of an ingrown toenail is often improper nail care.

It is usually painful and rarely successful to treat an ingrown toenail on your own. If the swelling and inflammation is significant, the nail corner must be cut back significantly. This usually requires a local anesthesia. Destroying a portion of the root of the nail by either chemical or surgical means so that the nail no longer grows against the nail fold should adequately treat recurrent ingrown toenails.

Fungal Infection of the Toenails

Onchyomycosis is a fungal infection of the matrix of the nail. Even though the toenail material itself is thickened and discolored, this is a symptom of an infection deep in the root of the nail. Removal of the nail does not cure the problem. While fungal infections of the toenail are unsightly, they don't lead to serious problems.

Fungal infections of the nail are not contagious. They become more common with advancing age. Medical conditions such as diabetes and AIDS increase the chance of developing these fungal infections, but many people without these risk factors develop them. Fungal infections of the nail should be diagnosed by a doctor and differentiated from trauma, age-related changes, lichen planus, and psoriasis.

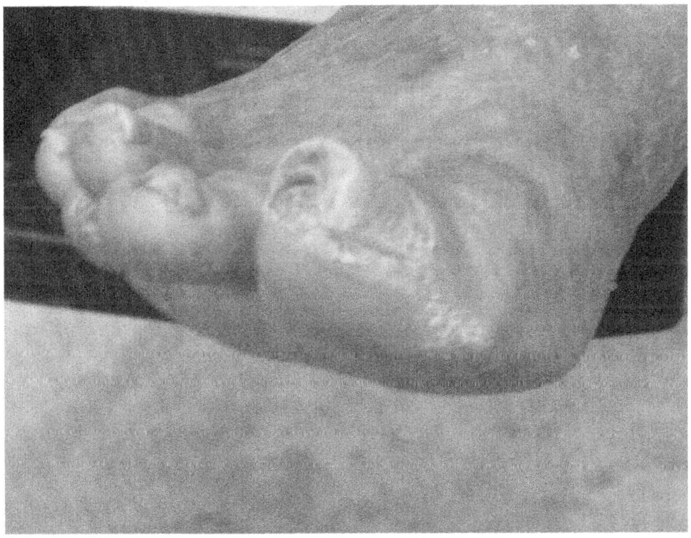

FIGURE 8.14 Thickened, deformed toenails as a result of fungal infection.

Not all cases of fungal infection of the toenail need to be treated. For many, it is a cosmetic condition that, although embarrassing, is unlikely to cause serious problems. Common home remedies include soaking the nails in peroxide, Listerine, over-the-counter fungal creams, and bleach. It is doubtful that these substances penetrate into the nail enough to be effective at the site of the problem. Topical application of medication is unlikely to affect the fungal infection deep within the nail root or matrix. Penlac Nail Lacquer® is a prescription medication that is applied to the nail and dries as a hard layer. This treatment is somewhat effective, but requires application for three months. The most effective medications are oral anti-fungals including itraconazole (Sporanox®) and terbinafine (Lamisil®). Although these medications usually have few side effects, laboratory tests should be monitored to ensure that the medication is not affecting the liver. These medications must be taken for a prolonged period. You will see the nail get better first at the root, as it grows in. It may take nearly a year for a complete recovery of your nail.

9

From Athletes' to Kids' Feet to Unusual Conditions

ATHLETES

- Athletic ambitions in a person with an injury can affect the choice of treatment.
- Although athletes can suffer any injury, certain stress injuries seem to be characteristic of athletic activity and the special stress that athletes put on their feet.
- The older athlete can pursue challenging and rewarding athletic goals, but training errors are not tolerated as well as in the younger athlete.
- Avoiding training errors centers on setting reasonable goals, broadening the types of training, and the methods of training to include balance, aerobics, flexibility, and strengthening of all areas of the body.

Athletic injuries are different than other injuries because they occur in an athlete. The needs of the athlete are different than the needs of the nonathlete. Athletes strive to make their body perform close to its maximum ability. Many times athletes' ambitions impose time-critical goals in the recovery. Although these goals certainly should take a back seat to the overall health of the athlete, they are still important to consider and should be respected.

Athletic injuries may look much like any other injury and may occur outside of athletic training. The athletic injury is a physical obstacle separating athletes from their performance. To some extent, this changes certain decisions that are made during treatment. It may drive treatment, when there is a proven advantage, toward more aggressive approaches that may accelerate a return to activity and eventually to play. However, this must be balanced with other potentially conflicting goals in the athlete's life because the athlete may need to work to support him- or herself, and may also be a husband, wife, father, mother, or student.

It may also mean there are many other people besides the athlete who may have a stake in the outcome of the injury. Among these people are coaches, teammates, possibly fans, and parents. All of these people may potentially have some input in treatment decisions. Although the desires of these parties should be considered, the interests and long-term well-being of the athlete is paramount in the decision-making process.

Stress Fracture

Stress injuries are particular to athletes. In any stress fracture, the key problem is that the bone is experiencing more force than it can repair on a daily basis. In order to identify the factors that caused it, look at the athlete's activity, how quickly it was taken on, and any mechanical abnormalities in the foot. Athletes are highly motivated and driven people. There is often a tendency to accelerate training beyond what is prudent. A key to preventing stress injuries and to returning to athletic participation after injury is a gradual progression of activity over a period of months from the current activity level to the goal activity level.

It is important to look for other contributing medical problems. These are rare, but can be a readily treatable part of the problem. One specific problem is in the female runner. Up to 20% to 30% of avid female runners can train so hard as to minimize their body fat percentage below a normal, functional level. When this occurs, the athlete can stop normal menstruation. Without the normal cycle of hormones that their body is exposed to, the bone can lose its density and become abnormally fragile. Although the solution to this is not to gain excessive weight or to discontinue running, dietary evaluation and adjustment of the training schedule may do much to alleviate this problem.

The navicular bone seems to be prone to stress injury in athletes. It lies at the top of the arch. When viewed from the side, it would lie directly below the front of the shin. The weight and stress from the first, second, and third metatarsals and their respective cuneiforms eventually are transferred to the body through a common joint with the navicular bone. Because the flexibility of bones that lead to the first, second, and third toes varies, the navicular bone can twist excessively, eventually overwhelming its limited potential for healing.

Navicular stress injuries can be devastating injuries. In some cases, the navicular bone can split and crush essentially ruining the critical joints in the midfoot. It must be seriously approached and monitored. Early surgery can be a reasonable solution to avoid prolonged recuperation from this injury.

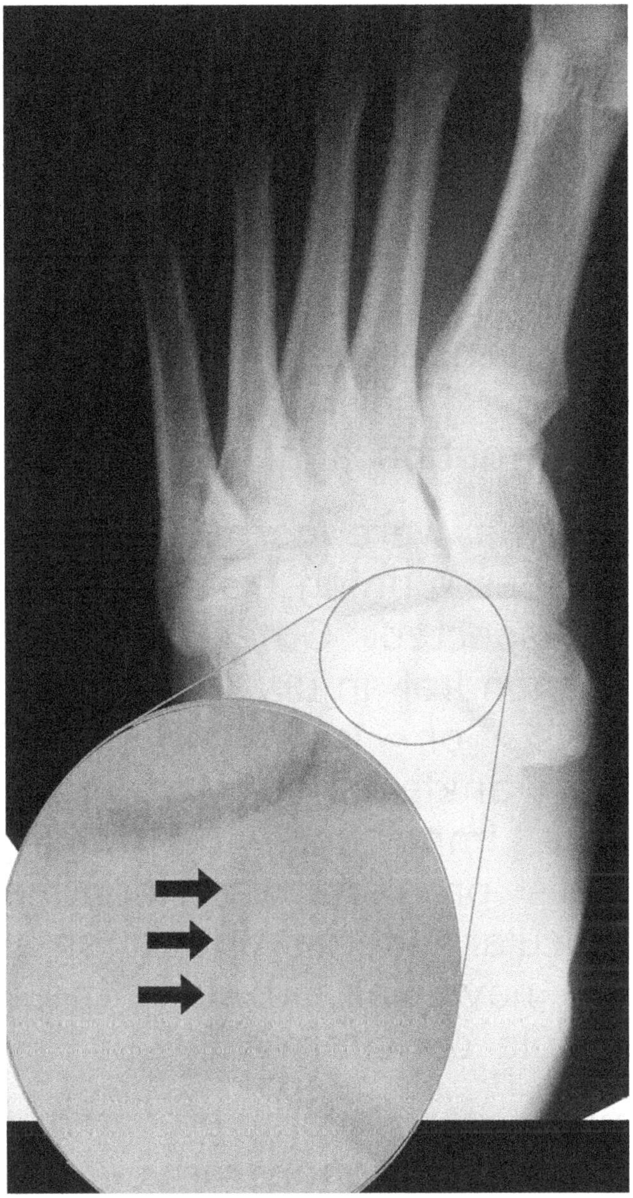

FIGURE 9.1 Navicular stress injuries can be subtle on x-ray, but must be treated aggressively to avoid major damage to the foot.

Emily's Story

Emily is an avid runner who completed her third marathon this year. She noticed after the marathon some ankle pain immediately that had improved in the weeks following the marathon when she took a slight break. However, she was beginning to ramp up her mileage now in preparation for another marathon in the spring and the ankle pain was getting worse.

Emily was thin and fit, as you would expect in an avid runner. Her tenderness was fairly specific to the inside of her foot, just in front of her ankle, while she still had full motion and her ankle was aligned.

Emily's radiographs were normal. Given the location of her pain and her running history, a navicular stress fracture was suspected. Other potential possibilities included osteochondral injury of the talus, posterior tibial tendonitis, or joint inflammation of the talonavicular or ankle joint. An MRI was ordered because of the importance of making a definite diagnosis if this problem was identified. The MRI showed a navicular edema and a small incomplete fracture in the navicular between the joints of the medial and middle cuneiforms.

Since the injury was incomplete and Emily was a recreational runner, nonoperative treatment was elected. Emily was placed in a walking boot and followed clinically and with x-rays. At three months, the pain had resolved and a CAT scan was ordered to confirm complete healing of the injury. She decided to continue running but at a more moderate level and does not compete in marathons any longer.

Exercise-Induced Compartment Syndrome

Another unusual phenomena that seems to be common in athletes is shin pain. Shin pain can be caused by many problems including stress fractures of the tibia or a form of tendonitis commonly known as shin splints. These are usually caused by overuse, increasing training at too high a rate. Another cause of pain that limits running is exercise-induced compartment syndrome.

Exercise-induced compartment syndrome causes pain, burning, and swelling in runners at some point during their run. The problem lies in the fascia that surrounds the muscles of the lower leg. This fascia is a tough lining that divides groups of muscles within the leg. To some extent, they also shape the legs. In some well-conditioned individuals, the exercising muscle can swell during running to the point that the pressure within these compartments increases. If it gets high enough, the blood supply to the muscles may shut off. This is intensely painful and forces the athlete to rest. The pain and pressure usually subsides after a short period of rest.

Marvin's Story

Marvin is a sergeant in the Army and was going to be leaving for security training. He started to increase his running in anticipation for this, but found that he was unable to run more than one and a half miles before he was forced to stop. Besides that he was fine.

When Marvin returned from security training, he was asked to run on a treadmill until he felt the symptoms he described. Before and after his run, a needle specially designed to measure pressure within his tissue was placed in a few of the muscle compartments in his leg. The measurements before and after were taken, and they indicated elevations in his tissue pressure indicative of exercise-induced compartment syndrome.

Because of Marvin's desire to continue to run with his fellow soldiers, he underwent bilateral compartment releases. The fascia overlying his muscles was opened through two incisions of either side of both of his legs. He started running about one month later and was able to pass the Army physical fitness test three months later.

The Mature Athlete

Youth in athletics has its advantage, as many of us know. Young tissue is resilient and overuse injuries often quickly and completely heal. In fact, in the young athlete, flexibility is not always a benefit. A certain degree of inflexibility may aid in performance. Many distance runners have abnormally tight hamstrings and Achilles tendons. It is possible that this tendinous tension may store energy during running and improve performance especially in endurance and jumping athletes. There is a cost to this, however. These structures are likely to eventually wear at a higher than normal rate. In fact, former elite runners are 30 times more likely to develop Achilles tendonitis than their more sedentary counterparts.[1]

A mature athlete is one who is beyond the peak age for her sport, which may be as young as 30 to 40 years of age. When compared to a younger athlete, a mature athlete is less able to tolerate high degrees of stress or recover from them as quickly. As a result, training errors and flexibility deficits are not tolerated well. Although high-level athletic performance is possible, training must be more consistent and diverse.

A training plan is crucial. An honest assessment of the degree of the athlete's physical fitness and identifying chronic injuries is important to establish a reasonable starting point. A realistic conditioning plan that progresses in intensity over a period of weeks and months should be outlined. Consistent, regular participation in the training plan is crucial to building tolerance to stress within the connective tissue.

An ideal plan should involve both strength and aerobic conditioning of the upper and lower extremities. Diversify your workouts to avoid overuse injuries. Cross training is helpful in minimizing overuse injuries while promoting aerobic fitness. Flexibility exercises that could be skipped in the young athlete are absolutely crucial in the older athlete.

Young or old, every joint and body has limits. Prolonged and dedicated training may extend these limits, but endurance can probably be extended only so much. Although there is no good evidence that exercise—including strenuous high-level exercise—causes osteoarthritis,[2] strenuous exercise does aggravate already existing osteoarthritis and may accelerate joint destruction. Moderate exercise can be beneficial in people with various degrees of osteoarthritis, but prolonged high-impact exercises should avoid prolonged high-impact exercises.

A joint replacement can be a life-changing procedure for a person with severe arthritis of the lower extremity. However, it does impose its own restrictions. Aerobic exercise is recommended for nearly everyone including people with joint replacements. High-impact exercises such as jogging, tennis, and hiking increases stresses to the plastic, metal, and implant-bone interfaces that can accelerate loosening and wear on the joint replacement. The danger of a hip dislocation may force people with these replacements to modify their stretching exercises and calisthenics. You can get specific recommendations from your surgeon. Swimming, power walking, and bicycling are excellent exercises that have not been shown to damage joint replacements significantly.

FOOT PROBLEMS IN CHILDREN

- Because the child's foot is growing, it heals remarkably well but is prone to injuries that are different than the adult foot.
- This susceptibility is present with both traumatic and overuse injuries.
- Atraumatic rotational and angular abnormalities in the legs and feet of a child are very worrisome to parents, but are rarely of any functional concern.
- Orthotics, bracing, therapy, and other interventions are usually ineffective at changing the alignment and appearance of the legs. Surgery is necessary only in very specific circumstances.

Pediatric Foot Fractures

A child's foot is not an adult foot in miniature. The main difference is that the child's foot is rapidly and continually changing. From the moment the child is conceived through the teen years, all of the tissues in a child's foot and the rest of their body are changing, developing, and maturing.

This means that the tissues are extremely active metabolically, burning nutrients at an accelerated rate to power its development, reabsorbing and remaking itself perpetually. The bony tissue has specialized areas called growth plates that allow the bones to lengthen with the child's growth. Although the growth process is marvelous, it also leaves the child's bones prone to specific and common injuries.

The growth plate is a zone of cartilage at the end of the bone usually within a centimeter from the joint or weight-bearing surface of the bone. As the child grows the cartilage expands to lengthen the bone through cell division. At the same time, the bony tissue on either side of the growth plate is consuming the cartilage and laying down bone. The rate of bone formation and cartilage formation continues at an even and measured pace until the end of adolescence when the sexual hormones signal to the growth plate to close and completely bridge the growth plate with bone. At that point, further growth in the length of the bone is no longer possible.

This process leaves the growing bone vulnerable to injury. Cartilage is not nearly as strong as bone in tensile strength. This means that when a bone is pulled apart the cartilage will break long before the bone or ligament will. In addition, the newly formed bone tissue at the end of the bone is not fully developed and hardened and is not as strong as the adult bone in compressive strength. When the child falls on the bone or stresses it suddenly, it will become injured with much less force than an adult bone even when accounting for its decreased size.

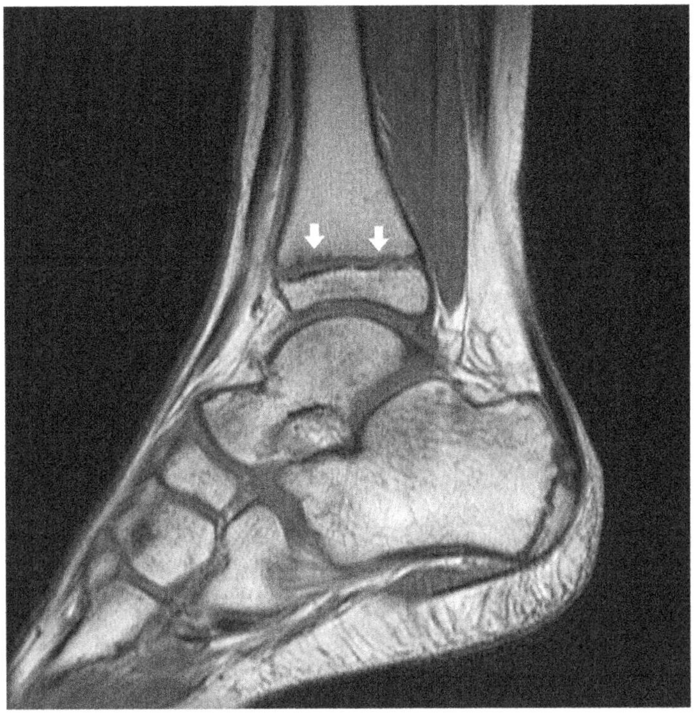

FIGURE 9.2 MRI of the hindfoot. Although injuries to the bone around the growth plates heal rapidly, the bone and cartilage represent a weak spot that injures easily.

Although the cartilage within the bones makes a child vulnerable to injury, the extremely high metabolism of the bones accelerates its recovery. Children return to activity two to three times faster than adults with a similar injury. Growth problems after fractures in the ankles are fortunately rare.

Injuries that disturb the joint or the growth plate that are left to heal in a displaced position are more much more devastating than similar injuries in an adult. If an injury through a growth plate is allowed to heal so that the bone on either side of the growth plate touches, the bone will deform because of uneven growth. It can lead to a short bone in comparison to the uninjured side as well as arthritis and joint deformity.

After an injury, persistently tender bones should be evaluated and usually x-rayed in a child. Although serious or dangerous injuries are rare, the window for appropriate treatment is brief, so prompt evaluation is strongly recommended.

The cartilage growth plate is also prone to injury through repetitive trauma. Traction and overuse injuries to the growth plates in children are extremely common. Although nearly any growth plate can become painful and irritated by repetitive stress, common areas are the heel, the arch, and the inside of the ankle. Sever's disease is by far the most common form of growth plate irritation. It is an overuse of the calcaneal apophysis, the growth plate at the tip of the calcaneus. Both the Achilles tendon and the plantar fascia attach to the growth plate at the end of the heel. The strong muscles and stout ligaments place a great deal of stress on it making it prone to injury. Calcaneal apophysitis can make walking more painful and make it hard to get out of bed in the morning. The muscles recoil when the leg is placed in a relaxed flexed position when sitting. When stretching these structures back out to length when initiating walking, extra stress is needed to bring them out to length. This stress is felt as pain.

This condition is treated by aggressive stretching, arch supports if the foot is flat, rocker-soled shoes, and rest. It is common for them to recur because these children usually have predisposing factors such as tendon tightness or extreme participation in sports. It is also notoriously difficult to interest children in a rehabilitation program. Casting the painful limb can successfully treat the injury.

Julia's Story

Julia is a nine-year-old girl who twisted her ankle when playing volleyball. She fell on the ground and could not walk afterward. Her parents saw her fall and said that she rolled on the outside of the ankle during the injury. Julia went to the emergency room and the x-rays were normal.

Julia's ankle was swollen and bruised along her heel. Her foot was tender about two centimeters above the end of the bone on the outside of the ankle, the fibula. Julia has sustained a fracture of the growth plate at the end of the fibula, a common injury. In the process of turning her ankle, she cracked through the growth plate instead of tearing the ankle ligaments as an adult would in an ankle sprain. Because cartilage is transparent on x-rays, the injury wasn't identified. Although Julia's injury is really a fracture, her ankle remained very stable, owing to the thick soft tissue around the bones and within the ankle.

Julia's splint was removed and she was placed in a prefabricated cast boot. She was allowed to begin walking on the ankle as the pain allowed her to. Julia returned for follow-up three weeks later. She was walking with no pain and was playing volleyball five weeks later. These injuries rarely cause significant growth plate damage that affects growth.

Mark's Story

Mark is an 11-year-old boy who is very active athletically. He is star forward in soccer. Mark noticed pain in his heels—right worse than left—but had continued to play. His parents noticed that he was limping during his game. It seemed to get better with some ibuprofen.

The following morning, Mark was unable to get out of bed. When he tried to get on his feet, it brought him to tears. He was brought to his pediatrician's office. Although he was feeling somewhat better, he still limped.

Mark's feet appeared to be normal. There was no bruising or swelling. He had normal motion and strength. When standing, his feet were mildly flat. He was slightly tender on the inside of his ankle along the inside. The bottoms and back of his heel hurt. When asked to touch his toes while keeping his knees fully extended, he was able to reach no farther than midshin. His x-rays showed a normal heel with calcaneal apophysis that was still open.

Mark was diagnosed with calcaneal apophysitis or Sever's disease, an overuse injury of the end of the heel. Mark was placed in a cast boot for four weeks. During this time, he was started on an Achilles tendon- and hamstring-stretching program, supervised by a physical therapist for the first four weeks. After four weeks, he was gradually returned to walking, jogging and finally running. He returned to soccer two months after treatment.

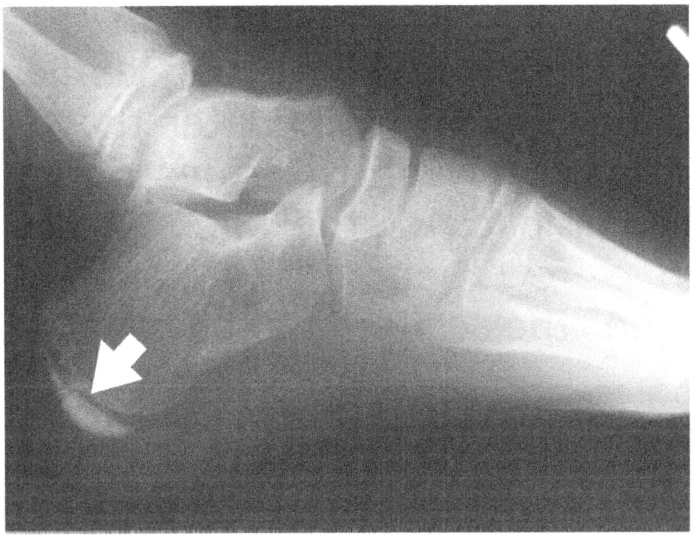

FIGURE 9.3 Lateral or side view of the Mark's heel. The calcaneal apophysis (white arrow) is a layer of cartilage that allows the heel to grow, but is prone to injury in athletic children.

Growing Pains

Children have a bewildering array of pains while growing up. In fact, musculoskeletal pain is one of the leading reasons that children are seen in the pediatrician's office. Parents are typically concerned that the pain represents a form of serious illness.

Fortunately, this is rarely the case. At the very least, they are usually distraught because they feel powerless while their children are in pain.

At some time during childhood, 30% to 60% of children have nontraumatic extremity pain.[3][4] The syndrome of "growing pains" has been identified for centuries and the cause is unknown. Growing pains are most common in children from age 5 to 14. They commonly occur at night or in the late afternoon and rarely interfere with activity although there has been the suggestion that heavy exertion earlier in the day may trigger the growing pains later that evening. This kind of pain is usually on the sides of the leg, in the shins, thighs, or back of the knee, and usually goes away within a few hours. The pain is often more frequent when the child has been more active or moody.

Although the cause of growing pains has not been identified, a number of interesting observations have been made. Children with more growing pains tend to be more flexible and a higher proportion of them have bunions and flat feet.[5] They seem to have a decreased pain threshold when compared to their peers.[6] They also seem to have a decreased bone mineral density within their bones suggesting that this is an overuse syndrome. It does not—as was once thought—coincide with periods of growth.

Parents and children need support and reassurance that the problem is not dangerous. Kids who have markedly flat feet may benefit from over-the-counter inserts. Stretching programs may also be helpful. You can try massage and anti-inflammatory medications such as naproxen before bedtime. The problem usually resolves itself.

Intoeing and Outtoeing

Parents worry about their children. This is only natural. Many parents have concerns about the appearance of the legs in their children. They worry about everything from proper growth, gate changes, to their child's ability to participate in sports. We all are different. Some children are clumsier than others. Some are faster. Some can jump higher. A gait that works well for one child may be very different than the gait of another. There are fortunately few abnormalities that significantly affect our children's potential to painlessly work and play. In the vast majority of these cases, there is little indication that braces, surgery, or prolonged therapy is helpful.

Common descriptions of the rotation of the legs in children are being "pigeon toed," when the toes are rotated to the inside, or having a "duck walk," when the toes are rotated to the outside. These abnormalities can be caused by rotation of the bones at the tibia, femur, or foot. The most common cause for intoeing is a twisting of the femur that begins in the uterus with the positioning of the baby. Often children with this abnormality will sit with their legs folded underneath them to the sides of their thighs, the "W" position. Parents describe their children as being clumsy because their toes hit their opposite leg as the leg is swung during running. This problem usually stops as your child's foot becomes smaller in relation to his overall body frame. Twisting in the tibia usually causes outtoeing. This abnormality often decreases as the child grows to maturity. Sometimes, children consciously compensate for their walk by adjusting the position of the hip during walking. Athletic abilities are usually not compromised with these problems. The foot progression angle is the angle between the foot and direction of walking. If the foot is within 15 to 20 degrees of pointing straight forward, this is normal and no treatment is typically necessary.

Bracing, inserts, and stretching are of questionable benefit. Surgery is considered only for severe and disabling problems, but is emotionally and physically taxing for both the parents and the child. It should not be considered when addressing a mild or moderate case.

Knock-Knees and Bowlegs

The angle that the thigh makes with the leg is also a common worry of parents. The angulation between the thigh and the shin can be measured on an x-ray. It can also be measured with a ruler by determining the distance between the knees in bowed legs when the ankles are placed together or the distance between the ankle when the knees are placed together in knock-knees.

It is typical for children to be slightly bowlegged at birth. If the legs are squeezed together until they touch, the knees are usually separated less than six centimeters. While the child is packed into the uterus prior to birth, the legs are crossed over the body causing them to bow. Over the first three years of life, the legs gradually become more valgus or knockkneed.

Knock-knees are almost never a sign of a significant problem. Most children go through a period of bowleggedness when they are toddlers. In most cases, it goes away by itself.

Blount's disease is a type of developmental illness of the knee growth plates that causes bowed legs. It can be identified through radiographs. Many of these children are overweight. Some believe that the increased weight of these children damages the growth plate on the inside of the knee. As a result, the knees do not grow properly and begin to bow worse. If the disease is untreated the problem can progress. As a result, careful follow-up is necessary if the bow deformity is severe or seems to be getting worse. Occasionally, this disease may require bracing or surgical treatment.

Toe Walking

A toe gait is essentially normal in a toddler for some time after learning to walk. Often children are brought in for evaluation when the toe-walking pattern continues when they begin preschool. Usually the children are not concerned about it and it does not usually cause pain. Rarely, this is a sign of a neurological problem, but more frequently no cause can be found.

There really is no easy and effective treatment for toe walking, but the good news is that the children develop functionally without treatment. Studies that have looked at bracing, casting, and physical therapy have shown no evidence of improvement after these interventions. In one study,[7] untreated toe-walking children followed for a period of years improve half of the time and remain unchanged in the other 50%. Surgical release of the Achilles tendon improves 75% of children and in 25% the gait remains unchanged or worse. Surgical treatment is done very rarely.

RHEUMATOID ARTHRITIS AND OTHER INFLAMMATORY ARTHRITIS

• Rheumatoid arthritis and many other similar conditions are caused by the body's immune system attacking the body itself.

• These diseases commonly result in joint and ligament destruction.

- Many medications have been developed to treat them, but these medications have side effects.

Inflammatory arthritises are a family of diseases in which the body's immune system attacks itself. It affects about 1% of the population and almost all of these diseases are more common in women than men. The causes of inflammatory arthritis are unclear. Some theories suggest that the immune system may react to an infection and make antibodies—proteins that tag things as foreign or dangerous—that also attach to the body tissues.

The most common inflammatory arthritis is rheumatoid arthritis. In rheumatoid arthritis, the immune system attacks the joint lining. This immune reaction results in the release of many inflammatory chemical messengers and proteins that eventually can destroy the joint. The fluid within the joint also breaks down and loses much of its lubricating property. Consequently, the cartilage thins and finally erodes away altogether. The ligaments, which are integrated within the joint capsule and are instrumental in ensuring that the joints maintain proper alignment and move properly, begin to stretch. The loss of the ligament's stabilization leads to typical deformities of the hands and feet of rheumatoid arthritis.

Rheumatoid arthritis is diagnosed by the presence of a number of characteristic factors, none of which alone diagnose it. Swelling or synovitis is present in two or more joints. Morning stiffness is experienced for more than an hour for six weeks or more. Most of the tests used to diagnose it are not only present in rheumatoid arthritis. Rheumatoid factor is a blood test that identifies the presence of specific antibodies. Rheumatoid factor is positive in 80% of people with rheumatoid arthritis but is also found in many other problems, including hepatitis, other viral diseases, and other autoimmune diseases such as lupus.

Medical treatment of rheumatoid arthritis and other inflammatory arthritis is directed at blunting the immune response. Nonsteroidal anti-inflammatory medications such as naproxen and ibuprofen can give some relief, but are not "disease modifying" anti-rheumatic drugs (DMARDs) because they do not stop the damage that rheumatoid arthritis does. Rheumatologists and other physicians can prescribe disease-modifying drugs, but they are strong medications with significant side effects including liver and bone marrow damage and skin rashes.

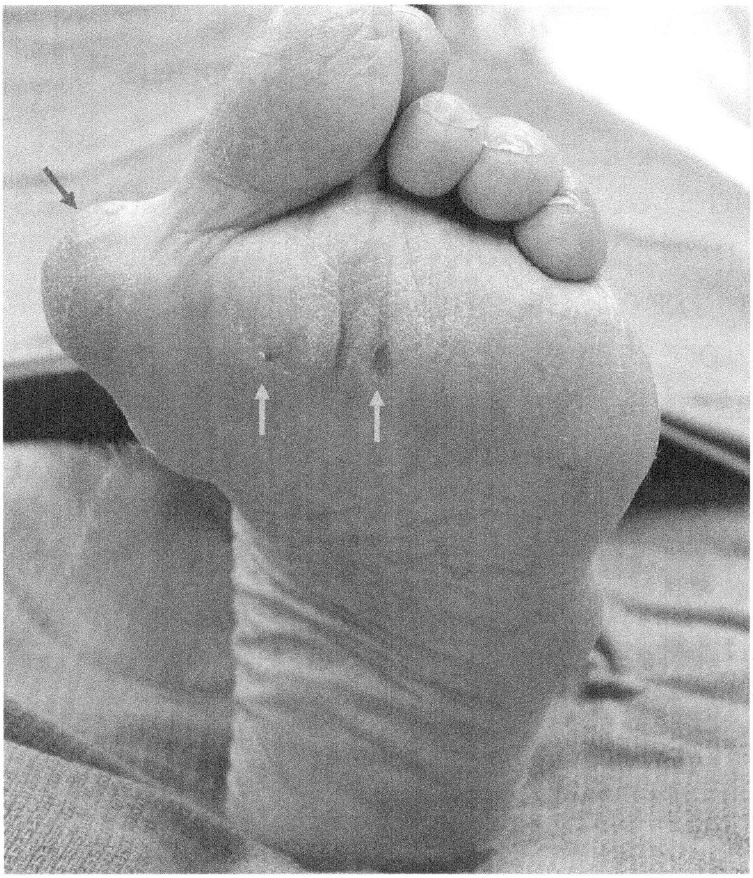

FIGURE 9.4 The bottom of the foot of a person with a typical rheumatoid forefoot deformity. A severe bunion is present (dark arrow) with marked prominence of the metatarsal heads of the second and third metatarsophalangeal joints in the ball of the foot due to dislocation of the joints (white arrows).

People with rheumatoid arthritis commonly have problems with their feet. Some of these foot issues are treatable without surgery. Often, damage to the ligaments results in severe bunions. The lesser toes develop hammertoe deformities that may dislocate the metatarsophalangeal joints. The dislocation of the metatarsophalangeal joint often makes the metatarsal heads so prominent in the ball of the foot that calluses and ulcers develop. Many people feel as if the metatarsal heads are coming through the bottom of their foot.

Rheumatoid foot problems can be treated as a forefoot overload problem from a rehabilitative standpoint. Stretching exercises and postural training can reduce pain and pressure, but are often not sufficient. A simple closed foam insert or orthotic can help make the foot more comfortable. The amount of comfort that gel inserts give is often disappointing. Adding a metatarsal pad can also relieve forefoot pressure, but if the arch is collapsed, the pad may be too bulky to be comfortable.

The most important aspect of making the shoe comfortable is to control pressure on the metatarsal heads. The most effective way of doing this is through the use of a stiff rocker-soled shoe. A soft upper or extra-width, extra-depth toe box can accommodate the bunion and hammertoes and protect the fragile skin along the bony prominences.

Midfoot and hindfoot problems may cause the foot to collapse into a flat-footed position. This can sometimes be controlled using an extended insert called a University of California Berkley Laboratories (UCBL) insert. More extensive foot issues require control of the ankle and midfoot using a hinged or fixed ankle brace, which extends into the arch such as a short articulated ankle-foot-orthosis (AFO) or a molded leather ankle brace called an Arizona brace, which you can read about in the resources section.

Surgery is often necessary in cases of rheumatoid arthritis. Often fusions of joints are used to realign them because of the tenuous condition of the ligaments. Many joint-preserving procedures are also being evaluated.

There are other inflammatory conditions that commonly affect the foot.

- Scleroderma: This often causes stiff deformities of the toes including bunions and hammertoes. The stiffening of the soft tissues can make the vessels prone to clotting when they are straightened.
- Psoriatic arthritis: This causes inflammation especially of the ankle and hindfoot usually well managed through medical means.
- Crystalline arthropathies: See Chapter 3, Gout.

DIABETES AND NEUROPATHY

- Diabetes is a disease of faulty control of sugar metabolism resulting in high blood glucose levels.
- High glucose levels are toxic to many tissues especially the nerves, immune cells.
- Neuropathy, impairment of the nerves, causes numbness and muscle weakness.

• Complications of diabetes and neuropathy include stress injury to the bones, deformity, and infection.

Diabetes can have a devastating effect on the feet. It is the leading cause of amputation in the United States. In addition, wound care clinics are filled with people living with diabetes-associated complications such as wounds and infections. Neuropathy is a medical term describing nerve damage. Although there are many reasons people can develop neuropathy, diabetes is by far the most common cause of nerve damage and the effects of the nerve damage is main method that diabetes injures the feet.

Why Does Diabetes Affect the Feet?

Diabetes mellitus is a group of metabolic diseases in which a person has high blood sugar. This insulin system that controls the glucose concentration breaks down in two ways. The first is that not enough insulin is produced. This usually occurs because the islet cells that are produced in the pancreas are destroyed. Many researchers suspect that the cells are killed when the body forms an immune response against the cells. A second method of interfering with this system is that the target cells no longer are able to recognize the insulin or the insulin is taken out of the system too fast. This is called insulin resistance and is more common in the type 2 adult-onset variety of diabetes. The high concentrations of glucose can actually attach to the proteins in the body. If long chains of these glucose molecules attach to the proteins, it can interfere with their function. This can affect proteins within the membranes of our cells especially in the nerves where proteins conduct electrical impulses and within our connective tissue where it may inhibit immune and repair processes. It affects in some way nearly every bodily function.

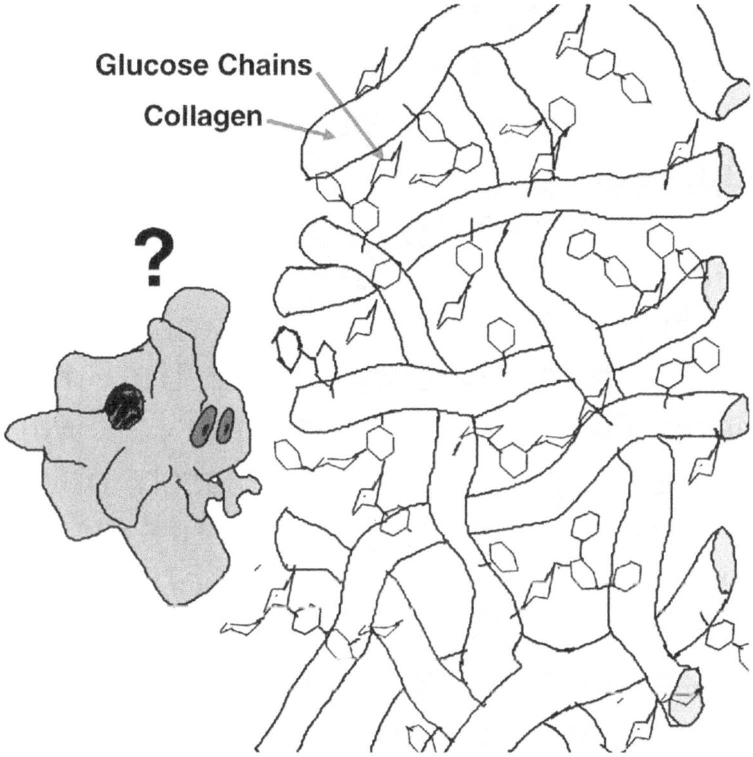

FIGURE 9.5 Immune and reparative cells may have difficulty traveling through connective tissue that is heavily bound with glucose chains. This may contribute to poor wound healing and immune suppression in diabetes.

Other methods of damage to cells that diabetes may cause are still being figured out. The high concentrations of glucose within the cells of the nerves may also produce the formation of other toxic metabolites of glucose. This poisons cell metabolism.

The longest nerves in the body are the nerves to the feet. The control centers of the sensory nerves or cell bodies are near the spinal cord in the middle of the lumbar spine. The axon or long thin filament that sprouts off the cell body travels in the nerve bundles to receptors in the tissue of the feet. These nerve cells are single cells that are several feet long. The longer the nerve is, the more opportunity exists to quench a signal along the long axon through gummed-up, poorly functioning membrane channels that conduct the nerve signals. If the damage becomes great enough, this will cause the sensory nerves to not work correctly resulting in numbness. The motor nerves, in addition to controlling the muscles, also nourish them. Damage to these nerves will cause the muscles, especially those in the arch of the foot, to waste away. The scarring that occurs as the muscles waste away affects the toes and foot. The nerves that travel to the sweat glands, and blood vessels are also damaged, leading to skin dryness, the inability to regulate heat and to control blood flow within the tissues. As a result, the skin can crack and become damaged.

The rate of damage caused by diabetes is variable. On average, signs of neuropathy often occur three to five years after the diagnosis of diabetes, although, occasionally, the neuropathy can occur before the diabetes is recognized. In other situations, it may not be present even after many decades of diabetes. The damage to nerves is related to the average concentration of the serum glucose and the length of time since the onset of diabetes, but other factors such as genetics and other medical problems undoubtedly affect this.

Diabetes also affects the blood vessels. People with diabetes develop damage to arteries earlier than people without diabetes. The vessels also become more permeable or leaky allowing the fluid and protein within the vessels to seep into the tissue causing swelling in the legs. Damage and scarring of the artery and vein walls leads to calcification and narrowing that can block them. These blockages can strangle the tissue of needed blood and result in pain, poor tissue healing of wounds, and potentially the death of the leg. In the veins, the scarring of the vessel walls and the valves within the veins that prevent backflow can increase the pressure in the veins. Varicose veins and rashes around the ankles occur. This situation also causes the skin to be easy to injure.

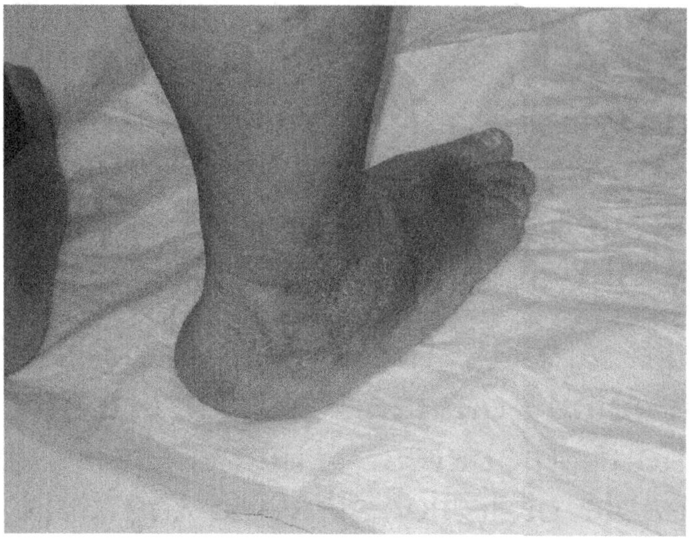

FIGURE 9.6 Dark discoloration of the skin around the ankles that is typical of severe vein damage in the legs, common in diabetes.

What Can I Do to Stop This?

Some of the damage that occurs in people with diabetes is not repairable even if the diabetes were to suddenly and completely go away. There is also a lot of damage that the body *can* repair.

The most important part of preventing diabetic complications like neuropathy is to control glucose levels within the blood. The more normal the glucose level is, the less damage occurs. Tight regulation of glucose levels through oral medications and insulin is key. A large study called the "Diabetes Care and Control Trial" was conducted until 1993. It specifically looked at intensive versus standard diabetes control and found that intensive, strict control of blood sugar reduced most complications of diabetes. Specifically, the incidence of neuropathy was reduced by 60%.[8]

Intensive glucose control is achieved through frequent monitoring blood glucose and administering insulin several times a day, in addition to diet and exercise. Your doctor can also test how well controlled your average glucose level is by ordering a test called a glycosylated hemoglobin test or hemoglobin A1C. This test measures the amount of glucose attached to the hemoglobin in your red blood cell corpuscles. It reflects the average concentration of glucose in the blood throughout the lifetime of your red blood cell, about 120 days.

If you are overweight, make a plan to get back to an ideal body weight. Normalizing your body weight in many incidences of type 2 or adult-onset diabetes can make diabetes much easier to control.

Finally, control and medicate other problems that can contribute to the development of medical complications. It should be no surprise that diabetes and smoking do not mix well. The effects of both together are worse than either alone. If you are diabetic and smoke, quit smoking now! Get any support or help from your doctor that you need including counseling, support groups, and medication.

What Else Can Cause Neuropathy?

Diabetes is a major cause of nerve damage. It is often assumed by doctors that if you have neuropathy, it must be because of diabetes, but there are other common causes of nerve damage.

Certain medications—especially medications used in chemotherapy or treatment of cancer and AIDS—can damage the nerves. Many are listed in Table 9.1.

TABLE 9.1 Medications Known to Cause Neuropathy

Antibiotics:

Ciprofloxacin

Dapsone

Flagyl

Metronidazole

Anti-Alcohol Drug

Disulfiram

Anti-Convulsants:

Phenytoin (Dilantin®)

Anti-Depressant:

Celexa (Citalopram)

Cymbalta (Duloxetine)

Effexor (Venlafaxine)

Effexor XR

Nortriptyline

Zoloft

Anti-Seizure:

Lyrica (Pregabalin)

Blood Pressure or Heart Medications:

Aceon

Altace

Amiodarone

Atenolol

Cozaar

Hydralazine

Hydrochlorothiazide (HCT)

Hydrodiuril

Hyzaar

Lisinopril

Micardis

Norvasc

Perhexiline

Perindopril

Prazosin

Prinivil

Ramipril

Zestril

Chemotherapy Drugs:

Cisplatin

Vincristine

Cholesterol Drugs:

Advicor

Altocor

Atorvastatin

Baycol

Caduet

Cerivastatin

Crestor

Fluvastatin

Lescol

Lescol XL

Lipex

Lipitor

Lipobay

Lopid

Lovastatin

Mevacor

Pravachol

Pravastatin

Pravigard Pac

Rosuvastatin

Simvastatin

Vytorin

Zocor

Dental Creams:

Zinc containing creams including Polygrip®, Fixodent®

HIV Drugs:

d4T (Zerit®)

ddC (Hivid®)

ddI (Videx EC®)

Other things that cause neuropathy:

- Alcoholism
- Amyloidosis (metabolic disorder)
- Autoimmune disorders
- Cancer
- Charcot Marie-Tooth disease and other genetic nerve disorders
- Chronic kidney failure
- Connective tissue disease (e.g., rheumatoid arthritis, lupus, sarcoidosis)
- Diabetes mellitus
- Herniated disc
- Infectious disease (e.g., Lyme disease, HIV/AIDS, hepatitis B, leprosy)
- Liver failure
- Radiation treatment
- Radiculopathy
- Surgeries that damage a nerve
- Vitamin deficiencies (e.g., pernicious anemia)

Pain With Neuropathy

Neuropathy can be painful. This is sometimes the earliest sign of nerve damage. The exact way that the feet are affected can vary from person to person, but it is often described as tingling or a "sun-burn" feeling. It is pretty common for the symptoms to be worse at night and can be so intense as to cause the lightest touch to be uncomfortable.

Although neuropathy can be painful, it is important make sure that other dangerous problems are not present before assuming that this is the diagnosis. Infections and stress injuries can also cause pain and need to be considered before simply taking medicines to treat the pain.

Initial treatment involves tight control of serum glucose through intensive management and frequent administration of insulin and other diabetic medications. Smoking cessation is crucial. Control of other associated medical conditions including lipid and cholesterol abnormalities and hypertension has been shown to help.

Topical treatments include capsaicin cream, which is available without a prescription. Care needs to be taken with handling this cream because, if it is accidentally gotten onto mucosal membranes such as the eyes, it can be intensely painful. Lidocaine patches and ointments are also sometimes helpful.

Many other oral medications used in the treatment of painful neuropathy were originally created to help with other neurological disorders such as depression and seizures. Anti-depressants such as amitriptyline, desipramine, and nortriptyline have been of some benefit but can cause sedation and cardiac arrhythmias at high dosages. Duloxetine (Cymbalta®) is perhaps the most widely prescribed antidepressant used for neuropathy. Anti-seizure medications such as gabapentin (Neurontin®) and pregabalin (Lyrica®) are helpful but can cause sedation and other significant side effects.

Ulceration/Absess

Calluses along bony prominences are common in people with diabetes. Contractures of the joints can change the way that weight is placed on the foot so that the skin thickens. If the thickened skin becomes very hard, it can produce tissue damage of its own. In general, this should be medically evaluated to determine whether regular removal is prudent. If the callus becomes deep, then bleeding can occur under the skin, which will give it a purplish or blackish color. This can progress to blistering and leakage around the callus.

Once a break in the skin has occurred, debris and bacteria can get in under the skin causing infection. If the damage penetrates into the deeper structures, especially along the fascia and tendons, or into the joints, an ideal environment is present to promote bacterial growth with relatively little exposure to the immune system that protects the body. Bacteria in these conditions can proliferate rapidly, making a smoldering ulcer into a deep absess. Antibiotics alone are rarely effective in curing an absess.

Gail's Story

Gail is a 39-year-old female who works in a pharmaceutical lab. She had diabetes for 12 years, which was sometimes in poor control. She then developed a callus under her fourth toe. She noticed that the callus had turned purple and some leakage had begun under it as well as smelly discharge and swelling into her arch. She was prescribed a broad-spectrum antibiotic, but, despite this, she began to experience fevers and recently was having confusion at home.

In the emergency room, Gail had a sore under the ball of her big toe that was swollen and red and extended into her arch. Pressure on the arch or around the toe caused fluid to flow through the wound. She was just in mild pain.

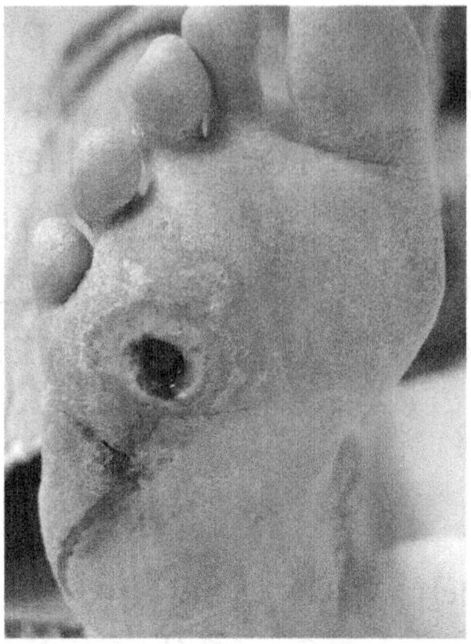

FIGURE 9.7 This ulcer was caused by pressure from a bony prominence in the front of the foot. From the depth of the wound, it probably has an underlying absess.

Her foot was operated on. During surgery, we found the infection had traveled into the arch area by following the tendons nearby. The infection had involved the joint underneath the ulcer. The infected tissue was removed, as was the cartilage around the joint.

Three weeks after surgery, her wound healed and she was allowed to resume her normal activities.

Stress Injury/Charcot Arthropathy

The neuropathic foot is prone to stress injury. These are some of the most troublesome and dangerous conditions that can occur in the diabetic foot. The neuropathic foot does not handle stress like a healthy foot. Changes in the shape of the foot and many protective mechanisms in conjunction with loss of sensations that alerts the mind to problems contribute to mechanical failure, specifically fracture and deformity.

It begins with swelling and pain. Often it is confused with infection because of its impressive swelling so that the diagnosis is many times delayed.

Charcot arthropathy can severely deform your joints. Joints and fractures can become unstable and collapse. The change in alignment can shift weight onto areas that are not meant to bear weight, which can lead to breakdown of the skin. This can endanger the foot and should be followed closely.

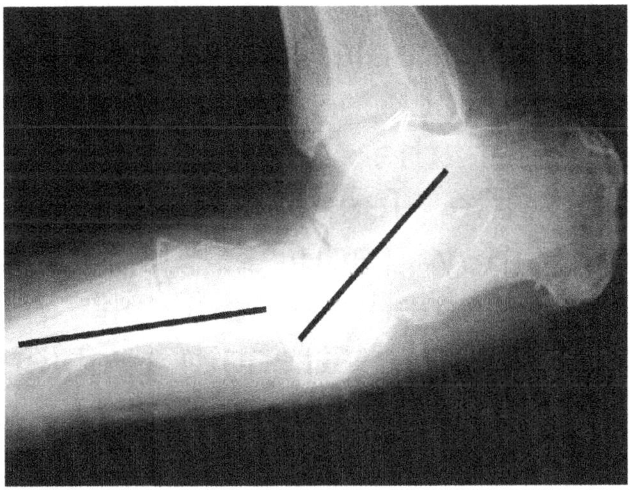

FIGURE 9.8 Untreated Charcot arthropathy leading to a near reversal of the arch, otherwise known as a rocker-soled foot. In a normal foot, the black lines would be aligned. The midfoot in this foot is nearly dislocated.

Charcot arthropathy heals a lot like other injuries. The swelling goes down and bone formation begins to stabilize the joints and fractures. The goals of treatment in Charcot arthropathy are to regain a stable foot that will safely fit into a shoe and will withstand walking without skin breakdown.

Initially this means protecting the foot from excessive motion and stress. This can be accomplished through bracing with a cast boot or through casting. Removing the motion that would occur with unprotected walking encourages bone formation and improves stability in the area of injury. As the stability improves in the foot, the bracing can be reduced; however, this takes months.

Rocker-soled shoes are sometimes a good idea for a person who has a stable, healed foot after Charcot arthropathy. Considerable weight relief is possible through the use of rocker-soled shoes.[9][10] Release of the portions of the Achilles tendon along with realignment of the foot surgically is sometimes necessary, but may require restriction of weight bearing. This is sometimes difficult in people with diabetes due to balance strength problems.

Arthur's Story

Arthur is a 56-year-old man who worked as a production supervisor at an automotive plant until he lost his vision due to diabetic damage to his retina. He was used to recurrent swelling in his ankles but the swelling became more than usual and he noted warmth as well.

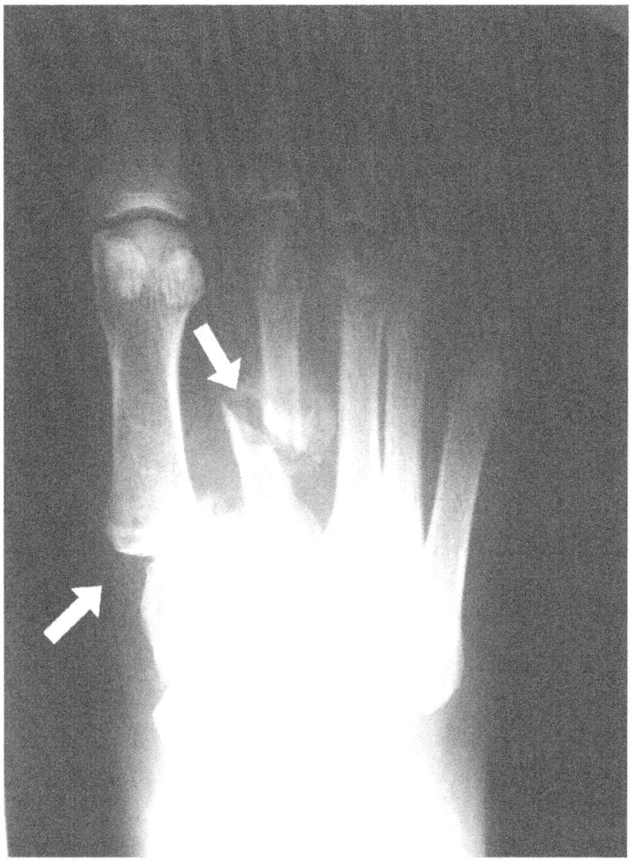

FIGURE 9.9 A midfoot fracture-dislocation in diabetes. There is a dislocation of the first tarsometatarsal joint and a fracture of the second metatarsal.

Arthur's foot was normally flat, but the flatness was accentuated. The arch area was unusually loose to any stress and a coarse grating sound was heard and felt when the arch was moved. The x-rays showed fractures of some of the metatarsals of his foot. Despite this, he was in very little pain.

Arthur was diagnosed with Charcot arthropathy. He was placed in a series of short-leg, walking casts for two months. The swelling and warmth gradually decreased and he transitioned to a prefabricated walking boot. Although the metatarsal fracture never completely healed, the pain and swelling abated and he was placed in a shoe with metal extensions that kept the ankle immobilized to protect it from pressure. His injury gradually became stiff and stable at about eight months and he returned to an extra-depth diabetic shoe and a low-impact aerobic-conditioning program.

FIBROMYALGIA AND OTHER PAIN DISORDERS

- Pain is a sensation that helps us protect our body and recognize danger.
- Fibromyalgia and reflex sympathetic dystrophy (RSD) is a disorder of faulty pain perception.
- Although difficult to treat, fibromyalgia and RSD can be helped by physical conditioning, psychological techniques such as stress reduction and counseling, and modest use of pain medications.

Pain: It's Not All Bad

Pain is the most feared sensation. There is good reason for this. Pain sensation signals that tissue damage is occurring and that our body is in danger. The wiring within our brain instructs us to avoid these situations and, through this very unpleasant sensation, it impresses that action must be taken immediately. This has some significant survival advantages.

Pain is also our teacher. It is present even in very primitive organisms such as small worms. Through our capacity to learn, this unpleasant sensation becomes associated with dangerous situations so that we avoid them in the future. A child, even before she or he has developed a high sense of reasoning, understands that touching a hot stove is to be avoided.

How Pain Works

Pain is sensed through nerves. The cell bodies of pain nerves are located within a small swelling in the nerves close to the spinal cord and the axons or the nerve fibers travel along with the other nerves that give touch sensation and motor control to the skin, muscles, tendons, and bones. The nerve fibers terminate in the tissue at a receptor that is able to sense tissue damage. The signals are relayed at the spinal cord to the brain.

There are two basic types of pain fiber. One is the myelinated, "fast" pain fibers that give pain a sharp, piercing quality. We are able to localize this pain well. This system of pain fibers allows us to perceive where a painful problem is. Myelin is a cellular wrapping that insulates the nerve fiber a lot like the plastic on an electrical wire insulates the wire and improves the efficiency of electrical conduction within your home. This allows these nerves to conduct nerve impulses very fast so that if you step on a tack, the information is sent to your brain so that you can avoid further injury. It initiates the withdrawal response to the painful stimulus.

The second type of pain fiber is controlled by unmyelinated, "slow" pain fibers. This nerve conducts much slower than the "fast" fiber and stimulation of this nerve gives a more dull, unpleasant, burning quality to the pain. This is a more primitive system of pain. The activation of other sensory inputs such as deep pressure and "fast" pain fibers inhibits "slow" pain fiber activity. This is why rubbing an injury helps to decrease pain. The "slow" pain fibers are thought by many researchers to be responsible for more chronic forms of pain. Pain from "slow" pain fibers basically tells the animal not to use the extremity. An animal in the wild that breaks its leg is quite likely to become lunch for the next lion that comes by, but it may have a chance at survival if it does not use the leg and allows it to heal in some roughly straight position.

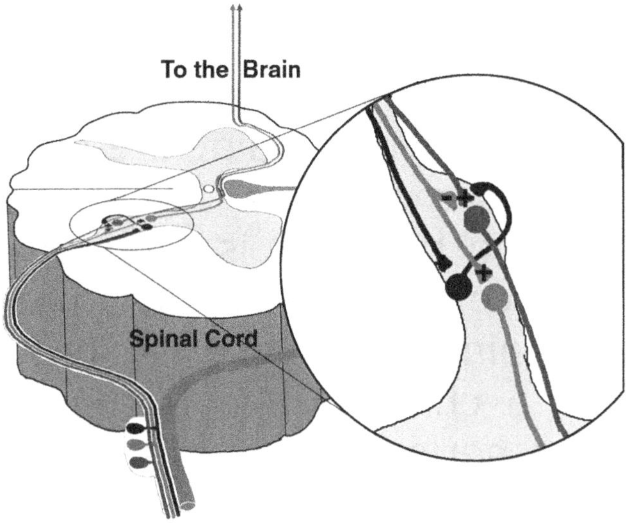

FIGURE 9.10 Activity of the "slow" pain fiber (dark gray) is inhibited directly by the "fast" pain fiber (light gray) activity and by pressure sensory fiber (black) activity. It is also inhibited by stimulation of inhibitory nerves. These interconnections modulate the pain sensation to the brain.

The perception of pain is then transferred to other nerve cells within the spinal cord and from there into various areas of the brain including the brain stem and cortex. Ronald Melzack and Patrick Wall introduced the gate control theory of pain in 1965[11] and suggested that pain perception is not simply to direct stimulation of pain fibers. The pain signals are altered by both negative feedback (signals that travel back into the spinal cord and other areas that inhibit or lessen the pain signal) and positive feedback (signals that travel into the spinal cord and other areas and make it easier to sense pain). Pain perception then is the total sum of pain fiber input modified by feedback from many sources including other sensory fiber input as well as from higher centers within the brain.

In the higher levels of the brain, the sensation of pain is interpreted and modulated in the thalamus and cortex, parts of the brain. It is affected by emotional states and other cognitive activities that may amplify or reduce the pain experience. A firefighter in the midst of saving a child from a burning building may be unaware of a serious burn. On the other hand, a depressed person may be unable to effectively cope and may amplify pain that would otherwise be easily tolerated.

The chemicals that transmit the impulses from one nerve to another are very important to the understanding and treatment of pain. The most important part may be that many of these chemicals are used predominantly in pain nerves. This gives medicine the ability to exploit these chemicals to modify pain perception. Among the chemicals that increase pain response are glutamate and neurokinins, and small protein neurotransmitters such as Substance P. Chemicals that inhibit pain include gamma amino butyric acid (GABA), norepinephrine, serotonin, and endorphins.

So what changes pain from a beneficial and crucial part of our defense mechanism into a disease that requires treatment? Leading researchers often describe it in terms of the plasticity of our brains. Plasticity is the ability of our brains to change in response to the way in which the brain has been stimulated and what it has experienced in the past. Prolonged pain can change the brain neurons, leading to an enhanced sensitivity and more efficient transmission of pain to the brain. It can occur by producing more of the neurotransmitters that allow us to relay pain within the nervous system and by producing more of the protein receptors for the neurotransmitters on the surface of the nerve cell. It can also occur by depleting the neurotransmitters that inhibit pain perception or producing fewer of the receptors that sense these chemicals. Over time the sensitivity of these pain pathways can become heightened so that painful stimuli can be overperceived by the brain and nonpainful stimuli can be interpreted by the brain as painful.

Fibromyalgia

Although no surgeon specializes in fibromyalgia, it is certainly seen frequently in surgical clinics. The incidence of fibromyalgia in the general population is generally quoted at 2% to 4%, but it is much higher among people seeking medical help for foot and ankle disorders. In one study,[12] the incidence was 10% in a group of people with general foot complaints and 20% in people with heel pain. It is a disorder that often dominates the person's life and sometimes disables them. Unfortunately, it is a problem that is poorly understood and difficult to treat.

Fibromyalgia is a syndrome of generalized body pain. The definition of fibromyalgia by the American College of Rheumatology was established for research purposes in 1990. It defined it as the symptom of widespread pain associated with tenderness in 11 of 18 defined points along the upper and lower extremities and spine for greater than three months. Fibromyalgia is often associated with a number of other symptoms including fatigue, depression, insomnia, anxiety, impaired memory and concentration, and headaches. The presence of these other symptoms undoubtedly contributes and complicates the treatment of the chronic pain. There is considerable overlap between fibromyalgia and other common pain syndromes such as myofascial pain syndrome, and chronic fatigue syndrome.

Although fibromyalgia literally means painful fibrous and muscle tissue, no consistent changes have been found in the connective tissue of people with fibromyalgia. In fact, no established underlying cause has been found for fibromyalgia. Possible causes for fibromyalgia that have been put forth include stress, hereditary and viral causes, deficiency in various neurotransmitters within the brain and psychiatric disturbances. None of these theories adequately explains fibromyalgia.

A recent comprehensive Internet survey on fibromyalgia was published[13] that demonstrated some interesting points. Much of this data may be skewed because the participants were recruited from the Internet and so demographically were people comfortable with this technology. Of the respondents to this survey, 97% were female. Most were middle-aged and overweight.

Seventy-three percent of people noted some inciting factor for their fibromyalgia. Many attributed the onset of the fibromyalgia to be associated with an emotional trauma or chronic stress, although many blamed a physical illness or trauma. A significant portion noted physical or sexual abuse either as a child or as an adult.

Fluctuation in the intensity of symptoms was found to be common with fibromyalgia. Most respondents suggested that many emotional stressors such as worry, family conflicts, and emotional distress worsened their symptoms. A majority noted increased pain with weather changes, physical inactivity, or injury.

The most popular methods of treatment were rest, distractions (such as watching TV or reading), exercises, massage, and medications. The treatments rated most effective were rest, heat, prescription pain and sleeping medications, anti-depressants, and aerobic and nonaerobic exercises such as tai chi, yoga, and stretching. Meditation and prayer were also rated high (6.0 and 5.0 on a 10 point scale, respectively). It is interesting that nearly all of the therapies, traditional and nontraditional, cited were rated between 4 and 6 on a 10-point scale. This suggests that there is little difference in satisfaction between treatment strategies. It also suggests that no one treatment is likely to please every person and that some trial and error is necessary to find the right strategy for an individual.

Medication usage is common among people diagnosed with fibromyalgia. All of the medications that were rated as helpful by more than 60% of the respondents were opiate narcotics such as hydrocodone and oxycodone or sedatives such as Valium® and Xanax®. Ibuprofen was rated as helpful by 51% of survey participants and was rated highest among the over-the-counter analgesics. Flexeril, described by most as a "muscle relaxant," was rated as helpful by 58% of participants. Anti-depressants such as Prozac® and Wellbutrin® were rated negatively and felt to be helpful in about 30% to 40%. Gabapentin (Neurontin®) a commonly prescribed anti-seizure medication and analgesic, was also not rated as helpful by a majority.

Where does this leave the person with fibromyalgia when approaching treatment?

Certainly, a few commonsense generalizations can be made. If there are signs of an associated psychiatric, orthopedic, or rheumatological disorder, it should be aggressively treated. Signs of depression should be evaluated by an appropriate professional and medication or cognitive therapies prescribed. Although signs of an underlying rheumatological or orthopedic disorder are often hard to separate from the pain and tenderness of fibromyalgia, careful examination of any new or predominant symptom should be performed and only attributed to fibromyalgia after appropriate and reasonable evaluation is completed.

An effort should be made to minimize stressors to the fullest extent possible. A careful assessment of interpersonal and financial problems should be done and solved when possible. This may involve family, financial, or marital counseling. Spirituality is something that many people find helpful. Even in people who are not spiritual, having a sense of purpose in life helps people find meaning in things even pain. This can make discomfort easier to tolerate.

A regular, realistic, and consistent aerobic and stretching program promotes weight loss and helps to combat pain. The goals of such a plan should be improvement of flexibility, aerobic conditioning, weight loss, and increasing stamina. The specific activity should not aggravate fatigue or pain symptoms. Certainly, positive interaction and participation with a friend or family member will improve consistency in a fitness program. In the best circumstance, the activity should be something that the person truly enjoys. Beginning the program at a level that can be reliably completed is better than overdoing it because this can actually worsen the symptoms and frustrate a person living with fibromyalgia.

Ensuring an adequate amount of uninterrupted sleep is vital. Avoiding excessive caffeine or caffeine before bedtimes can promote this. Other good sleep habits such as avoiding working or reading in bed, long midday naps, or strenuous exercise late in the evening are also helpful. Reserve the bed area as a place for sleep rather than a work area or place to iron out marital difficulties. Sleeping medications are not a substitute for good sleep hygiene, but can be used for short periods to promote a regular sleep routine. Remember that most sleep medications are addictive sedatives with considerable possible side effects if taken for a long period.

A well-balanced diet high in fiber, fruit, and vegetables, and low in saturated fats, simple carbohydrates, and salt will promote weight loss and improve many of the other medical problems such as diabetes and hypertension common in people with fibromyalgia. For unclear reasons, obesity is often associated with fibromyalgia. Interestingly, two studies have shown a remarkable decrease in pain and tender points in people after they undergo bariatric surgery.[14][15] Weight loss may give equivalent results.

Medications and other medical treatments are helpful as an adjunct, but are not cures for fibromyalgia. The use of narcotics for long-term chronic pain control is associated with a decrease in tolerance of pain. Some pain researchers have found that narcotics provide little if any improvement in important factors such as quality of life and social function.

COMPLEX REGIONAL PAIN SYNDROME

Complex regional pain syndrome (CRPS) is a condition in which pain is experienced within an extremity that is vastly out of proportion to the injury and usually involves a single region of the body such as a foot or hand. The pain is often so severe that it may cause the person to avoid any contact of the extremity to the point of making examination difficult. As the older name, reflex sympathetic dystrophy or RSD, suggests it is associated with signs of increased sympathetic sensitivity. The sympathetic nervous system is a set of nerves that use adrenalin and its related substances as a neurotransmitter. This system is often referred to as the *fight or flight* mechanism because it is most known for its ability to prepare the body to defend itself. The signs of sympathetic stimulation and sensitivity that are often seen with CRPS are temperature changes, sweating, swelling, and abnormal regulation of blood vessel dilation often resulting in bluish or purplish discoloration. With time, the effects of the nerve dysfunction compounded by the lack of usage lead to wasting of the muscle, demineralization of the bone, contractures of the joints, and shiny tight skin. Loss of hair in the extremity is also common. It is important to realize that this syndrome is not the same for everyone experiencing it. It affects about 0.03% of the population.

Cases of CRPS typically last for years or decades. Most people with CRPS are 35 to 45 years old and women are predominantly affected by a 4 to 1 margin. An injury such as a fracture, sprain, contusion, or surgery is usually what begins the syndrome. Twenty percent of people with CRPS will develop it spontaneously. Numerous cases of CRPS have been reported to run within families and people who have developed CRPS are much more likely to develop it in another extremity after a second trauma.

The cause of CRPS is unknown, but many of the topics that we have discussed above including increased production of adrenalin receptors by the nerve cells and intensification and enhanced efficiency of pain pathways through plasticity has been implicated. Evidence points to changes in multiple areas of the nervous system including the peripheral nerves, connections within the spine spinal and reorganization of sensory perception within the cerebral cortex that lead to the pain. Inflammatory factors and changes within the neurologic system have also been suggested.

There are no currently available laboratory tests to diagnose CRPS. Typical radiographic tests used in CRPS such as MRIs and bone scans commonly demonstrate the changes in blood flow, bone activity, and swelling that are associated with CRPS. It is difficult to say whether any of the changes commonly seen help to define the best approach for treating the disorder, but can be used to rule out other problems such as fractures that may be difficult to see on routine x-rays, serious ligamentous damage, or tumors.

Functional MRIs (MRI studies enhanced with chemicals that illuminate the brain's activity) of the brain show specific changes in the manner in which the brain perceives pain after the development of CRPS and are related to the degree of pain that is experienced. These changes have also been reported in fibromyalgia. Studies looking into these changes are enhancing the knowledge of CRPS and may sometimes lead to better treatment or, better yet, prevention of this disorder.

Many of the techniques outlined in the fibromyalgia section apply to CRPS. Depression and sleep disorders are common in both problems. There is little quality medical scientific study that is helpful in guiding treatment of CRPS. Medications commonly prescribed include steroids, opiates, as well as many other classes of medications and typically have disappointing to mediocre results. In an effort to reduce bone metabolic hyperactivity, many agents commonly used in the treatment of osteoporosis such as calcitonin (usually administered as a nasal spray) and bisphosphonates (such as Fosamax® and Boniva®) are used and have demonstrated some success in treatment. Despite the implication that the sympathetic system is involved in the production of CRPS symptoms, medications that can be used to block the effects of adrenaline have not been helpful in alleviating symptoms.

Direct interruption of the sympathetic nerves that lie along the side of the spinal vertebrae by using anesthetic injection has been a technique used for decades in the treatment of CRPS. There is scientific support for this, but the number, timing, and indications for the injections is still not clear. Most of the study to date has involved the upper extremity with much less investigation on lumbar sympathetic blocks for the lower extremity. Sympathetic nerve blocks used preoperatively in people who must undergo surgery and have a history of CRPS are effective at lowering the rate of aggravation of this problem. Permanent destruction of the sympathetic nerves either by surgical stripping of these nerves from the arteries or by chemical or thermal damage of the sympathetic nerve cell bodies or ganglia along the spine is also sometimes done. Spinal stimulation through the use of an electronic electrical device is used in cases that fail to respond to other forms of treatment.

One of the more exciting forms of treatment currently being evaluated and thus still somewhat experimental is the use of ketamine. Ketamine is an inhibitor of glutamate in an important cell membrane receptor in pain nerve cells and it also has an effect on opiod cell receptors. Unfortunately, it is also a controlled substance and has a history of recreational abuse. In some small pilot studies, it has been reported to have an impressive and long-lasting effect on pain in CRPS. Further study is necessary before it can be recommended.

AIDS

- HIV/AIDS has become a chronic disease with long-term survival in modern society.
- People with HIV/AIDS commonly suffer from nerve damage that may be caused by the virus, the drug treatment or both.
- HIV neuropathy can be difficult to treat.
- People with HIV/AIDS are prone to many exotic and common infectious diseases.

Acquired immunodeficiency syndrome or AIDS is a disease that hampers the immunity by destroying a variety of white blood cells. It is transferred from person to person by contact with bodily fluids. A virus call human immunodeficiency virus (HIV) causes it.

The disease in its epidemic form was first recognized in 1977 although there is evidence that it has been around for much longer. Currently, there are about 40 million people worldwide with HIV and more than one million in the United States. Although HIV/AIDS has in the past been considered fatal, new treatment techniques and medication protocols now allow people with HIV/AIDS to live long, productive lives. The life expectancy for a person newly diagnosed with HIV infection is more than twenty years. This amounts to a major victory in medical science. However, it poses problems because these people present unique medical challenges that must be treated and managed indefinitely.

Although HIV/AIDS is a systemic infection, there are many ways in which the foot can be affected. Perhaps the most common effect is in damage to the nerves or neuropathy. Twenty to 40% of people infected with HIV/AIDs have neuropathy. The most common manifestation of this is painful peripheral neuropathy. The symptoms of this problem are tingling, numbness, and burning pain that can be extreme. Muscle weakness and even joint breakdown has been reported.

The cause of HIV associated peripheral neuropathy is not yet known. The virus is known to infect nerve tissue directly. Damage to mitochondrial DNA has been implicated. Mitochondria are small structures within our cells that generate energy. Damage to these structures in the nerve cells may starve the cells of energy and leave the nerves unable to function.

Although HIV drugs are nothing short of a huge breakthrough in the treatment of HIV, they are very strong medicines with significant side effects. Many of these drugs work by interfering with viral DNA production within the infected cells. However, it can also affect normal DNA synthesis in the body's own cells. The potentially toxic effect of HIV drugs on nerves has been evaluated, but the findings are inconclusive. In some studies, exposure to HIV drugs is associated with neuropathy and in others, no correlation could be found. The neuropathy seems to be associated with a decreased CD4+count, implying that it is more common in people with advanced destruction of their immune system.

HIV neuropathy is more difficult to treat than many other neuropathies. Many drugs that work on other neuropathies including gabapentin, pregabalin, and amitryptaline have been found to have little effect on HIV neuropathy. High-potency capsaicin cream and marijuana are currently being studied and seem to show promise in controlling the symptoms. There are no current studies on the effectiveness of opiod pain medications or duloxetine specifically in HIV neuropathy.

The other major HIV complication in the foot is due to suppression of the immune system. People suffering from AIDS are extremely prone to infections. Infected ulcerations and bone infections from a variety of uncommon organisms such as tuberculosis and fungi are possible. Skin warts caused by papalloma virus can grow out of control. Onchyomycosis, a nail infection that results in discoloration and thickening, is much more common in people with HIV. Certain otherwise rare cancers such as Kaposi's sarcoma can be found on the feet as in other parts of the body. Any unusual skin lesion should be evaluated carefully by a knowledgeable physician.

THE EVERYWHERE FOOT PAIN

This is perhaps the primary motivation for the creation of this book. It is a common problem seen in a foot clinic and is one of the most frustrating problems for physicians and patients alike. People with this disorder often inaccurately are diagnosed with fibromyalgia, reflex sympathetic dystrophy, chronic fatigue syndrome, and neuropathy (even when their nerve tests are normal). Often, they are ignored and put off. Even worse, they are inappropriately (by physicians with the best of intentions) surgically reconstructed for the symptoms of the problem when the underlying condition is ignored.

Roxanne's Story

Roxanne had been to many physicians who had ordered x-rays, MRIs, and other tests over the years. She had had a plantar fasciotomy, a surgery to treat plantar fasciitis heel pain. Since then, she had been to physical therapy twice and had three separate pairs of orthotics. None it had done any good.

She was having problems at work, too. Her boss was initially sympathetic to her problem and had allowed her unscheduled time off when the pain was really bad. However, she was getting the feeling that his patience was wearing thin.

Finally, the question was asked, "Where does it hurt?"

"Oh, everywhere." Her hand waved to the ball of the foot, arch, heel, around the ankle, and up the back of her calf.

The "Everywhere Foot Pain" is a vexing, but common, problem. A host of diagnoses are often offered to explain the pains and even surgical solutions are sometimes suggested or carried out in the hope of getting a handle on the problem. However, this is where the physician and the patient needs to stop concentrating on the foot and look at the person attached to the foot. A head-to-toe evaluation is necessary, because the problem is rarely solely the foot.

There are several problems that can present as "Everywhere Foot Pain":

- Neurological problems
    - Lumbar radiculopathies—"pinched nerves in the back," "slipped discs" (a very rare cause of foot pain).
    - Compression on the peripheral nerves such as tarsal tunnel syndrome (usually associated with characteristic tingling).
    - Peripheral neuropathy most commonly from diabetes.
    - Complex regional pain syndrome.
    - Fibromyalgia.
- Rheumatological problems

• Almost any of them, but they're usually obvious by swelling in the joints.

• Neuropathic/diabetic arthropathy (aka Charcot arthropathy), also usually obvious if worked up properly.

• Forefoot overload syndrome.

Forefoot overload syndrome alone makes up a majority of the cases. Many more are caused from multiple problems such as fibromyalgia and forefoot overload syndrome. The remaining few are a smattering of other diagnosis with a liberal number in the "unknown" category.

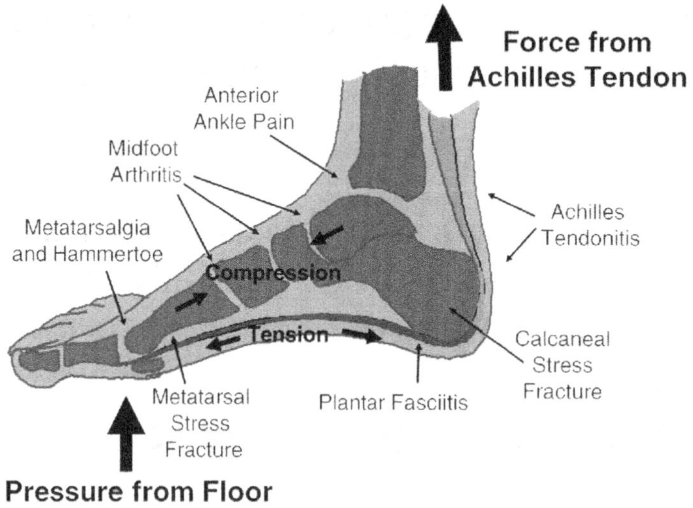

FIGURE 9.11 Common areas for pain in forefoot overload syndrome.

We bring back this figure from Chapter 3. Forefoot overload syndrome affects multiple areas in the foot.

Sometimes it seems like a house of cards. One problem leads to another, that leads to another.

When it comes to MRIs and other radiographic tests, unless the findings fit the symptoms, it is likely to be unrelated to the problem. When a great deal of fluid or swelling is localized around the joints, rheumatological tests, or better, an evaluation by a rheumatologist is reasonable.

If a specific diagnosis (not diagnoses) or nerve disorder is found, the treatment should be directed toward this problem. If no specific disorder is found, the principles of treatment have been reviewed several times in this book:

- Weight loss.
- Postural training.
- Regular stretching and conditioning exercises.
- Firm rocker-soled shoes.
- Occasionally, over-the-counter arch supports, sometimes and temporarily heel lifts.
- Minimize the medications especially the narcotics.
- *Very, very rarely* surgical reconstruction.

NOTES

[1] Kujala UM, Sarna S, Kaprio J. Cumulative incidence of Achilles tendon rupture and

tendinopathy in male former elite athletes. *Clin J Sport Med.* 2005 May;15(3):133–135.

[2] Dorr LD. Arthritis and athletics. *Clin Sports Med.* 1991 Apr;10(2):343–357.

[3] Evans AM, Scutter SD. Prevalence of "growing pains" in young children. *J Pediatr.* 2004 Aug;145(2):255–258.

[4] Bishop JL, Northstone K, Emmett PM, Golding J. Parental accounts of the prevalence, causes and treatments of limb pain in children aged 5 to 13 years: A longitudinal cohort study. *Arch Dis Child.* 2010 Sep 30.

[5] Viswanathan V, Khubchandani RP. Joint hypermobility and growing pains in school children. *Clin Exp Rheumatol.* 2008 Sep-Oct;26(5):962–966.

[6] Uziel Y, Hashkes PJ. Growing pains in children. *Pediatr Rheumatol Online J. 2007* Apr 19;5:5.

[7] Eastwood DM, Menelaus MB, Dickens DR, Broughton NS, Cole WG. Idiopathic toe-walking: does treatment alter the natural history? *J Pediatr Orthop* B. 2000 Jan;9(1):47–49.

[8] [No authors listed] The effect of intensive treatment of diabetes on the development and progression of long-term complications in insulin-dependent diabetes mellitus. The Diabetes

Control and Complications Trial Research Group. *N Engl J Med.* 1993 Sep 30;329(14):977–986.

[9] Schaff PS, Cavanagh PR. Shoes for the insensitive foot: The effect of a "rocker bottom" shoe modification on plantar pressure distribution. *Foot Ankle.* 1990 Dec;11(3):129–140.

[10] Praet SF, Louwerens JW. The influence of shoe design on plantar pressures in neuropathic feet. *Diabetes Care.* 2003 Feb;26(2):441–445.

[11] Melzack R, Wall PD. Pain mechanisms: a new theory. *Science.* 1965 Nov 19;150(699):971–9.

[12] Harvey CK. Fibromyalgia. Part II. Prevalence in the podiatric patient population. *J Am Podiatr Med Assoc.* 1993 Jul;83(7):416–417.

[13] Bennett RM, Jones J, Turk DC, Russell IJ, Matallana L. An internet survey of 2,596 people with fibromyalgia. *BMC Musculo Disorders.* 2007;8:27.

[14] Hooper MM, Stellato TA, Hallowell PT, Seitz BA Moskowitz RW. Musculoskeletal findings in obese subjects before and after weight loss following bariatric surgery. *Int J Obes (Lond).* 2007 Jan;31(1):114–120.

[15] Saber AA, Boros MJ, Mancl T, Elgamal MH, Song S, Wisadrattanapong T. The effect of laparoscopic Roux-en-Y gastric bypass on

fibromyalgia. *Obes Surg.* 2008 Jun;18(6):652-625.

10

Rehabilitation for the Foot

Exercise therapy is an incredibly useful tool to treat foot pain and other foot disorders. The work that you put into your rehabilitative program will pay off, but the treatment success will not happen without consistent dedication to your routine. No one else can do it for you. The rewards of this hard work are reduced pain, fewer injuries in the future, and avoiding the pain, debility, and risk of complications inherent in surgery. This chapter guides you through a rehabilitation program designed to treat the most common foot problems.

When committing to a rehabilitative program for a foot problem, the course of treatment should span a period of months. It will require weeks to months to accomplish the goals of treatment such as improvements in strengthening muscles, improving flexibility, and balance. Although some improvement may occur quickly, a rehabilitative program must accomplish some of these goals before the pain will subside. Stopping the program prematurely can result in recurrence of the problem.

Before beginning any rehabilitation program, it is always best to consult with your physician and physical therapist, as there may be conditions that make it difficult or dangerous to perform some of these exercises. This book is not a substitute for careful physical examination and medical evaluation. It is meant to supplement what your physician and therapist may not have covered with you.

REHABILITATION FOR FOOT OVERLOAD SYNDROMES

Stretching exercises are a key element of the rehabilitation of many chronic foot problems. These exercises are directed toward improving posture and treating contractures that are associated with these disorders. Optimally, they should be done three times a day. The set should take about fifteen minutes to complete.

Stretching

Neck twist: The head should begin looking forward with the head centered over the shoulders. Roll the head maximally from one shoulder to the other in a circle, contacting the back of the head to the neck, and chin to the chest. First, in a clockwise then counterclockwise fashion. Often clasping your hands while extending your elbows behind your back can make it easier to avoid shrugging, which decreases the effectiveness of the stretch. Do three rotations.

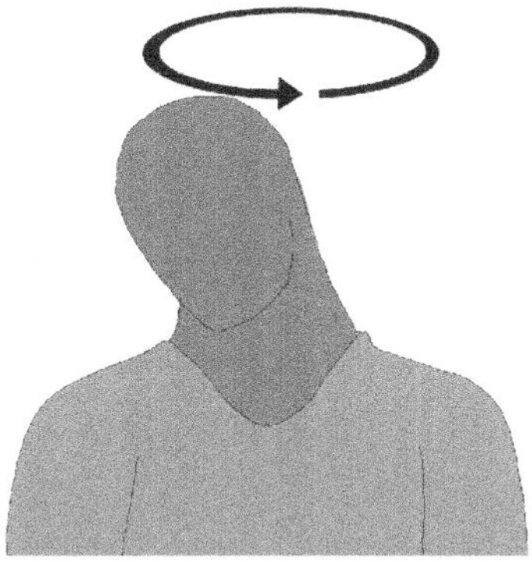

FIGURE 10.1 Neck twist

Crossover shoulder stretch: Extend the arm straight in front of you with the elbow, wrist, and fingers extended. Then cross the arm over the body, using the opposite arm to increase the stretch in the back of the shoulder by pulling the arm closer to the other shoulder. Repeat with the other shoulder. This stretch loosens up the periscapular muscles and the posterior capsule of the shoulder joint. Hold for 10 seconds, repeating two times with each shoulder.

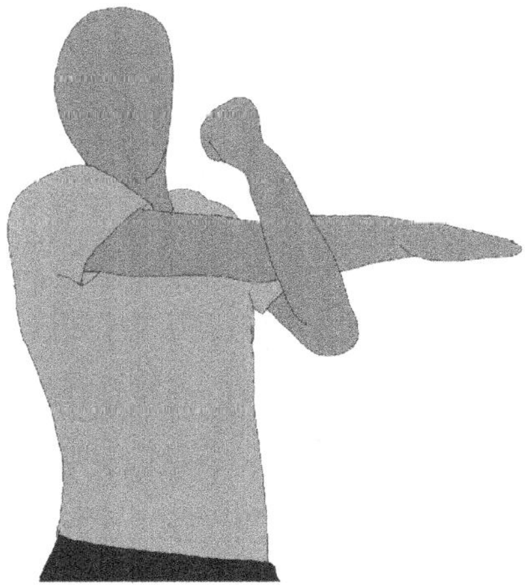

FIGURE 10.2 Crossover shoulder stretch

Shoulder rolls: Begin to roll the shoulders maximally down, forward, up, and back in a circular motion, taking approximately five seconds to complete a revolution. Repeat reversing the sequence. This continues to work on the muscles around the scapula and warms up the trapezial muscles. Do three rotations.

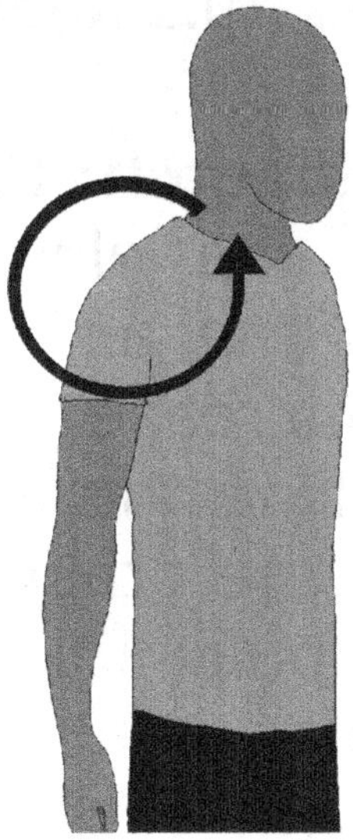

FIGURE 10.3 Shoulder rolls

Scapular stretch: Clasp your hands behind your back, initially with your elbows bent, palms together, and fingers intertwined. Gradually, extend your elbows, drop your hands toward your buttock and close your palms together, drawing your shoulder blades together. This stretch works on the anterior shoulder capsule and the periscapular muscles. Hold for 10 seconds, repeating two times.

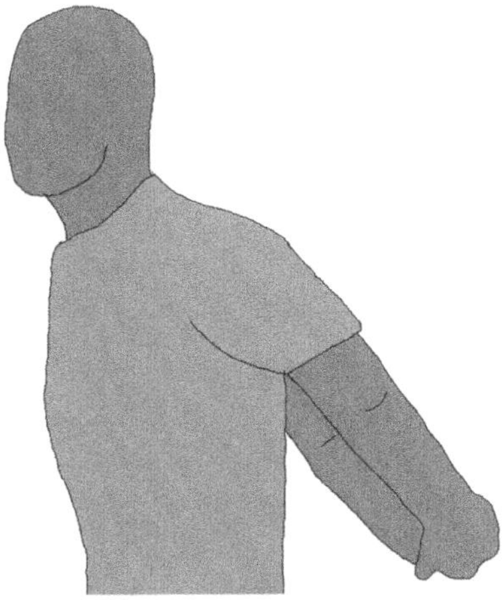

FIGURE 10.4 Scapular stretch

Lumbar stretch: Get on your hands and knees. Initially, pull the middle of your back as high as possible, like a hissing cat. Then allow the back to drop, simultaneously extending your neck. Each repetition should take 10 seconds. Repeat two times. With this exercise, we are beginning to get the back moving and getting used to using the lumbar flexors and extensors.

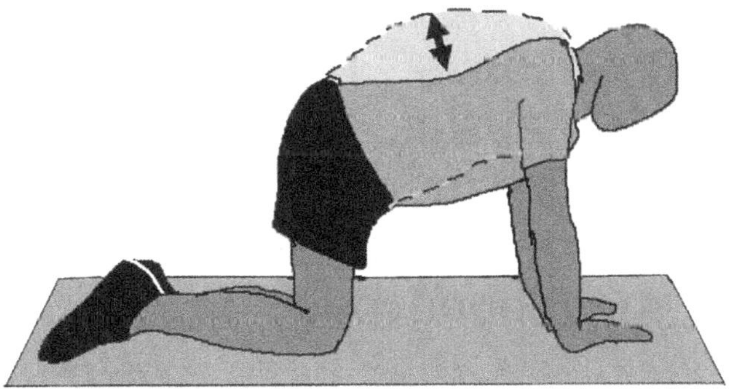

FIGURE 10.5 Lumbar stretch

Hip stretch: Begin on your knees extending your hips and back until resistance or pain is felt. Maintain position for 10 seconds, repeating two times. This is an excellent stretch for the back, shoulders, and front of the hip.

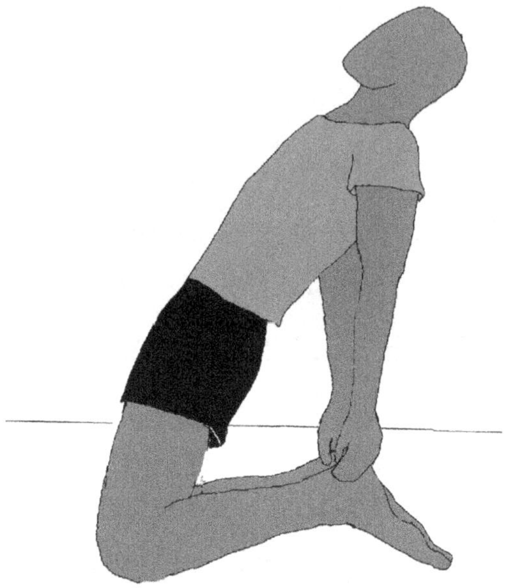

FIGURE 10.6 Hip stretch

Figure four stretch: Lie on your back with your knees bent. Place one ankle on the opposite knee, allowing the knee on the side being stretched to drop toward the ground as much as possible. Hold the position for 10 seconds, repeating two times. This stretches the hip capsule and the adductor muscles along the inside of the thigh. For an extra stretch, tuck both legs into the chest while maintaining the legs in earlier mentioned position.

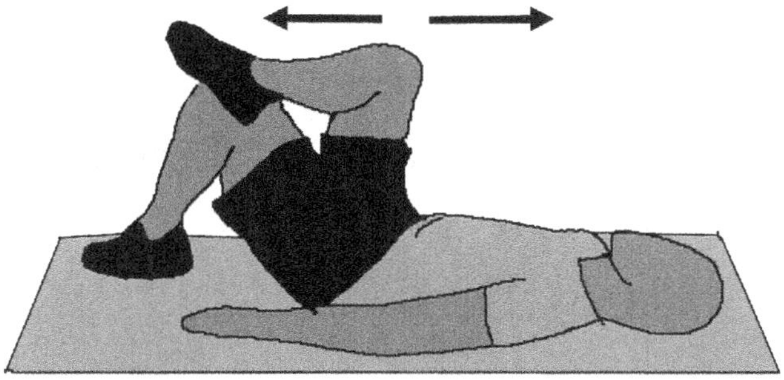

FIGURE 10.7 Figure four stretch

Hamstring stretch: Lie on the ground with knees extended in front of your body. Flex the hip, keeping the knee straight and the ankle extended. If possible touch the toe or calf. Alternatively, this can be done in the standing position by touching the toe or grasping the knee or calf while keeping the knee straight. The stretch can be done both with back and neck extended to increase the pull on the hamstring. This stretch works on the hamstring, the posterior hip capsule, back, and neck depending on the method. Repeat three times, holding the position for 10 seconds.

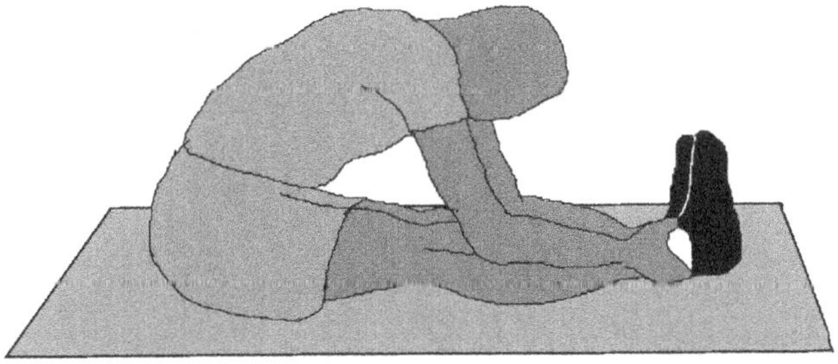

FIGURE 10.8 Hamstring stretch

Outer thigh stretch: Place on heel over the contralateral thigh. Twist the contralateral hand over the knee and onto the contralateral knee or calf.

Gently press the knee over the contralateral thigh, stretching the hip. Hold for 10 seconds and repeat, alternating legs two times. This stretch focuses on the lateral hip muscles especially the iliotibial band.

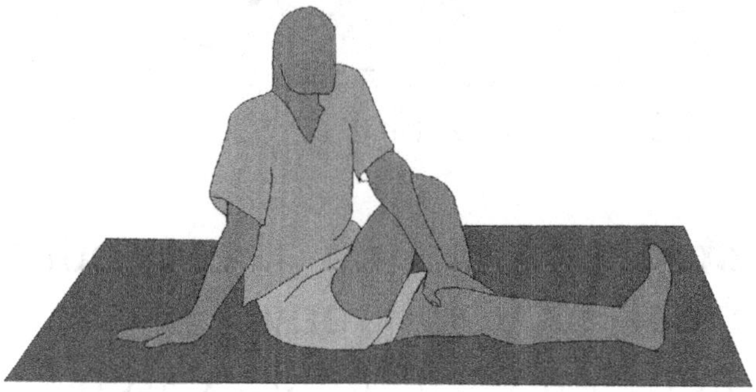

FIGURE 10.9 Outer thigh stretch

Inner thigh stretch: Begin on your hands and knee. Gradually, widen your knees, allowing your pelvis to approach the floor with your hips and knees at a right angle. When pain or firm resistance is felt, maintain the position for 10 seconds, repeating two times. This stretches the hip adductors and flexors.

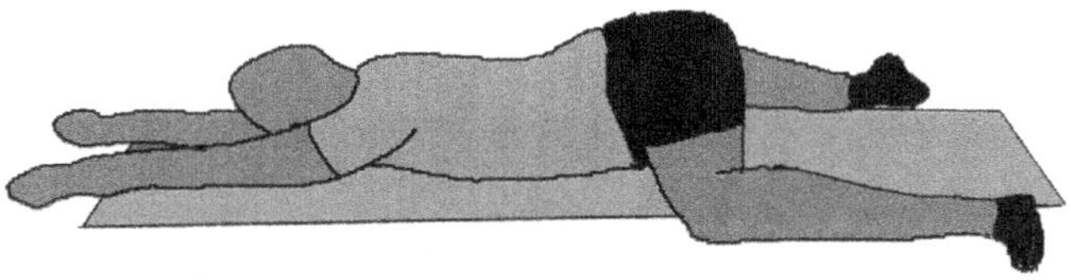

FIGURE 10.10 Inner thigh stretch

Calf stretch: Stand near a wall or other sturdy surface and place both hands on the wall. Extend one or both legs behind you and extend the ankles maximally, keeping the heel firmly on the floor and feeling a pull in the back of the calves. The toes should be pointing straight ahead or slightly to the midline. Maintain this position for 10 seconds, alternating feet and repeating two times.

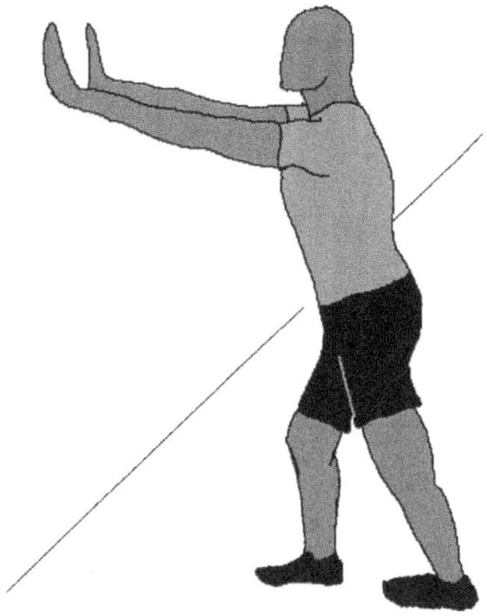

FIGURE 10.11 Calf stretch

Arch stretch: Stand approximately 12 inches in front of a sturdy wall and place the foot against the wall, extending the big and smaller toes at the MTP joint. Lean toward the wall until a stretch is felt in the posterior calf and arch. Hold for 10 seconds and repeat with the other side. Repeat two times with each leg. This stretch isolates the plantar fascia although it works as well on the Achilles.

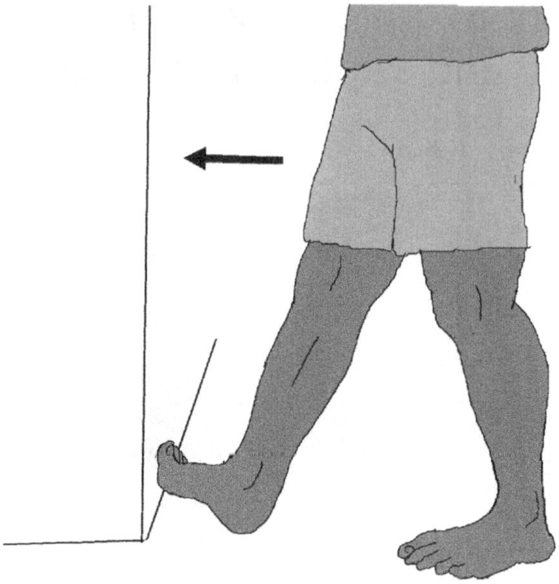

FIGURE 10.12 Arch stretch

STRENGTHENING EXERCISES

Poor conditioning both within the foot and throughout the leg from the back to the ankle leads to fatigue and overuse of the ligaments and joints in the foot. If it can be tolerated, these exercises should be done barefooted to improve balance and to work the small foot muscles. The strengthening program should be done three to five time a week and should take twenty to thirty minutes. Begin with the level one exercises and progress as you can tolerate.

Level I

Superman: Begin on stomach with arms in front of you. Extend back and legs, keeping arms extended parallel to head. Hold for 15 seconds and repeat three times. This strengthens that hip, back, and neck extensors.

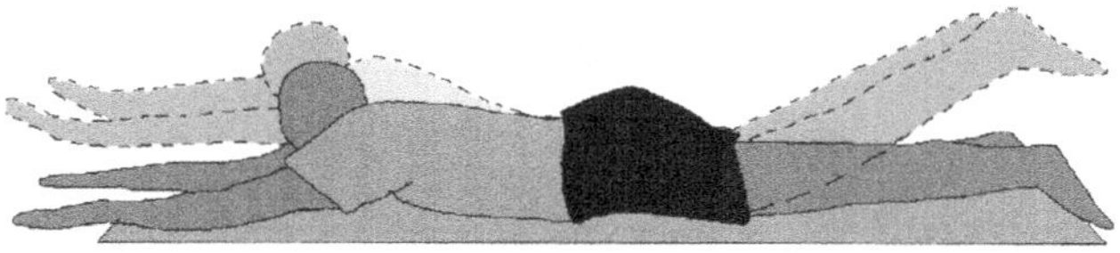

FIGURE 10.13 Superman

Abdominal crunch: Lie on your back with your knees partially bent. Locking your feet under an immobile object such as a couch is optional. Flex your trunk forward essentially drawing your lower rib cage toward your pelvis. Hold your position for three seconds, 30 repetitions. This exercise conditions the abdominal flexors that help centralize abdominal weight and organs.

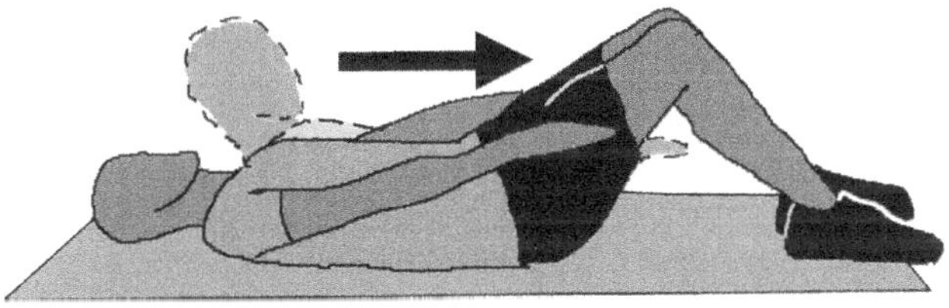

FIGURE 10.14 Abdominal crunch

Hip extensions: Begin this exercise on your hands and knees. Simultaneously and maximally extend your hip while extending your contralateral shoulder and extending your neck. Hold this position for five seconds. Then flex your knee and hip and flex your neck and draw the arm toward your chest. Repeat 15 times with each leg. The hip extensors and muscles around the scapula are both conditioned through this exercise.

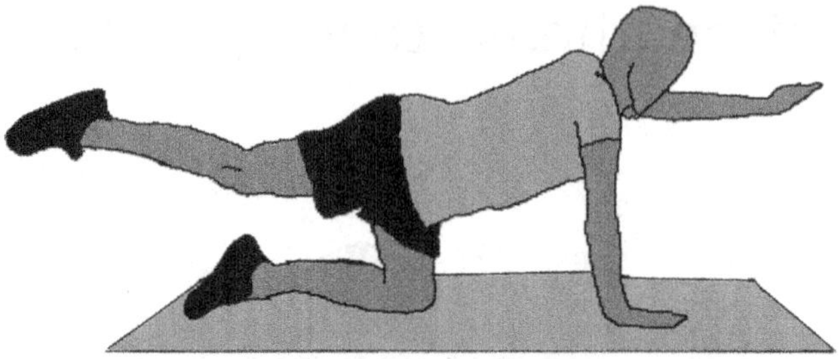

FIGURE 10.15 Hip extensions

Side step up: Stand on a block, stair, or step with one leg. Allow the other to touch the floor. Raise the lower leg up above the level of the other leg so that the waistline alternately tilts down then up. Hold the raised position for three seconds. Work up to 20 repetitions with each leg. This exercise works on the hip abductors that are critical for balance.

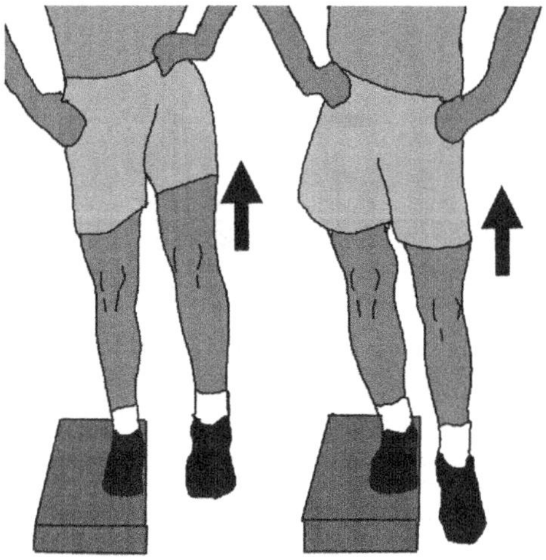

FIGURE 10.16 Side step up

Quad set: While lying on your back, tighten the quadriceps muscle and lock the knee in extension. Lift leg from the hip. Alternatively, place a rolled towel under the knee to support the knee. Hold for five seconds and repeat 20 times with each leg. This exercise works specifically on the quadriceps muscle.

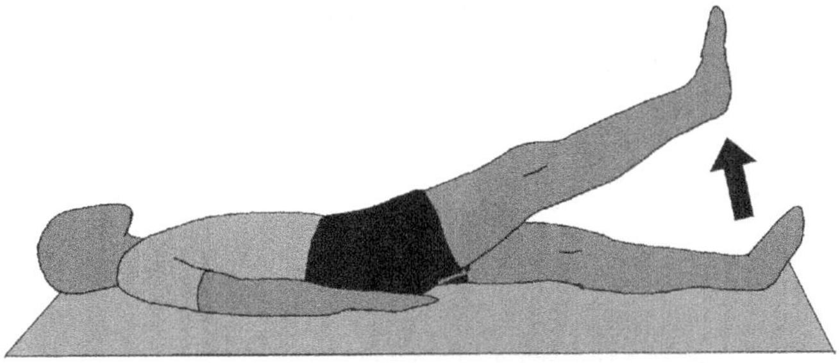

FIGURE 10.17 Quad set

Eccentric calf strengthening: Begin with toes on an elevated surface such as a board about two inches in height. Raise the heel and then, over 10 seconds, slowly lower the heel. Repeat 10 times. Exercises such as this increase the endurance of damaged tendons as well as strengthen the Achilles musculature and the inversion muscles of the ankle.

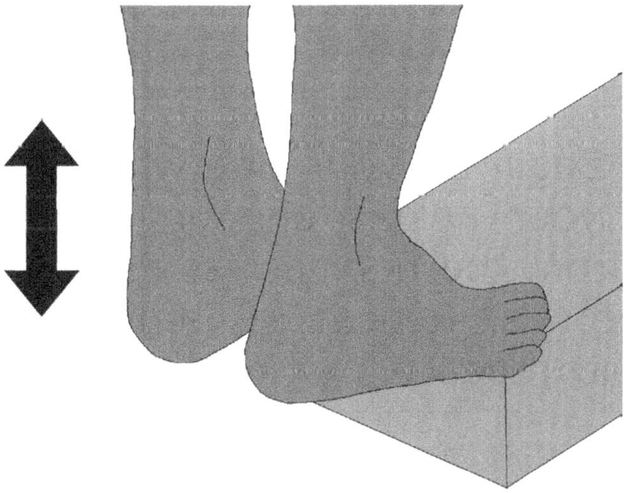

FIGURE 10.18 Eccentric calf strengthening

Toe raises: Begin seated and lift the toes off the floor maximally while keeping the heel on the ground. Hold the toe up for 10 seconds and repeat 10 times. An ankle weight may be wrapped around the foot to add resistance.

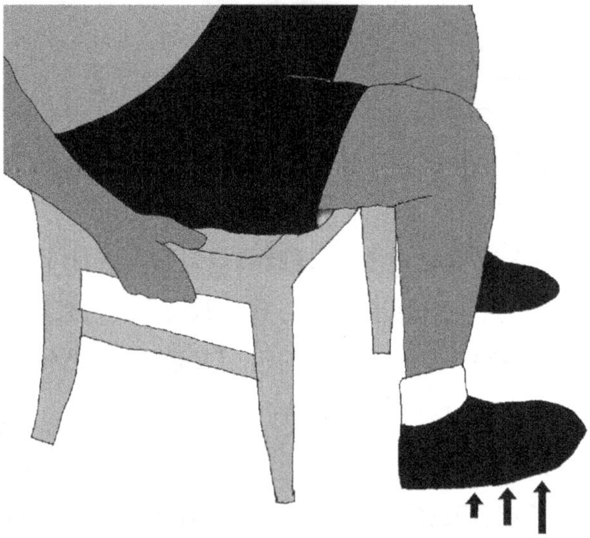

FIGURE 10.19 Toe raises

Level 2

Side plank: Begin on your side while leaning on your elbow. Lock your ankles one on the other. Lift the pelvis away from the floor as far as possible and hold for three seconds. Repeat 15 times, then switch to other side and repeat.

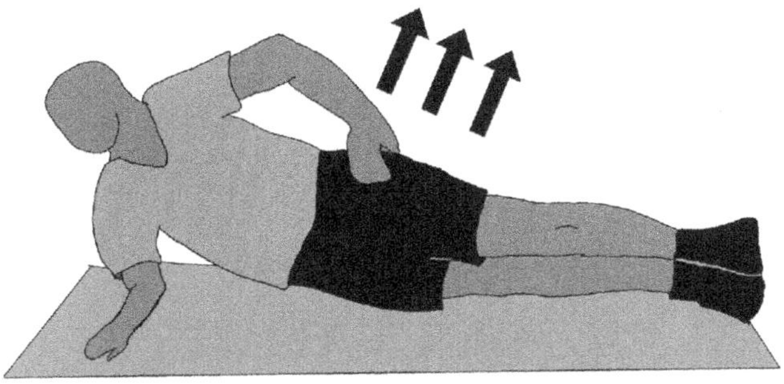

FIGURE 10.20 Side plank

Oblique crunch: Lay on your back with your arms on your hips or behind your head, knees bent. Alternating sides, pull your elbow toward your opposite knee and hold for two or three seconds. Repeat 15 times on each side. This exercise tones the oblique abdominal muscles that pass from the rib cage and lumbar spine to the pelvis.

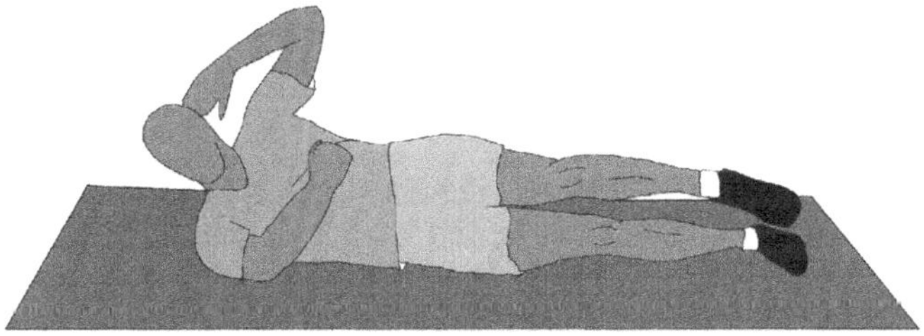

FIGURE 10.21 Oblique crunch

Standing kickbacks: Stand next to a wall, banister, or rail and lean slightly toward it using the wall for support. Extend the hip maximally backward and hold for three seconds. Repeat 15 times on each side. This exercise works out the extensor muscles of the hip and lumbar muscles. It also can help increase balance.

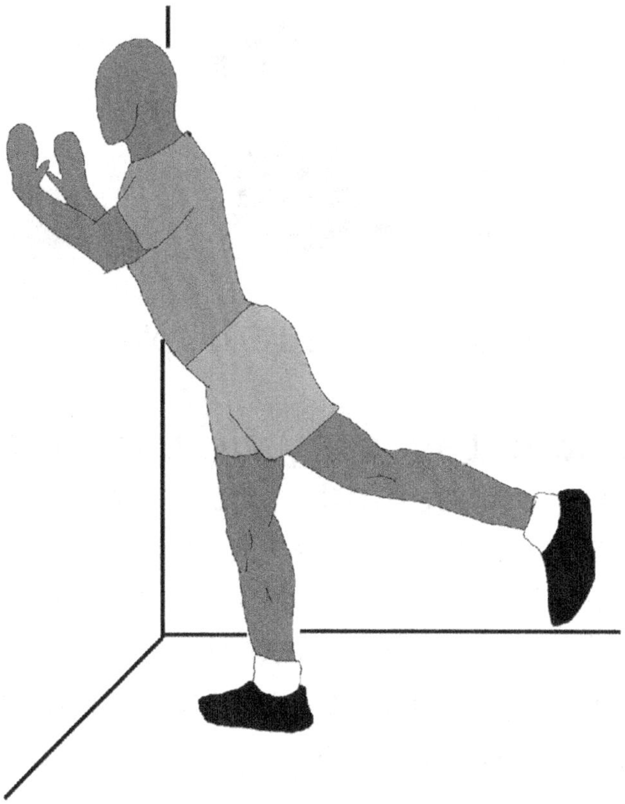

FIGURE 10.22 Standing kickbacks

Lunge: Begin standing. Take a large step forward or backward, and squat down, leaning against the forward leg until the hip and knee are at right angles with the floor. Hold for three seconds. Fifteen repetitions for each side. This helps with quadriceps strength as well as hip extensor strength. It also assists in regaining balance.

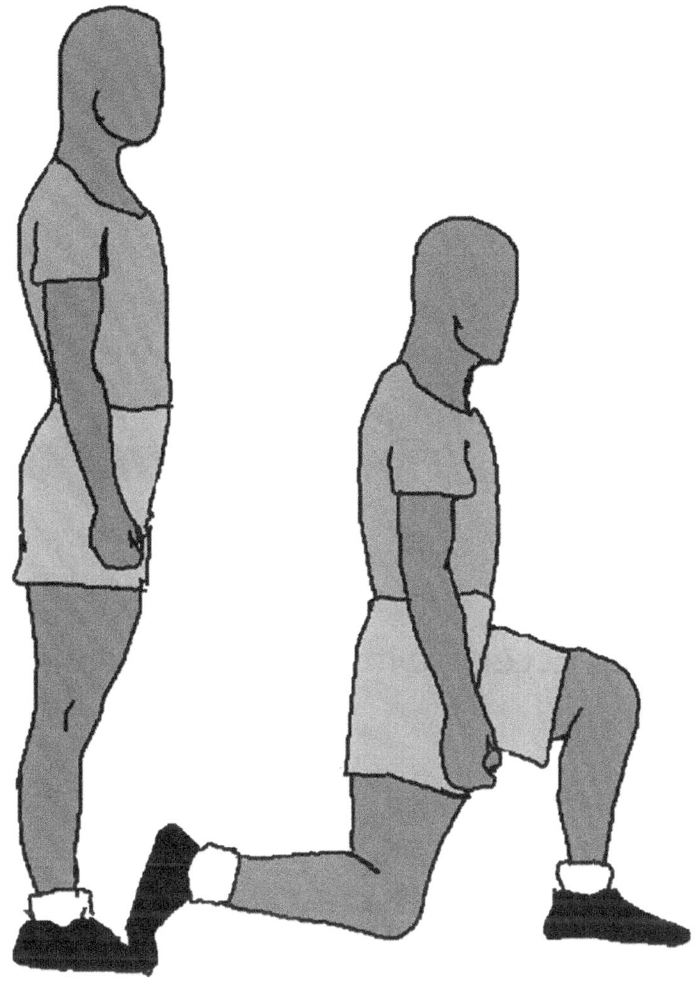

FIGURE 10.23 Lunge

Eccentric inversion, eversion, extension: Using a cable or ankle weight on the forefoot, maximally invert the foot and slowly allow the weight to evert the foot over a 10 count. Repeat 10 timcs. This exercise can also be used to strengthen the eversion and extension muscles by changing the direction of the tension. For eversion muscles, the pull should be from the inside of the foot. For extension muscles, the direction of tension should be the bottom of the foot.

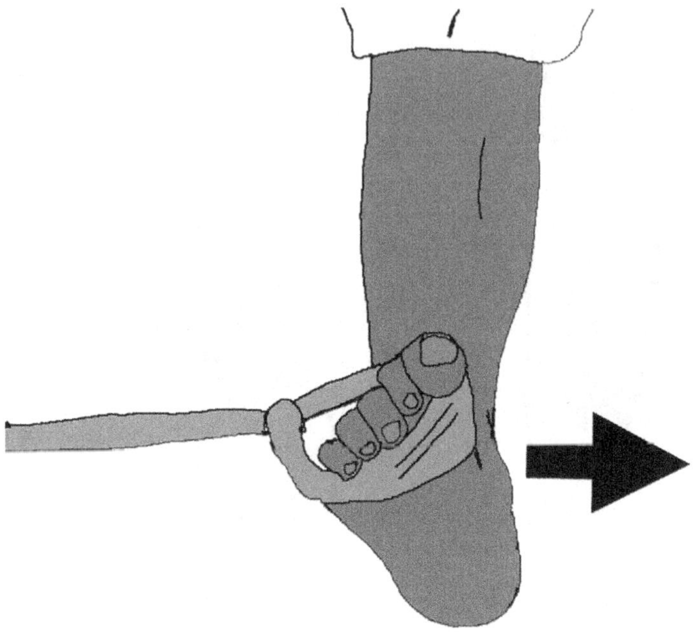

FIGURE 10.24 Eccentric inversion, eversion, extension

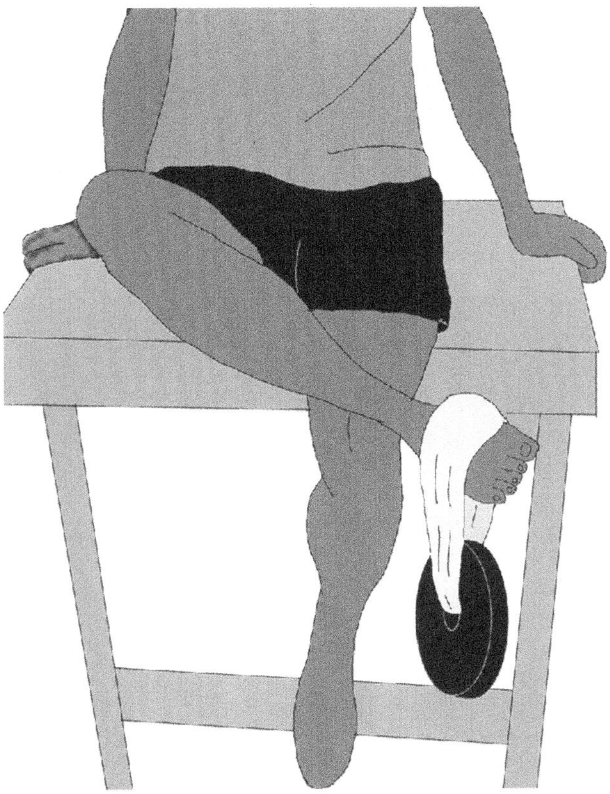

FIGURE 10.25 If a band or cable is unavailable, a free weight or other form of resistance can be used.

Level 3

Wall sit: Lean on the wall with your back and with the feet about two feet from the wall. Lower yourself by flexing the hips and knees until the knee, ankle, and hip are at right angles. Hold this for 30 to 60 seconds. This exercise works the lumbar, abdominal, hip extensors, and quadriceps muscles.

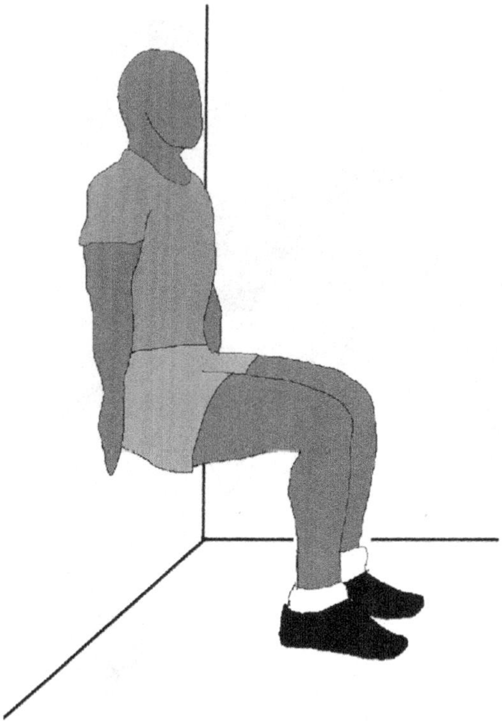

FIGURE 10.26 Wall sit

Tree: While balancing on one foot, bend over at the waist while extending on one leg simultaneously. Keep the ankle flexed as if you are standing against an imaginary wall behind you. Hold for 30 seconds.

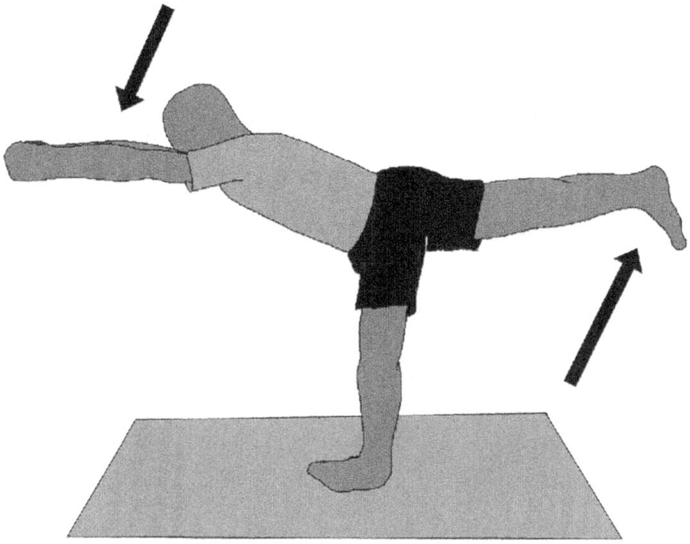

FIGURE 10.27 Tree

Jackknife: Begin this exercise on the floor on your back with the knees partially bent. The more bent the knees, the more difficult it is to use the hip flexors to elevate the torso. Straighten one knee and contract your stomach muscles until you touch that leg. This can be at the knee, ankle, or toe depending on your abilities. Hold for two to three seconds. Alternate legs, doing 30 repetitions. This is a great exercise for the abdominal muscles.

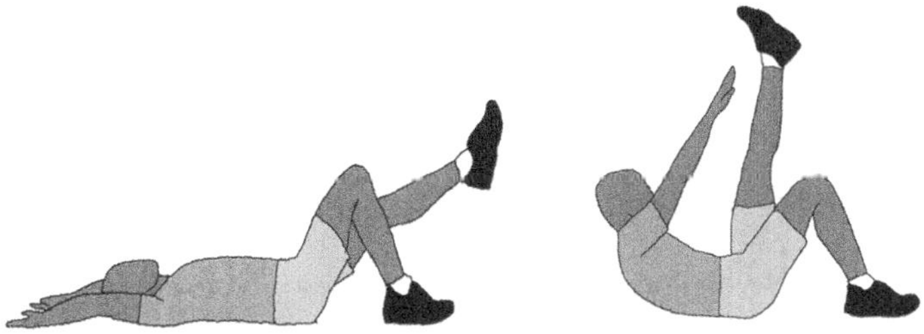

FIGURE 10.28 Jackknife

Side plank: Begin at plank position, which is basically, the "up" position for a push-up. While locking the ankles together, shift your weight on to one shoulder, lifting the other off the ground and extending the elbow. Hold for two to three seconds and return to plank position. Alternate arms and complete 10 repetitions with each arm. This exercise concentrates on the abdominal muscles and the periscapular and back muscles.

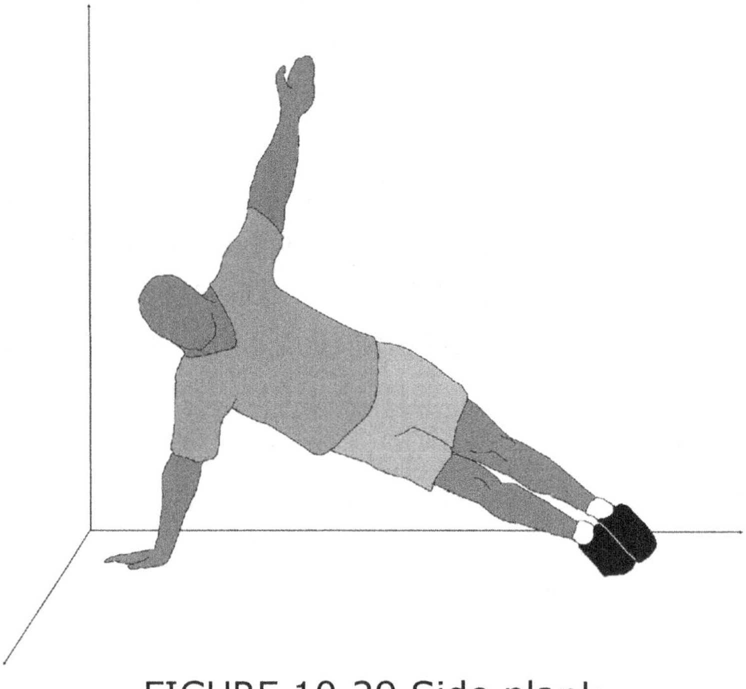

FIGURE 10.29 Side plank

Kneeling knee curl: Begin in kneeling position on knees and palms. Bring the knee and forehead together by flexing the hip, knee, and neck while lifting the leg off the ground. After holding for a second, maximally extend the neck, knee, and hip and hold for two to three seconds. Complete 15 repetitions and repeat on the other side. This works on the hip and neck extensors as well as the quadriceps.

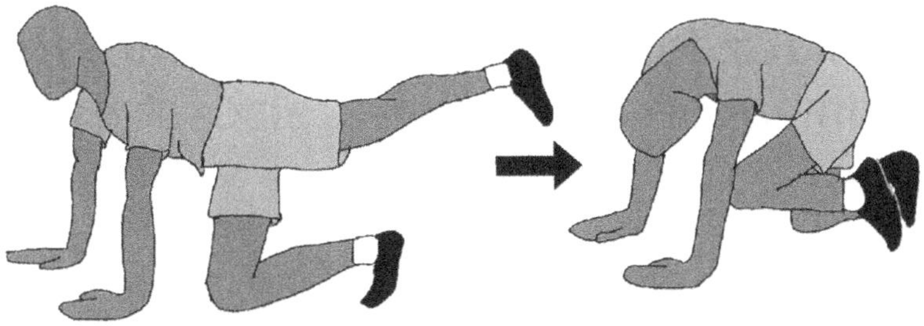

FIGURE 10.30 Kneeling knee curl

Bridge: Begin on your back with the legs bent. Lift your pelvis maximally off the floor, while keeping your shoulders on the floor and relaxing the neck. Hold for five seconds. Repeat 30 times. This is a good exercise for the hip extensors and lumbar muscles in addition to the quadriceps.

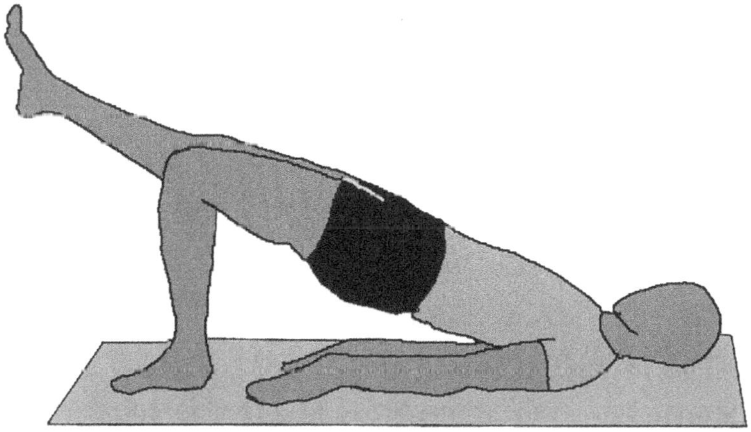

FIGURE 10.31 Bridge

Single leg squat: Begin this exercise facing the step. Lift one leg directly behind you and bend the other. The goal is to bend the weight bearing leg to 90 degrees, but do not go lower than you can comfortably balance. Hold the squatted position for 3 to 10 seconds and work up to 20 repetitions. This exercise works on balance. The quadriceps muscle on the weight bearing side, the lumbar and hip extensors on the nonweight-bearing side are also strengthened.

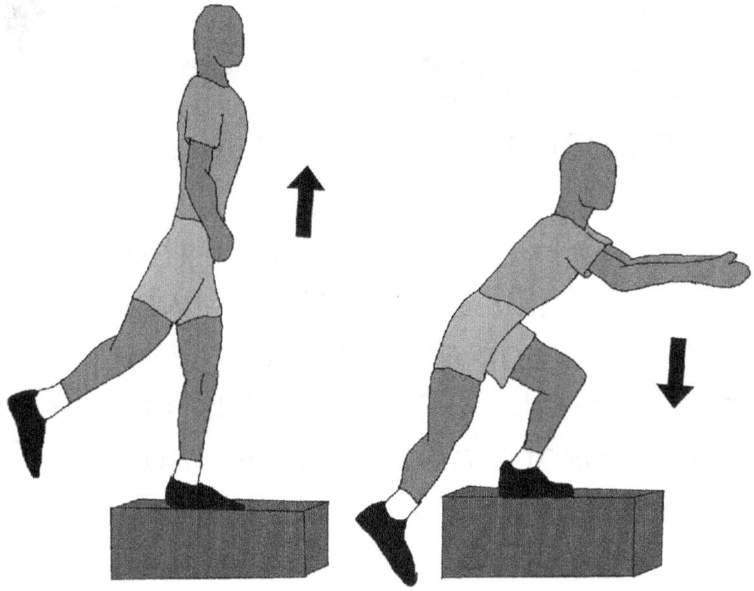

FIGURE 10.32 Single leg squat

Lunge heel raise: Begin in the lunge position with the forward knee bent and the back knee straight. Eighty percent of the weight should be on the forward leg. Keep the torso extended over the pelvis. Flex the foot maximally onto the toes and hold for five seconds. Repeat 10 times. Switch legs and repeat. This exercise focuses on the Achilles musculature.

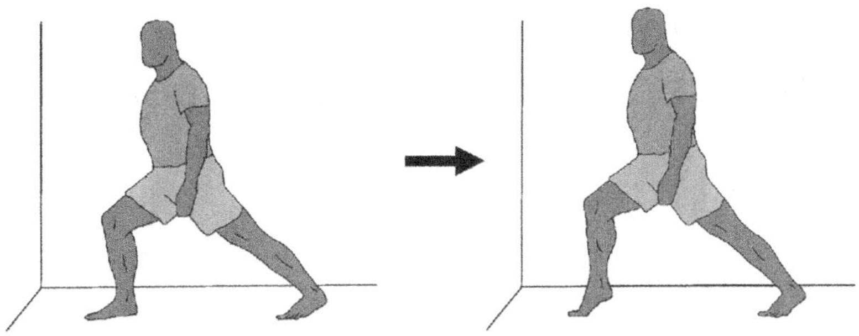

FIGURE 10.33 Lunge heel raise

Lunge toe raise: Once again, begin in the lunge position. Extend the foot and knee together and hold for five seconds. The intensity of this exercise can be increased by leaning forward over the forward leg or by holding weights. This exercise works the quadriceps and extensor muscle of the foot (anterior tibialis) that is crucial for offloading the forefoot.

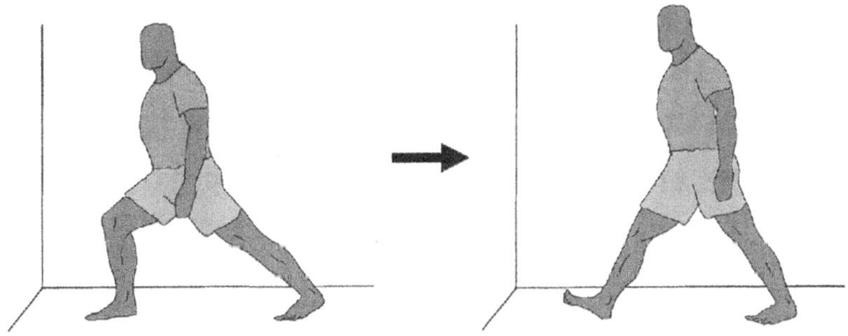

FIGURE 10.34 Lunge toe raise

Pigeon toe raise: Begin this exercise standing with the feet slightly apart. Rotate the feet inward so that the heels are farther apart than the big toes. Maximally raise the heels off the ground and hold for three seconds. Repeat 30 times. Weights in the hands will increase the intensity of this exercise. It works out the Achilles musculature, the inversion muscles of the ankle (posterior tibialis) and the peroneal muscles.

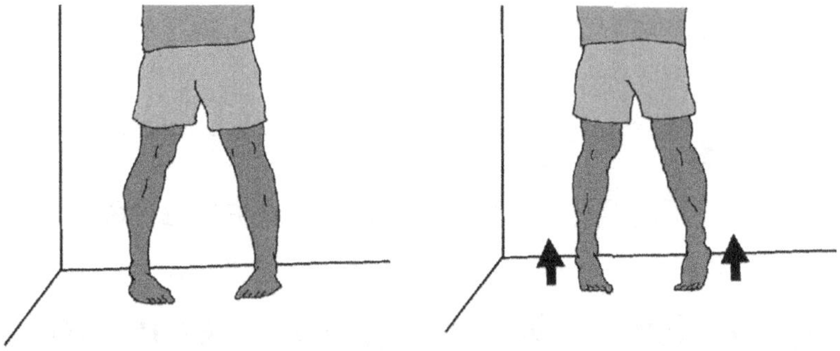

FIGURE 10.35 Pigeon toe raise

BALANCE EXERCISES

Nowhere else is a therapist more helpful than in the treatment of balance and instability disorders. The goal of a therapy program is to train the muscles and the brain to take over the job of the damaged and poorly functioning ligaments. Unfortunately, if the ligaments have healed at a length that is long enough to allow for your ankle to roll easily only surgery is capable of restoring this. That being said, the muscular retraining can help safely and securely allow the foot to be positioned in the proper way so that ankle re-injury is less likely.

In the initial stage of recovering from an ankle sprain, not all exercises are possible. Regaining a comfortable full range of motion is critical to recovery and preventing re-injury. Muscular strengthening exercises in inversion, eversion, flexion, and extension of the ankle should be introduced soon afterward. These initial exercises may incorporate tension such as with ankle weights attached to the foot or elastic bands. The exercises for the later stages of rehabilitation of ankle instability will be shown in this section. Many useful ones have been illustrated in the section above and involve weight-bearing control of the ankle. These include the tree, single leg squat, lunge toe, and heel rise. These can be added to the exercises below. Initially, it may be better to have something to support yourself. A banister on a stair, table, desk, or chair may be useful. Make sure that you have mastered the easy moves before attempting the harder ones. The key is to prevent re-injury.

Other exercise programs that can be useful for control and flexibility after an ankle sprain are yoga, Pilates, and, later, martial arts maneuvers of varying degrees of difficulty. Advanced activities can also include various types of dance aerobics or "boot camp" programs.

Bracing is often helpful early in the treatment of ankle sprains and may be useful when returning to sports after the injury.

Finally, there are instances where, despite aggressive and well-executed rehabilitation, ankle instability continues. Surgical repair of the ligaments can be very helpful in these instances

Step twist, heel raise: This exercise can be done in several ways. It can be begun as a simple double-leg heel raise using the handrail of the stairs as a support and progress to a single-leg heel raise. The full exercise is to rotate on the balls of the foot initially in a clockwise and then in a counterclockwise direction. This helps develop control of ankle motion to the inside and outside as well as improving strength and endurance. Do this 10 to 20 times.

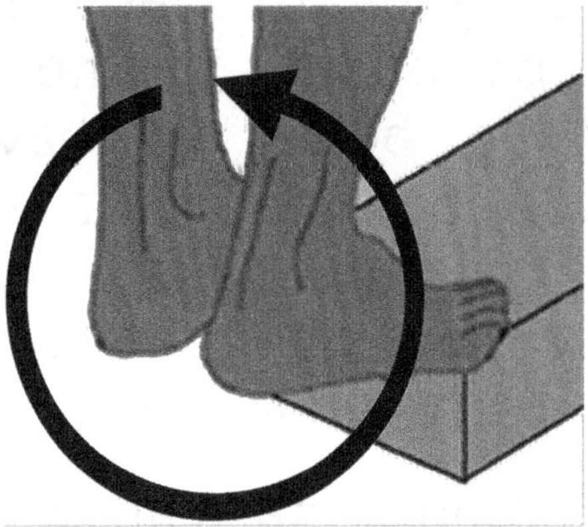

FIGURE 10.36 Step twist, heel raise

Side jump: This exercise is a jumping exercise that tests control of the lateral ligaments by leaping from side to side. The landing should be single legged. Initially, it should be tried with a relative short leap and can be gradually increased as confidence and strength is gained. Do this 30 times, alternating feet with each leap.

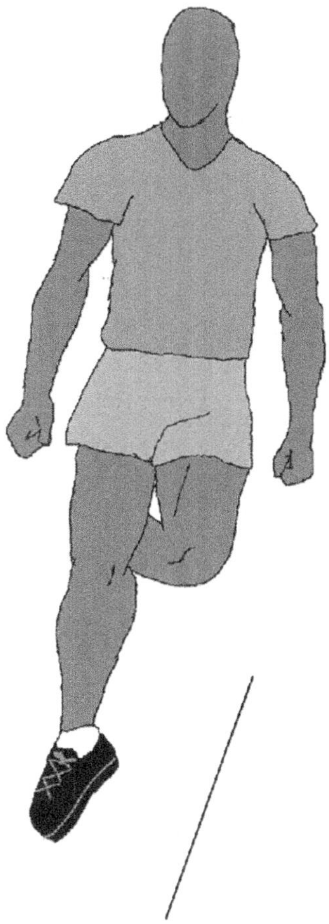

FIGURE 10.37 Side jump

Four-quadrant hop: This leaping drill is done on a single foot and tests control in all directions. Begin with 30 seconds on one foot and switch to the other. Increase the distance hopped as confidence increases.

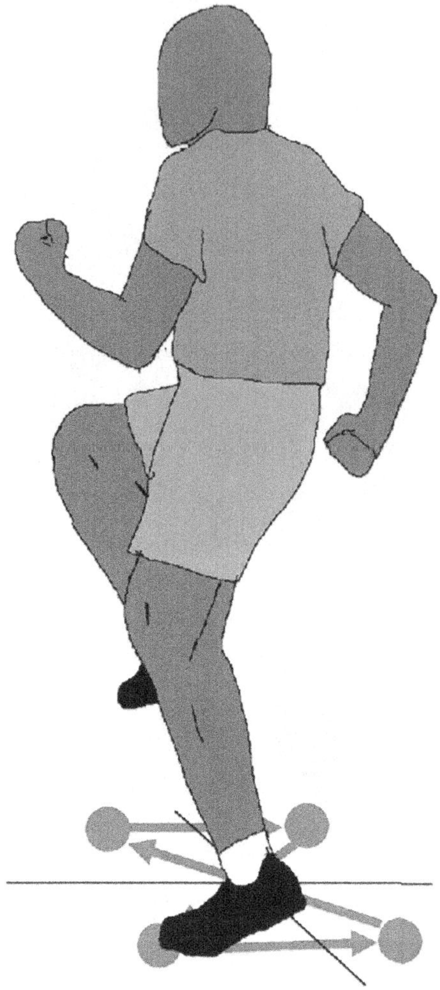

FIGURE 10.38 Four-quadrant hop

Other exercises:

- Forward jump/bounding stride: Jumping forward 12 inches or leaping from one foot to the other.
- Practicing jump shot: Get on the court and shot around. It is fun and it gets the ankle used to thrusting from the upper body.
- Passing medicine ball between two people.

- Bringing medicine ball from between legs to over your head.
- Use of balance board or mat: A balance mat is a heavy foam mat for jogging. A balance board is a board with a hemispherical surface.
- Both can help the ankle get used to uneven surfaces.
- Running and touching marks separated by distance: The "suicide" from gym class.

POSTURAL TIPS AND DRILLS

Let's start by breaking down proper posture, body part by body part.

Neck: Keep neck centered over shoulders. Keeping the head forward is a common cause of neck strain and muscle strain on the shoulder muscles. It also displaces the head forward, which weighs approximately 12 pounds and increases pressure on the forefoot. Concentrate on maintaining your eyes level with the horizon and chin up.

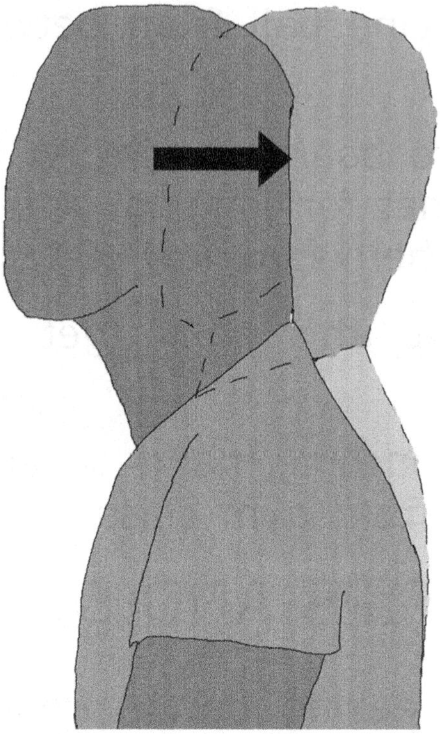

FIGURE 10.39 Neck

Shoulder: Retract shoulder blades to bring the arms and shoulders over the midportions of the chest. Avoid heavy shoulder bags especially when they are held in front of the abdomen.

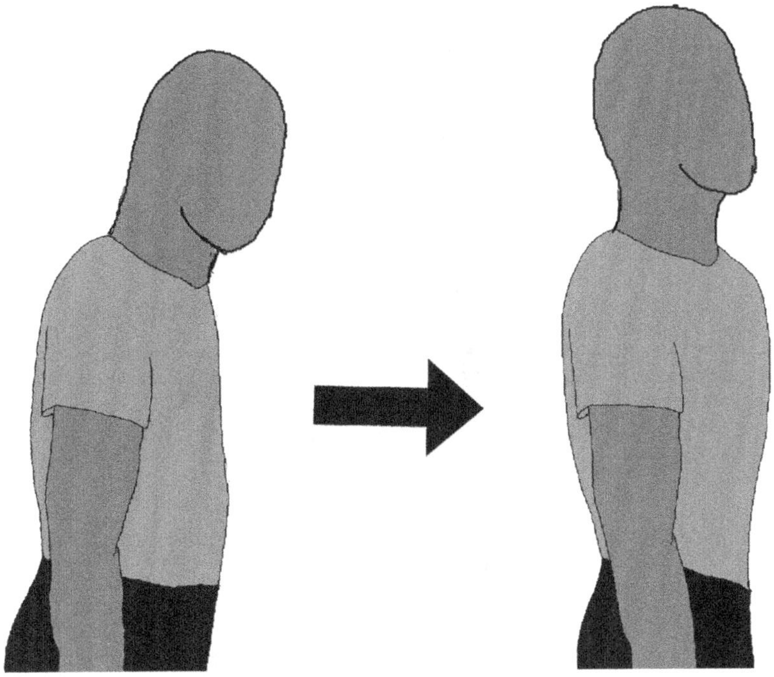

FIGURE 10.40 Shoulder

Back/hip: The back should be extended enough to place the chest over the center of the hip, but should not be hyperextended. The hip has to be rotated forward. This will feel like tucking your body under your torso or pulling your buttock under yourself. The hip has a limited range of flexion and extension. You can position this range in front of you or behind you. If you keep it in front of you, it will be much easier to take a full step and unload the foot.

Abdomen: Abdominal muscles should be toned to bring the abdominal contents within the pelvis. The typical belly that people develop is to a large extent more due to poor muscular conditioning than obesity.

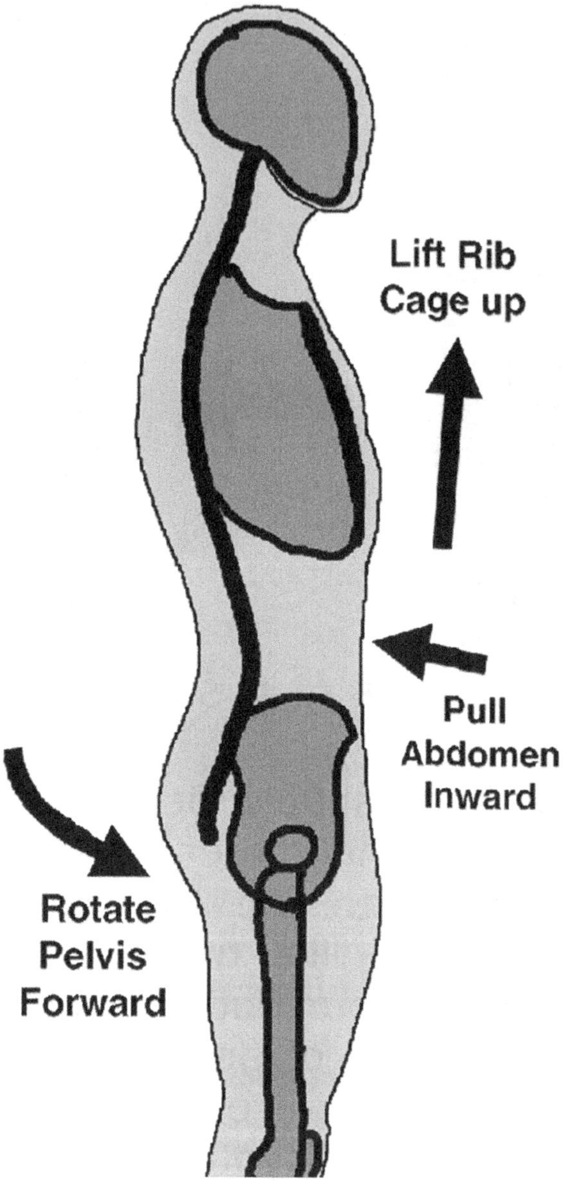

FIGURE 10.41 Abdomen

Knee: If the rest of the body is in proper alignment, you should have no difficulty avoiding excessive flexion. Flexion in the knee whether from stiffness after a surgery or tight hamstrings automatically affects the hip and the forefoot negatively.

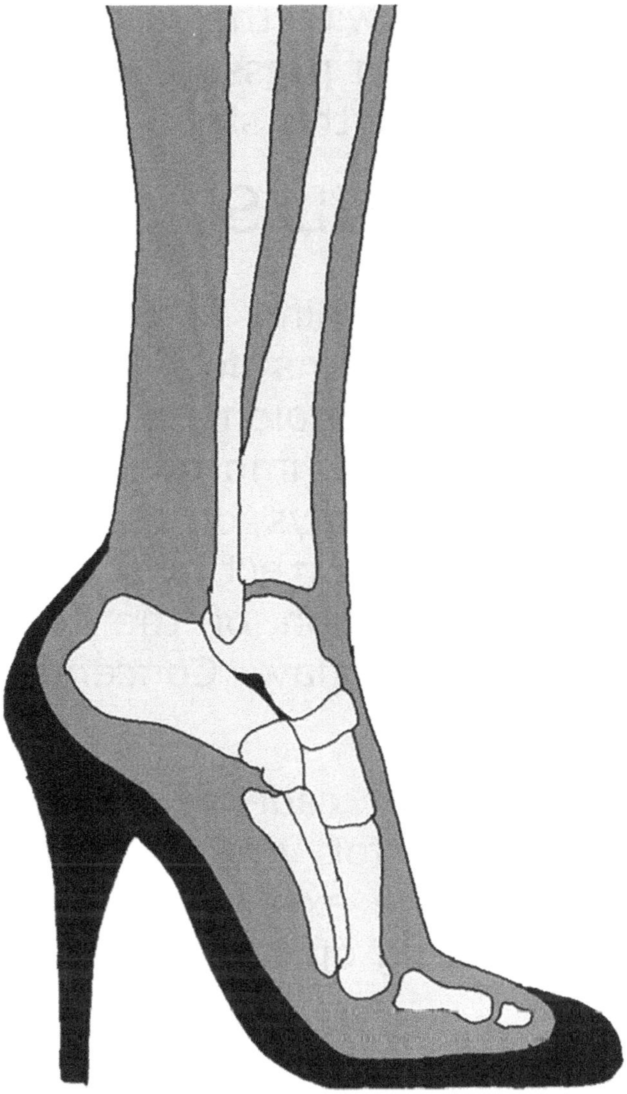

FIGURE 10.42 Foot and ankle

Foot and ankle: High-heeled shoes do affect the posture and shift the weight of the body onto the front of the foot. Certainly, high-heeled shoes are not likely the cause of all foot problems. That being said, they certainly can be counterproductive when you already have a foot problem. Choose shoes with a flat or slightly elevated heel. During walking, concentrate on contact with the heel at the beginning of the step and delaying pressure on the forefoot for at least the first half of the step.

AMBULATION DRILLS

Practice is crucial to learning to offload the forefoot. Learned ambulation patterns do not change overnight and take consistent and prolonged practice. The good news is that you can see improvement very quickly. Walking along long hallways or distances is a great opportunity to practice correct posture and gait and will reduce the aggravation of the foot problem as you get through your day. Concentrate on these points:

- Control the speed or cadence of your gait to the one that is natural for you. Trying to walk faster than this will require extra force that is usually in the form of thrusting off the forefoot. Be conscious of this.
- When beginning the step, make contact with the heel. There should be some delay from the time that the heel strikes the floor until weight is placed on the midfoot and forefoot.
- At the end of the step, concentrate on extending your ankle instead of pushing off the forefoot. If this is exaggerated, it will look like a limp. It is not necessary to exaggerate this.

- Pretend that you are walking on eggshells while you are walking. This will help you will avoid harsh treatment and overload of the foot and its supporting structures. Remember: Don't break the eggshells.
- Center your body over your feet. The most common problems are slumping shoulders, flexing neck, and most importantly positioning the pelvis.
- Positioning the pelvis is essentially tucking your butt in. It may feel like thrusting your pelvis forward. You will feel the reduced weight on the front of your foot immediately.
- The back should not be hyperextended during this. It should be flat to slightly curved. Usually if the back is hyperextended, the pelvis is flexed.

OTHER TIPS

People who suffer from forefoot overload syndromes commonly have increased pain after getting up from a seated position. This occurs because the soft tissue around the aggravated painful area is allowed to relax. When you get up to walk, this soft tissue must stretch to its working length. When a forefoot overload syndrome pain is present, the extra tension within the soft tissue greatly aggravates the pain for several steps. To prevent this, try keeping your foot on the floor and your heels behind your knees. This keeps the soft tissue stretched out so that the pain is less during those first few steps. It is also helpful to do an Achilles or plantar fascial stretch when getting up.

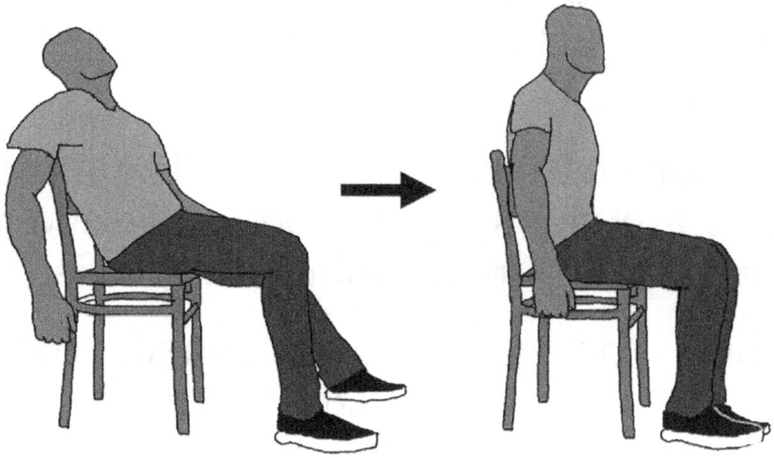

FIGURE 10.43

RETURNING TO NORMAL ACTIVITY

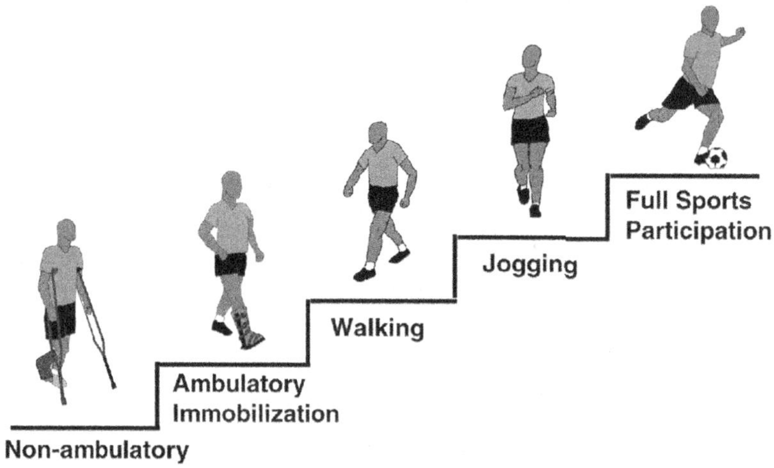

FIGURE I0.44

Returning to activity after an injury or surgery should be done one small step at a time. First, no matter how good you feel, discuss with your physician the activity restrictions to make your recovery after surgery or injury successful. Within these restrictions, carefully begin a structured and progressive return to normal activity. After surgery or injury, there may be weight-bearing restrictions or bracing that is necessary to protect the repairing tissue. After your physician has decided that the tissue has healed to a degree that should allow for return to normal activity, it is time to begin. First, with your physician, determine at what level you are now.

Each level brings with it challenges. Conditioning to maintain general fitness is usually possible with some creativity and adaptation at every level. Maintaining conditioning while recovering has the advantages of helping to control weight, improving mood, reducing fatigue, preventing other painful conditions, and quickening your return to athletics after recovery. Transitioning along each level should be begun with the consent and supervision of your physician.

Level 1: Nonweight Bearing

Not all injuries or surgeries begin with a period of nonweight bearing, but this is the lowest level of activity. This degree of activity restriction is often necessary after tendon tears and repair and many serious fractures. The first goal is to learn to safely be nonweight-bearing on the leg. Close coordination with your therapist and physician is necessary to determine the best method of restricted weight bearing. Several options are possible.

The standard is crutches. A walker is a second option. The walker can be modified in several very helpful ways. Most commonly the front pegs can be replaced with wheels. Although this can make it slightly unstable if it is suddenly used for balance, it makes it easier to push forward without completely lifting the walker. The walker can also be modified with a seat to allow for resting in case of exhaustion. One concern in the use of the walker is the safety of the uninjured leg. In people with nerve disorders such as diabetic neuropathy, the hopping or pounding that the "well" leg experiences can be damaging to the that foot. Use of a walker can also be difficult for people with upper extremity problems such as shoulder pain and weakness.

Several new devices have come on to the market recently. Most allow kneeling and gliding to get around. These devices include scooters and walkers with platforms. The advantage is that they require much less effort to ambulate, allow for resting with minimal effort, and drastically decrease the impact on the "well" foot. The disadvantage is that they can also be unstable. Because the body is being propelled at a distance above the wheels, it may be possible to push these devices over especially when an obstacle such as a rock or step is met. The steerable devices can tip if they are turned sharply. This seems to be common especially when in the house where a tight-turning radius is sometimes necessary. These devices are commonly not covered through insurance. In some cases, they can be rented economically. The secondhand market can also be a reasonable source of these devices, but it is advised that they be evaluated by an occupational therapist, pedorthotist, or other medical equipment professional prior to use to insure that they are safe.

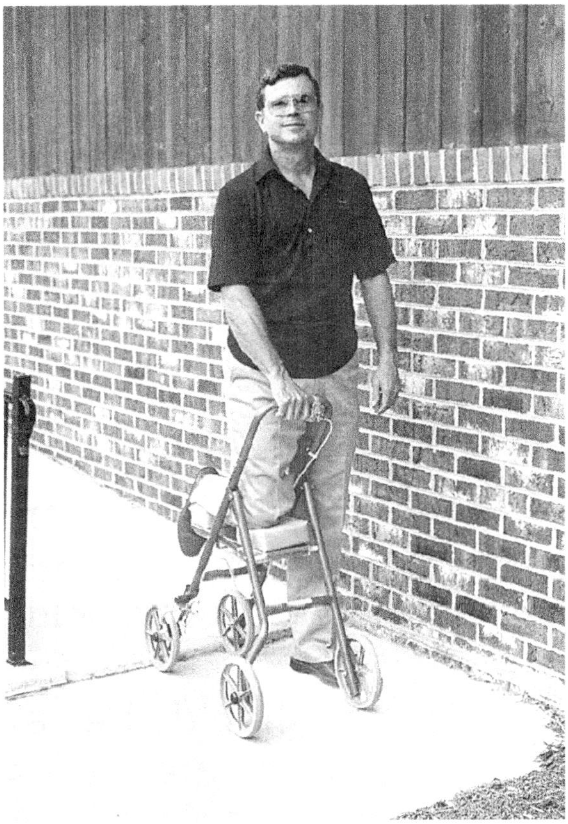

FIGURE 10.45 A kneeling ambulatory assist device. (Courtesy Roll-A-Bout Corporation)

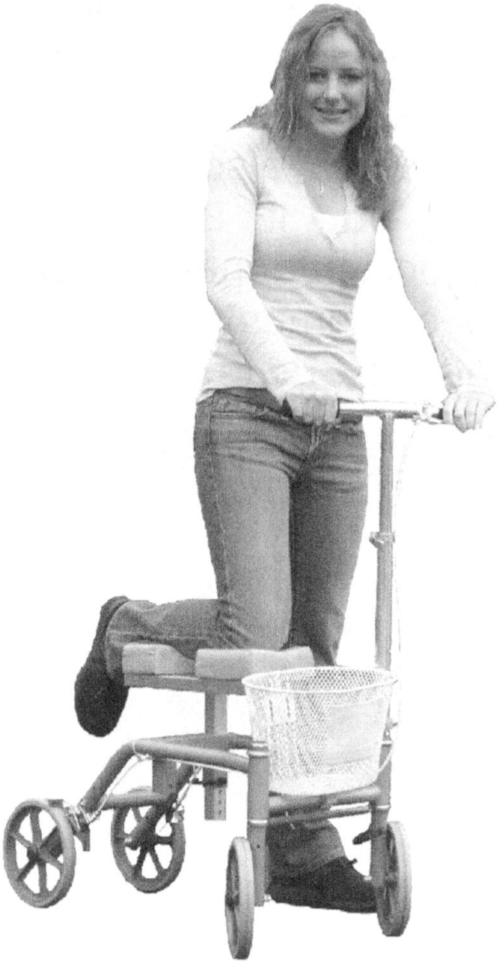

FIGURE 10.46 A steerable kneeling ambulatory assist device. (Courtesy Roll-A-Bout Corporation.)

Use of the wheelchair should be avoided as the primary means of getting around when possible. Reasons for using a wheelchair include severe weakness and poor balance, inability to follow weight-bearing restrictions due to dementia or other cognitive problems, severe neuropathies, and severe injuries on both legs. They are sometimes necessary when prolonged walking or standing is anticipated. Wheelchairs can be powered for people with upper extremity injuries, but special permission from insurance companies is often necessary to authorize this.

Conditioning of the other three extremities, the back, and the hip and knee on the injured leg, is important during nonweight bearing. Not only does this aid in balance and mobility during the nonweight-bearing period and help reduce fatigue, but it may prevent back and hip pain that is common during recovery. It will also help you prepare for normal activity and to resume a more normal gait after resuming ambulation.

The particular conditioning exercises that can be safely resumed and specific instructions for your particular situation from your physician are critical. To some extent the aerobic conditioning options open to you will be dependent on the strictness of the restrictions on your leg. The simplest option is ambulating for a distance on your crutches or walker or other assistive device. This activity will be considerably more strenuous than walking typically is when your foot is normal. A recumbent bicycle or a rowing machine might be appropriate exercise machines if the injured foot is allowed to rest on the ground. Using these machines without the use of one leg can be frustrating in comparison to using them in a two-legged manner, but is an effective means of promoting aerobic fitness. Several aquatic options may be reasonable including aqua jogging. Some treadmills are designed to permit jogging without full weight bearing through the use of a pelvic sling, but these are very expensive and are not widely available. An aerobic upper extremity-conditioning program can be productive. This can be a calisthenics program or light resistance weight-lifting program. There are even upper extremity ergometers that are basically bicycles for your arms. Beginning an upper extremity calisthenics program that accomplishes true aerobic conditioning requires some dedication, consistency, and patience but can be rewarding. It is a useful part of maintaining fitness during an injury.

Transition Level 1 to Level 2

Weight bearing is usually resumed gradually and should be done in close consultation with your doctor or therapist. The first step is called foot-flat weight bearing. The old description of "toe-touch" weight bearing is misleading, because the entire foot should be applied to the floor, not just the toe. Usually, it is begun by placing the foot with any immobilization devices such as casts, cast-boots, or other braces on the floor along with the crutches. When applying "foot-flat" pressure only the weight of the leg is rested on the injured foot. The remainder of the weight should be applied to the arms through the crutches. Usually pain is a good gauge of the degree of healing. Increasing pain is a sign of overdoing it and should be avoided. It is important to realize that even after adequate healing of the ligaments, bones, and tendons in the leg, a degree of achy pain can continue for some time. Although you should recognize this pain and mention it to your doctor, avoid becoming too emotional or frustrated about it. These kinds of feelings only serve as a roadblock to recovery. The best attitude is to recognize it as a normal and typical part of getting better and to accept it.

As more weight is allowed, begin weight bearing in the brace, if any, that you are in. We instruct our patients to get a bathroom scale and take their body weight and divide it into half. Place that amount of pressure on the scale, sensing about what that feels like. Now on your crutches or walker, begin to walk while allowing this amount of weight on the foot. Extend your crutches forward about the length of one step with your injured foot. Place 50% of your weight on the foot in the brace and 50% of the weight on your hands through the crutches, then step with the well foot. Try to walk otherwise as normally as possible.

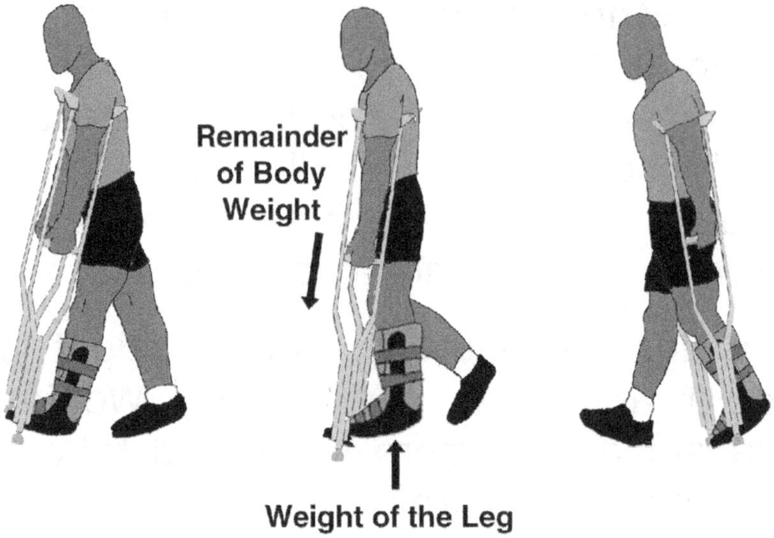

FIGURE 10.47 Foot flat weight bearing involves applying only the weight of the injured leg to the ground and shifing the remainder to the crutches. It is a useful start when resuming ambulation.

In several days or a few weeks, if the foot is nearly pain-free, advance the amount of pressure on it to 75%. If this is fairly tolerable, after a few days or weeks, place full pressure on the foot using the crutches or walker as balance or support if necessary. The next step is to abandon using the crutches with full weight on the foot/brace.

Level 2. Immobilization

Walking with an immobilization device such as a cast or cast boot is somewhat unstable. Walking without the flexibility of the ankle is not a normal gait. If balance is temporarily lost, it is much easier to fall because repositioning the ankle under the body is difficult. If recurrent falls are experienced, a walker or cane may help with balance.

The extra depth in the sole of the cast or cast-boot makes the injured leg long in comparison to the other leg. During walking, this causes the body to vault over the leg and increases the amount of wobbling in the pelvis and low back. This can lead to pain in the back and hip. To some extent, this can be reduced by wearing a thicker soled shoe on the uninjured leg.

Many more conditioning options exist when full weight bearing is allowed. Usually, impact aerobic exercises are not possible yet. A stationary bicycle is an excellent conditioning device in early recuperation. Other options include walking and using an elliptical jogging or stair-climbing device. Weight-bearing aerobic exercises with any degree of impact should be delayed until full weight bearing is comfortable throughout the day and pain medication has been discontinued.

This is a common time to develop forefoot overload problems. Ankle stiffness and weakness in the extensors and everting muscles of the ankle is common after severe injuries and surgical procedures. Rehabilitation is key to combating them. Prevention is better than treatment of these problems, so it is best to begin this as a routine after an injury. The exercises and stretches listed earlier are a good starting point and we recommend including them as a part of your rehabilitation. Postural exercises should be begun to normalize gait.

Transitioning From Level 2 to Level 3

Weaning out of the brace is often also a gradual process. Usually, we recommend removing the brace while at home for an hour or two during sedentary periods of the day. This length of time can be gradually increased by two-hour increments as tolerance to ambulation without the brace is increased. It is important to be nearly pain-free and comfortable before advancing this. When brace-free activity is possible for long periods, begin to venture outside of the house without the boot.

Depending on the specific injury, a flexible ankle brace or rigid rocker-soled shoe may be helpful in increasing activity while out of the brace. This works by controlling the motion in painful areas while starting to walk again. If swelling prevents the use of a standard shoe, a shoe may be selected with a more flexible upper. The shoe should also be fitted at the end of the day when swelling is greater. Loosen the laces completely before placing the foot in the shoe. Removing the liner from the shoe can also increase the room within the shoe slightly.

Level 3. Walking

Walking is the next milestone in recovery. The use of similar shoes on each leg reduces the stress on the back, hips, and knees. Activity also gradually increases during this period. One of the challenges during this period is to expose the injured and recovering tissue to increasing stress to encourage remodeling of these structures to normal strength and resilience. It is also important to gradually increase the stress on the foot to prevent stress injuries, because the strength of the bones, tendons, and ligaments may be weakened through underuse and unable to repair the damage caused by overly aggressive exercise.

Conditioning options become more numerous and are widely available at most exercise and therapy facilities. Stationary bicycles, treadmills, elliptical jogging machines, and stepping machines are devices that can be used with gradually increasing duration and vigor. Walking or hiking is also an excellent way to improve conditioning. The exposure to sunlight provided by outdoor activity also improves mood.

Uneven surfaces may still be difficult to negotiate without aggravating the foot. Ankle braces or other hinged immobilization devices may be helpful in preventing this discomfort. Avoiding turf, gravel, and areas with ground obstacles can also prevent re-injury and aggravation of the foot.

Transitioning From Level 3 to Level 4

Increasing physical activity beyond simple walking is a reasonable goal for most people after even severe injuries. A frank discussion with your physician should center on how realistic this is in your specific circumstance. Some injuries will result in problems that may not allow this without risking deterioration of the injured structures.

Activity should be gradually increased initially using low impact exercises through moderate- and high-impact exercises until jogging is possible. Initially, the jogging should be done in modest doses. One kilometer or one-half of a mile seems like a reasonable length in most cases. This may be done in combination with other lower impact exercises to allow for a full aerobic challenge. A reasonable rule of thumb is to avoid increasing the intensity or the length of the jogging by more than 10% per week. If aggravation of the injury or pain increases, then the level of activity should be decreased to a comfortable level for a week or more. Increasing the intensity of your workout can be attempted again after this period.

Level 4. Jogging

The goal at this level depends on the desires of the individual. For many, no further progress is necessary. Some seek to return to competitive athletic activity.

Transitioning From Level 4 to Level 5

The last step is to progress toward sports. Sports generally require some lateral/medial motion of the ankle and this activity is very different from the straight-ahead motion such as in running. Some of the drills that are done may require instruction and monitoring by a physical therapist or trainer especially if you expect to return to a high level of play. Initially, drills that stress changes in direction in addition to advanced strengthening exercises should be mastered. It is important to regain proprioception. Proprioception is the ability of your brain to sense the position of your foot and to effectively and subconsciously control its motion. Regaining functional proprioception involves retraining your brain and leg. Although many of the exercises will help with this, the expert supervision of an experienced trainer or therapist is crucial. When this is financially not possible, many martial arts programs of varying intensity can teach balance, as can several calisthenic programs.

Level 5. Full Sports Participation

The path to full sports participation can be laborious and frustrating, but slow step-wise rehabilitation is necessary to make it smooth and injury-free. It is important to maintain flexibility and conditioning.

Difficulties

Recovery from an injury or surgery is never "normal." It is typical for people to experience a wide range of sensations and worrisome symptoms. It is sometimes hard to understand why this experience varies widely from person to person, but, after years of experience of watching and listening to people as they recover, it varies greatly. Explain your abnormal sensations clearly to your physician, but do not be surprised if little is done. In the absence of a clear sign that these symptoms represent a serious condition, most of them resolve by themselves without treatment.

Among these concerning symptoms are varying degrees of fleeting pain, especially sharp, stabbing pains. The toes may not move as you would expect them. This is due to swelling around the tendons and goes away within several weeks. The foot may feel unstable because it is not positioned during walking properly. Swelling around the joints may make moving the ankle require more effort. When this occurs, it can make it easy to re-injure so that protection of the foot is important. Swelling can persist in normal circumstances for months and some may be permanent. Color changes in the leg such that the leg turns deep red, purple, or gray are common when the foot is swollen and below the waist level such as when sitting. If the color returns to normal when the leg is elevated, this does not usually represent a serious circulatory disorder.

Resources

Shoes, Orthotics, and Braces

Keon Mansoori
Advanced Orthopro, Inc.

The use of shoe wear and other orthotics and prosthetics is a powerful method of treating a wide variety of painful foot problems. When such a device is prescribed or recommended, it is an invaluable part of the treatment plan. There are a wide variety of orthopedic devices that can be used to place the foot in the optimal position to heal painful structures or to aid in recovery from injury. Through interaction with you, the physician, and other foot care professionals, the painful foot can be treated effectively using these devices.

ANATOMY OF A SHOE

Inappropriate and poorly fitting shoes contribute to foot problems. Common issues such as hammertoes and bunions develop partially from shoes that crowd or position the foot in a way that overloads important structures. Appropriate shoes can be a key, if not the most important method of treating foot pains.

The shoe is not simply a device that prevents damage to the foot such as when you step on glass. It controls the way that the foot interacts with the ground, the pressure distribution on the sole of the foot, and even the body posture. The shoe can be a complicated and finely engineered device.

Typically, the shoe is composed of several elements. Each of these elements can be manipulated to change the mechanics of walking. These elements are the upper, the sole and the heel.

The upper is the portion of the shoe that covers the top of the foot. It is usually sewn to the sole. The upper's primary function is to attach the sole of the shoe to the foot. Most of the problems with the upper involve the fit with the foot. Deformities such as bunions and hammertoes can become painful if parts of the upper press abnormally on them. Important mechanical characteristics of the upper include its cut, materials from which it is made, the closure system, and its volume.

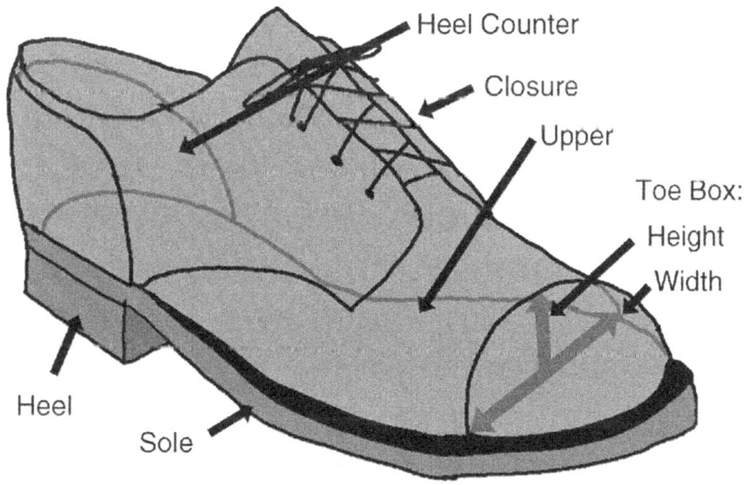

FIGURE 1 Diagram of a shoe and its parts.

Ideally, the material used in the upper should be compliant, durable, and cosmetically appealing. Leather is the traditional and still the most common material used. It is useful because it is compliant, breathable, and durable. Various types of leather exist that can range from the very soft (kidskin or deerskin) to the more rigid (cabrio). Synthetic materials such as plastic and artificial leather are poorly compliant and can often cause pain if not fitted precisely. Many shoe companies market neoprene or spandex uppers, materials that are extremely soft and compliant. However, some sacrifices in durability and support are made when using these materials. Attention should be directed to the stitching pattern on the upper of the shoe, as areas that are heavily stitched will not expand easily. If the stitching is over a prominence such as a bunion, it may cause pain.

The cut describes the portion of the foot covered by the upper. The cut affects how secure the attachment of the shoe to the foot and ankle will be and can also affect its ability to stabilize the foot. Commonly preferred standard shoes are cut just beneath the ankle. If ankle stabilization is desired, a higher cut shoe may be chosen such as is often seen in high-topped basketball shoes. In the cut of some shoes such as clogs and certain sandals, the upper ends at the arch. This type of shoe will not attach firmly to the foot and, therefore, the shoe will be less effective at controlling the foot. This is not always bad, as the lack of material around the heel can be used to reduce pressure on the back of the heel. It also allows the shoe to dry more effectively in between shoe usage.

The most common closure system is laces. Laces are useful and practical in many ways. They are very secure and can be tightened to the desired degree easily. Lacing can be adjusted to avoid bony prominences on the top of the midfoot, raised to loosen the toe of the shoe, or lowered to avoid the front of the ankle when prominences and tenderness are there. The longer the laced area is on the top of the shoe, the more secure the attachment to the foot will be.

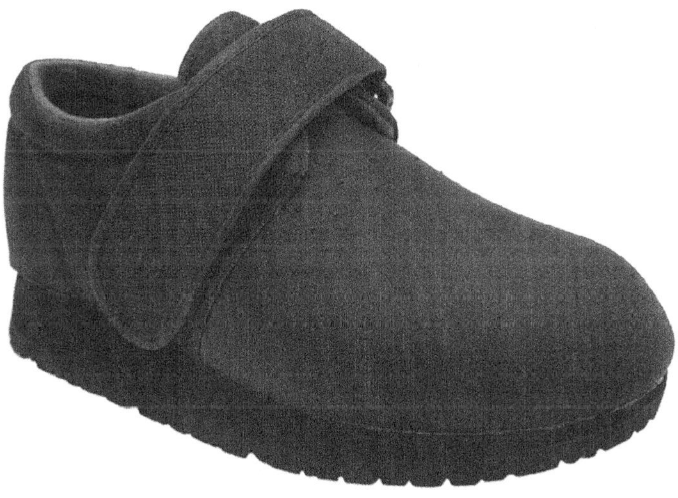

FIGURE 2 Pedors Classic Shoe. An example of a shoe with a Spandex upper and Velcro strap designed for foot deformities that are otherwise hard to fit with a shoe. (By permission, Pedors Shoes)

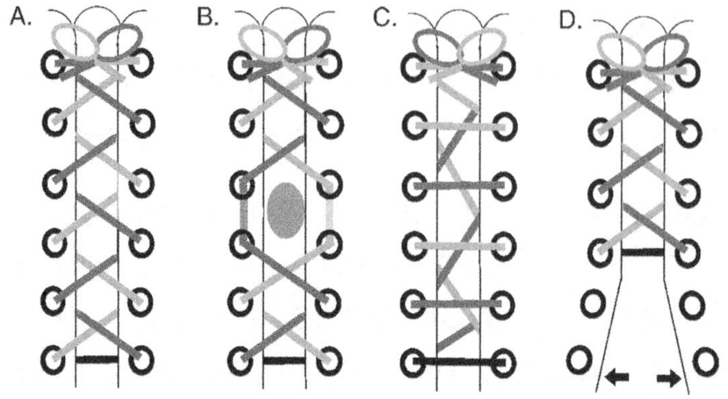

FIGURE 3 Lacing alternative that can be used for foot problems. (A) Standard lacing pattern. (B) Skipping an eyelet to avoid a painful bump or spur. (C) Decreased friction pattern to allow for easier tightening. (D) Lacing stopped prior to the bottom of the eyelets to accommodate bunions and hammertoes.

Another way of closing the shoe is by using straps secured either with buckles or Velcro. This method can be better when hand dexterity or strength is impaired. It also decreases the amount of and redistributes the pressure over the top of the foot. The straps are difficult to replace and do wear out more quickly. They may limit the life of the shoe.

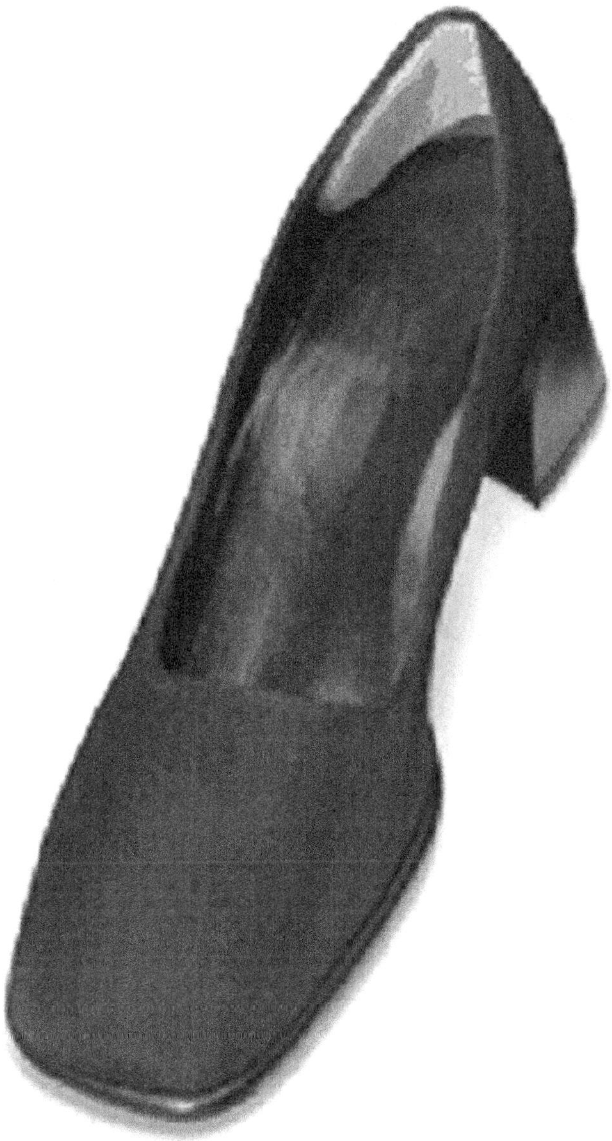

FIGURE 4 An adhesive felt pad could be applied to the heel counter to make the fit snugger and to make it less abrasive. (By permission, Hapad, Inc.)

The foot should be at its biggest when shoes are fitted. This is generally at the end of the day. The shoe should be proper length and width. Many people undersize their shoes. Generally, one-half inch should be left between the end of the toe and the end of the shoe. The shoe should follow the general contour of the foot and be of appropriate width. Often, commercially available shoes if sized to the forefoot will be loose in the heel and midfoot area. If this is the case, switching to a different style, placing a soft three-quarter length insert (one that doesn't go to the ball of the foot) or a heel snugger into the shoe are possible strategies to improve this. If one area is particularly tight, the shoe can often be stretched using a ball-ring stretcher usually available for purchase or at shoe repair stores or by a prosthetist/orthotist.

The sole of the shoe is what controls the way that the foot interacts with the ground and where and how pressure is placed on the foot. The stiffness and the shape of the sole of the shoe are perhaps the most important factors. These factors come together to protect the foot not only from objects that may cut into the foot, but they can also help to disperse pressure when it is abnormally high in areas in the foot during walking. Usually, the stiffer the sole of the foot, the more that it can disperse pressure. The more flexible the sole is, the more it is like walking barefooted and concentrations of pressure will be more likely. The shape and width will affect how the joints are stressed and how stable the shoe is. A shoe that is wider will resist motion from the side so that it is more difficult to twist or injure the foot. This has practical limits.

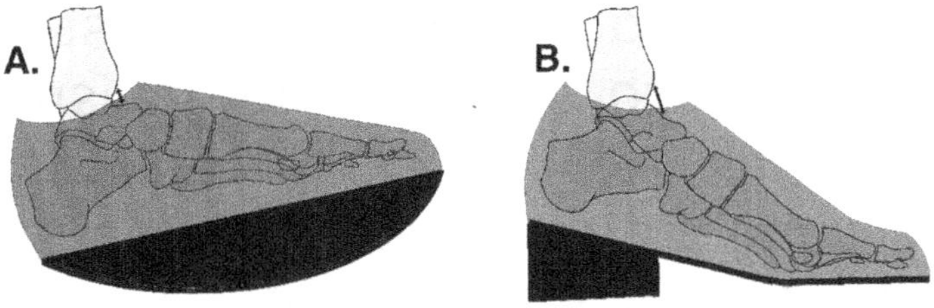

FIGURE 5 (A) In a negative heel (shoe in which the forefoot is higher than the heel), the front of the ankle closes (arrow), which may be painful in an ankle with restricted motion such as in arthritis. (B) In a shoe with a heel, the front of the ankle opens (arrow), which may place the ankle in a better position if the motion is restricted.

Heel height affects the foot in many ways. A flat or negative heel (a shoe with the heel at or below the height of the forefoot) may be difficult with someone with ankle stiffness. As heel height increases, the front of the ankle opens accommodating ankle stiffness, but weight shifts to the front of the foot. People with various forms of forefoot overload should expect to experience more pain when wearing a shoe with a very elevated heel. Often a pointed, higher heel is too narrow in its imprint with the ground. This may decrease the stability of the foot in someone with balance problems to the point that they could fall and twist or break their ankle. On the other hand, the heel can be buttressed to increase stability in someone with an ankle that gives out on them.

Socks deserve attention. Socks aid in shock absorption and protect the skin from irritation caused by the stitching of the shoe or chemicals within the upper. Socks also help absorb moisture from sweat. If the shoe were allowed to absorb this moisture, it would enhance the growth of microorganisms such as bacteria, leading to foot odor and irritation. Unbleached, white cotton socks are ideal because they lack dyes and are hypoallergenic. The sock, like the shoe, should be sized appropriately. People who have feet that swell should avoid socks with a tight calf or ankle band to avoid creasing the ankle and increasing the swelling.

SHOE SELECTION

There is a proper way to buy shoes. The first step is to decide what your needs are. If you know exactly what you want and feel comfortable in nearly any shoe, then almost any shoe store will be adequate for you. Go to the store with the best prices or buy from the Internet. If you are hard to fit or have difficulty finding comfortable shoes, you may want to consider going to a shoe store with a certified shoe fitter. A certified shoe fitter's credentials are not extensive. Most of the training could be finished in a weekend. However, it indicates two things. First, it indicates that the individual salesperson has some interest in shoes and is willing to become trained to safely fit shoes and to recognize some of the basic problems that might interfere with shoe fit and satisfaction. These salespeople are serious about their job and have made a commitment to understanding shoe selection. They may be able to give some knowledgeable advice. The second is that the shoe store expects more from its salespeople than being able to run the cash register and is willing to pay a little extra for that extra service. It also means that these shoe stores will charge more. In most instances, it is worth it, but you must decide for yourself.

Shop for shoes at the end of the day when your feet are the most swollen. Both feet should be measured and the shoes should be fit to the largest foot. Up to 60% of people will have a one-half shoe size or more difference in the size of their feet. It is easier to fill the extra space around the smaller foot than to try to create space around the larger foot. If the difference in shoe size between the feet is greater than 1 1/2 shoe size, there are retailers and Internet shoe companies that will sell different-size, individual shoes. Be sure to wear the socks that you normally wear and bring your orthotic or brace if you use one. If you do wear an orthotic or brace, make sure that the liner in the shoe is removable. Removing the liner will help maximize the space within the shoe.

Explain to the salespeople what problems you have had in the past. If they give you that faraway look, go somewhere else. Stand up in bare feet to allow them to evaluate your feet and give them any recommendations that your physician has given you.

Despite the impatient stares that the salespeople will sometimes give you, spend some time walking in the shoes in the store. Do not count on them "breaking in" or becoming more comfortable with time. Shoes with a wide forefoot and a narrow or normal heel are available, but finding these shoes is sometimes difficult. Usually, a knowledgeable salesperson can steer you toward them when appropriate. Buy shoes that are appropriate for your intended activity.

Most of this book's discussion is about the type of shoe to buy for painful feet. This is very different from the selection of shoes for healthy feet. Although for many problems of the feet, stiffer is better, this does not mean that this is a good recommendation for healthy feet. A painful foot is usually suffering from some type of overuse. The foot is being stressed more than it is able to tolerate. This is a function of both the stresses that are being expected from it and its resilience. Therapeutic shoe wear will protect a foot. Although the stress reduction that occurs may improve pain, it also shields the foot from stress that may over time reduce its strength and resilience. As you recover from a foot problem, it is advised that you return to more normal, but still sensible, shoe wear gradually if the pain and your doctor's advice permits this.

Athletic shoe selection is very different from selecting shoes for painful feet. Many companies have spent a great deal of money on researching and developing athletic shoes that are appropriate to specific sports. Many of them have come up with different solutions. Much of the engineering is based on philosophy. Good, general advice is to find the shoe that fits and feels comfortable in the particular sport.

ORTHOTICS

Although shoes can be very helpful, occasionally other methods are necessary to stabilize the foot and reduce pain. An orthotic is a device that fits within the bottom of the shoe. There are two different types. A functional foot orthotic promotes stability in the joints of the foot. This device seeks to controls abnormal foot motion and stress. An accommodative orthotic is used to equalize pressure on the bottom of the foot.

Orthotics may be off-the-shelf or custom. Off-the-shelf orthotics are premade in a factory. Some off-the-shelf orthotics are designed to correct specific problems. A physician or orthotist can often help guide this selection. They are considerably cheaper than custom arch support.

Custom arch supports are fitted and made for a specific individual. Usually, an impression of the foot is made from a foam box or plaster cast. Adjustments may be added based on the orthotist's visual impression and physical examination of the foot.

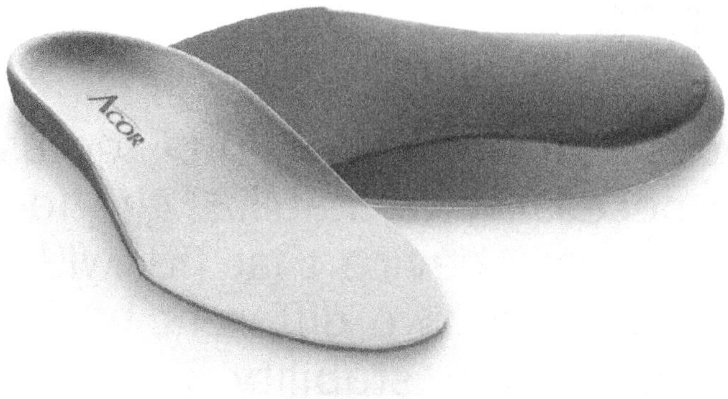

FIGURE 6 An off-the-shelf orthotic. In some situations, an orthotic such as this can be a cost-effective choice. (Courtesy ACOR Orthopedic Inc)

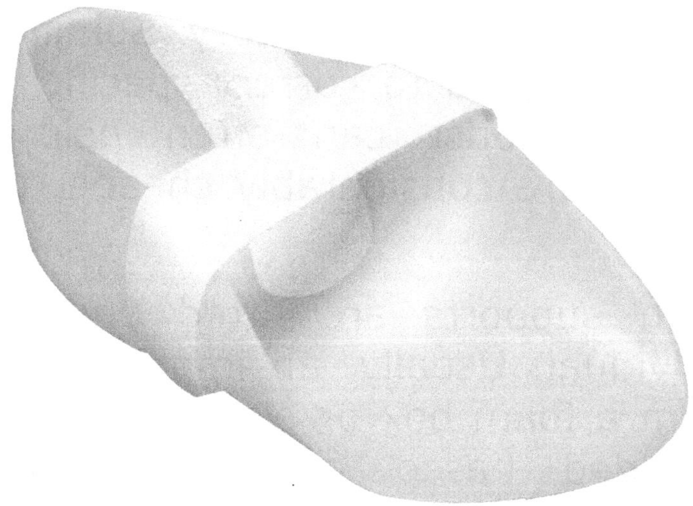

FIGURE 7 Semirigid orthotics can be modified to control the heel to compensate for more control and often have the optimal qualities of durability and comfort. (By permission, Advanced Orthopro, Inc.)

Using the impression, the orthotic is fabricated from various materials. More rigid orthosis are less susceptible to wear, but can be uncomfortable. Other materials such as plastazote and Celon® may become deformed with prolonged use and loose its effectiveness. Materials that are intermediate in stiffness such as cork and Pelite® often have the optimal qualities of resilience and shock absorption to function effectively for years. Custom orthotics can be modified to control the heel and arch position by extension along the side of the hindfoot.

Custom inserts are useful when the foot is not typical in shape or when a specific problems needs to be addressed. It is also successful in treating specific disorders and instabilities. If a particular bone within the ball of the foot is prominent, the orthotic can be modified to offload this area. If the ball of the foot is painful, a metatarsal pad can be added to shift the pressure away from the painful area. Tilting the heel through the use of wedges can position the foot in mild to moderate degrees of misalignment. Further control can be obtained by cupping the heel with an insert that surrounds and pushes the heel into a specific position.

In some cases, commercial shoes can be modified by pedorthotists to help with foot problems. A metatarsal bar can be applied to many commercial shoes to decrease the pressure placed on the forefoot. Certain shoes can be taken apart and modified with a rocker sole or a steel shank placed within the sole to stiffen it. A wedge or buttress is sometimes applied to the heel or sole to help correct ways in which the foot tilts abnormally or is unstable. If modification of a commercial shoe is being considered, discuss the selection of the shoe with the pedorthotists before buying it, as some shoes are inappropriate for these modifications.

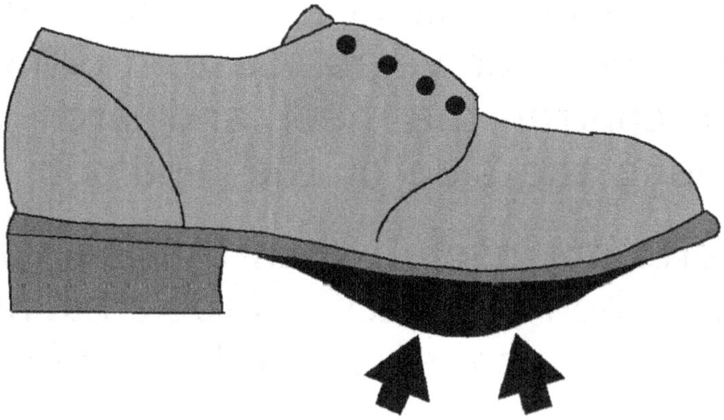

FIGURE 8 Metatarsal bar (arrows) fixed to the sole of a shoe.

BRACES

Some foot issues and painful conditions require more than an orthotic. Braces add to the control of the orthotic by incorporating more leverage on the ankle. Although braces can seem menacing to those who are not used to them, a well-made, properly fitted brace can improve foot and ankle function remarkably.

Premade over-the-counter braces can be very useful. Most commonly prescribed braces are used for ligament instabilities such as recurrent ankle sprains, but they can be used for any situation when mild restriction of the ankle's motion may be helpful. This includes Achilles tendonitis, ankle pain, ankle arthritis, mild degrees of fallen arch, and ankle arthritis. Although in many situations the braces are just not powerful enough to completely control the problem, in others, the over-the-counter brace can be an inexpensive and helpful part of improving pain.

Many commonly dispensed stirrup braces that are used in emergency rooms are not comfortable or practical. The air bladders in them seem to irritate and cut into the skin and often are too bulky to allow for use of a standard cut shoe. The other braces have a low-cut profile to allow for use of most sport shoes and are inexpensive. It is also easy to apply and relatively comfortable and durable. Several companies make lace-up braces that are also practical, although they can be more troublesome and complicated to apply.

The most common type of custom ankle brace is the ankle-foot-orthosis (AFO). An AFO can be helpful in many circumstances from ankle arthritis to fallen arch. The AFO is essentially an orthotic that extends onto the ankle and calf. An AFO is used to compensate for muscle weakness or damage, to immobilize painful joints such as in arthritis, or to stabilize unstable joints. An AFO can do this because of its added leverage.

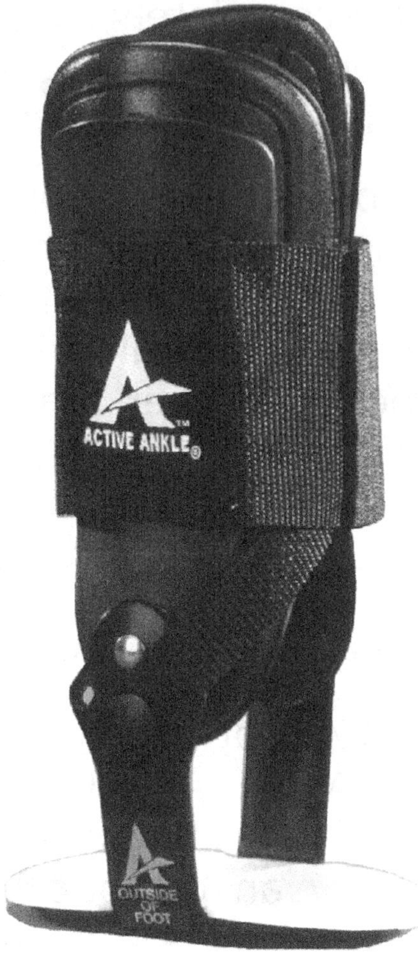

FIGURE 9 A comfortable, low profile, stirrup-type of ankle brace. (By permission, Active Ankle)

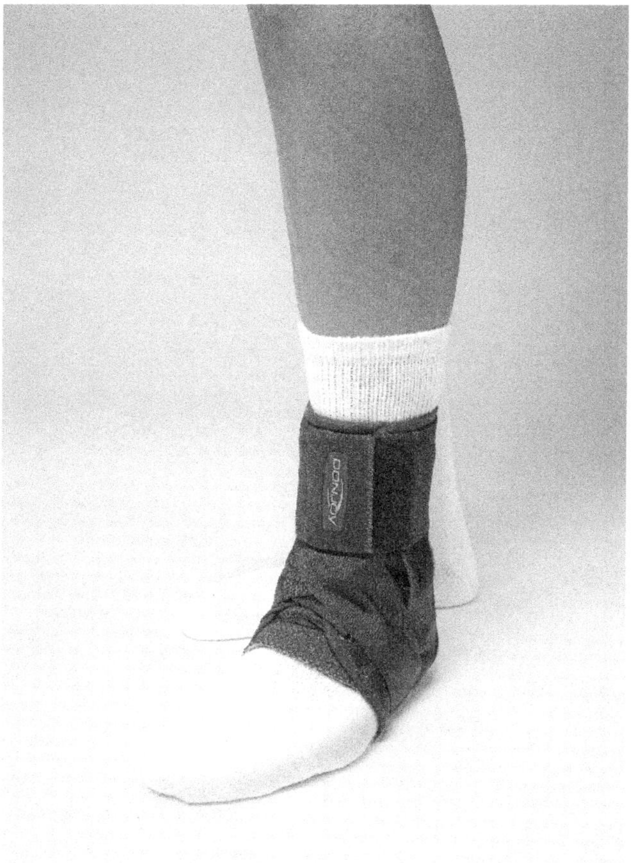

FIGURE 10 A lace-up orthosis (the RocketSoc). A lace-up ankle brace that supports the ankle using straps. (By permission, DonJoy Orthopedics)

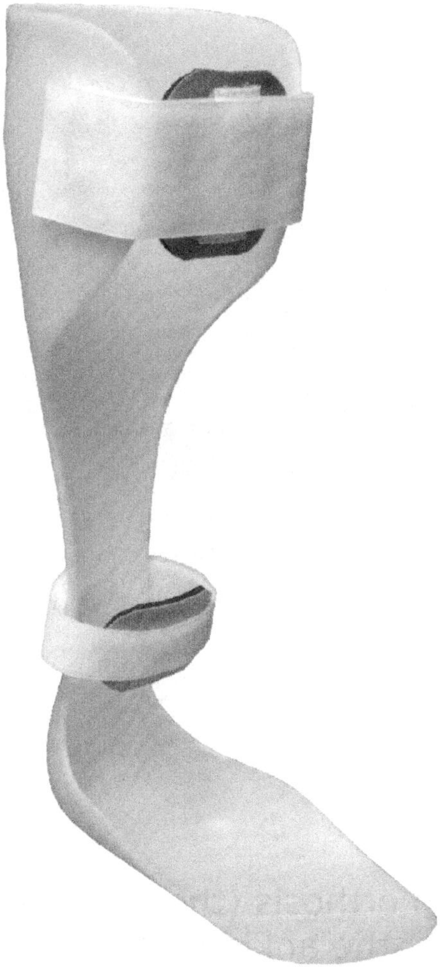

FIGURE 11 A fixed AFO. (By permission, Advanced Orthopro, Inc.)

Although off-the-shelf AFOs are available, many times they do not fit properly to allow for comfortable effective use. A custom AFO is formfitted to the foot and ankle, which decreases the possibility of skin irritation and breakdown. A custom AFO is fashioned from a cast mold of the leg. The joints of the leg are positioned in the appropriate position, preferably with the sole of the foot at a right angle to the ankle and the heel in alignment with the leg. A model is made of the leg and the brace is fitted to this mold. The brace is usually made of polypropylene. Adjustments are often necessary to ensure proper fit and comfort.

AFOs can be modified in several useful ways. One of the most common is to add a hinge to the ankle to allow for motion. This type of AFO is called a short, articulated AFO and can be the best choice for several problems. This device stabilizes the arch and ankle using leverage on the ankle while allowing for motion within the ankle, incorporating the advantages of a custom orthotic and the support of an AFO. This helps to normalize the step and decreases the amount of limp commonly seen in fixed ankle AFO usage. The motion of the hinge can be limited by various stops or the strength of certain motions increased with springs.

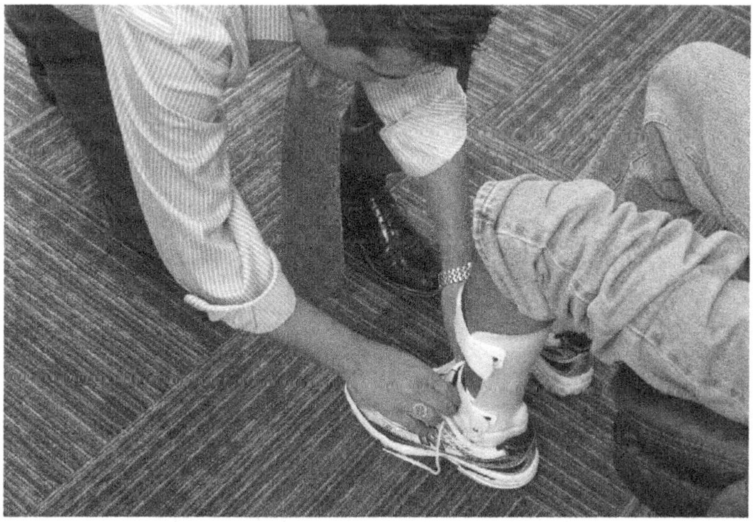

FIGURE 12 An orthotist fitting a short articulated AFO. These braces may take adjustments to achieve proper fit. A close relationship with an attentive orthotist is key to satisfaction with these devices. (By permission, Advanced Orthopro, Inc.)

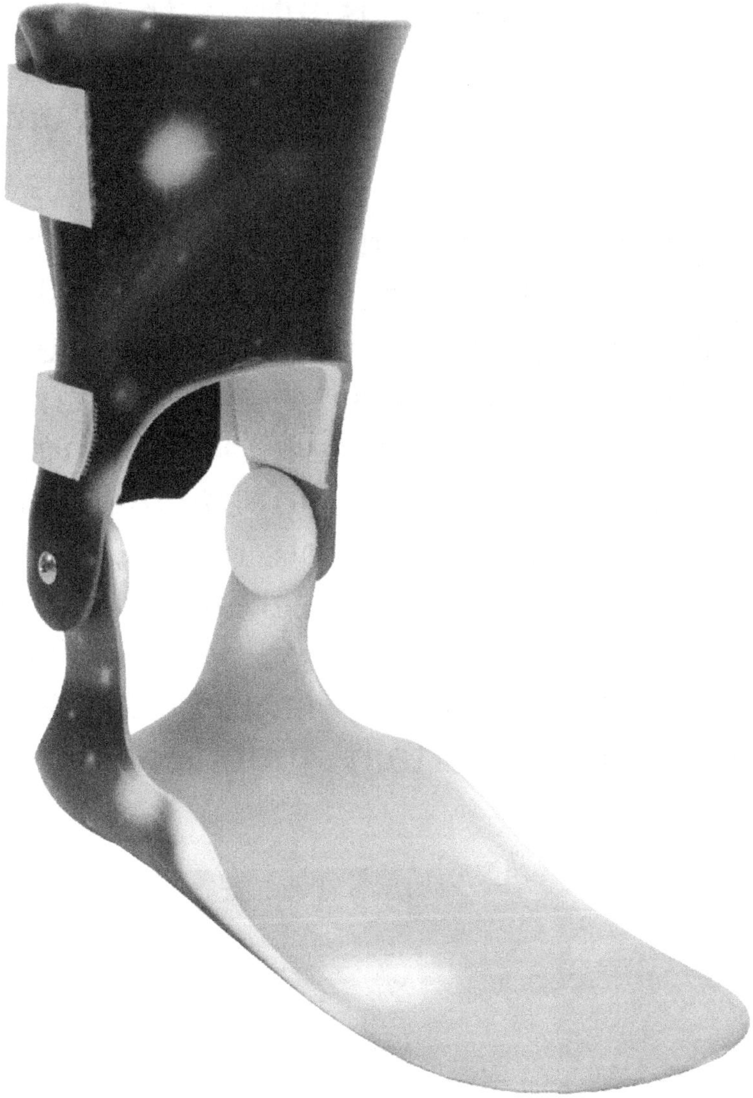

FIGURE 13 A short articulating AFO. (By permission, Advanced Orthopro, Inc.)

A common condition requiring a brace is foot drop. In this condition, the muscles controlling the upward movement of the foot do not function properly, usually because of nerve or tendon injury. When this occurs, the foot does not extend when it is lifted from the floor. It is difficult to clear the floor as the foot is swung through. It then comes down with a distinctive slap. In this case, an AFO may be helpful. It positions the foot appropriately so that it clears when swinging it during a step.

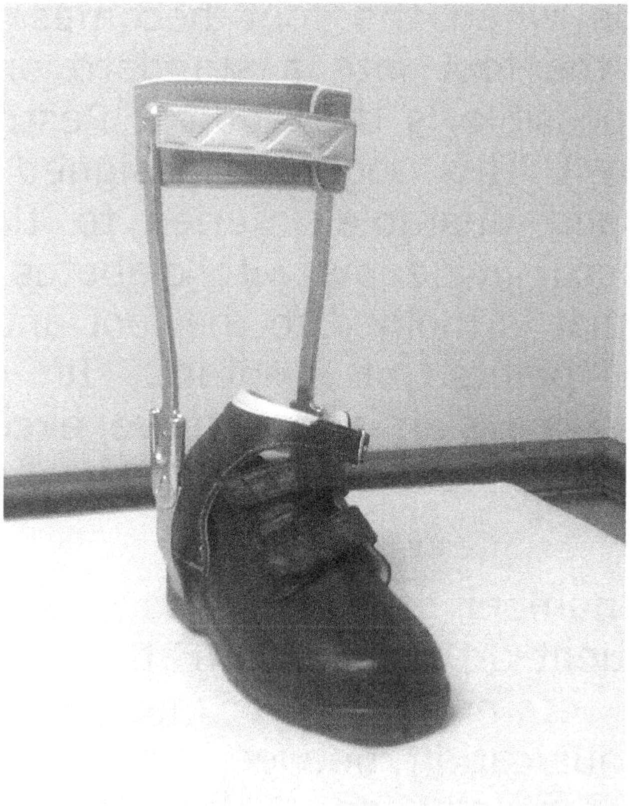

FIGURE 14 A double-upright brace attached to a shoe. This brace has the fit of a shoe with the ankle support and control of a brace (by permission, Advanced Orthopro, Inc.).

A similar effect can be achieved by modifying the shoe with a metal bracing bar on either side of the ankle. This extension is attached to the sole of a shoe. The calf is controlled using a cuff around the leg. This has the advantage of minimizing the rigid material in contact with the leg and foot, reducing the opportunities for skin breakdown. It also accommodates for swelling better than an AFO. The disadvantage is that the brace is permanently attached to one pair of shoes, limiting shoe selection.

A final option when the foot becomes so abnormal that placing the foot into a standard or prescription shoe is not possible is the Charcot Restraint Orthosis Walker (CROW). This boot was designed for feet that have developed unstable injuries to the joint that sometimes occur in people with diabetes. It is a hard plastic boot that is molded to the foot and is stabilized by multiple points of contact. It can prevent breakdown of the skin and achieve excellent control of very abnormal feet in situations when little else will help.

There are a number of effective tools available to the physician-patient-orthotist team that can assist in recovery and accommodation of multiple foot problems. Proper communication between all members of this team allows for selection of the optimal method of treatment for any particular problem.

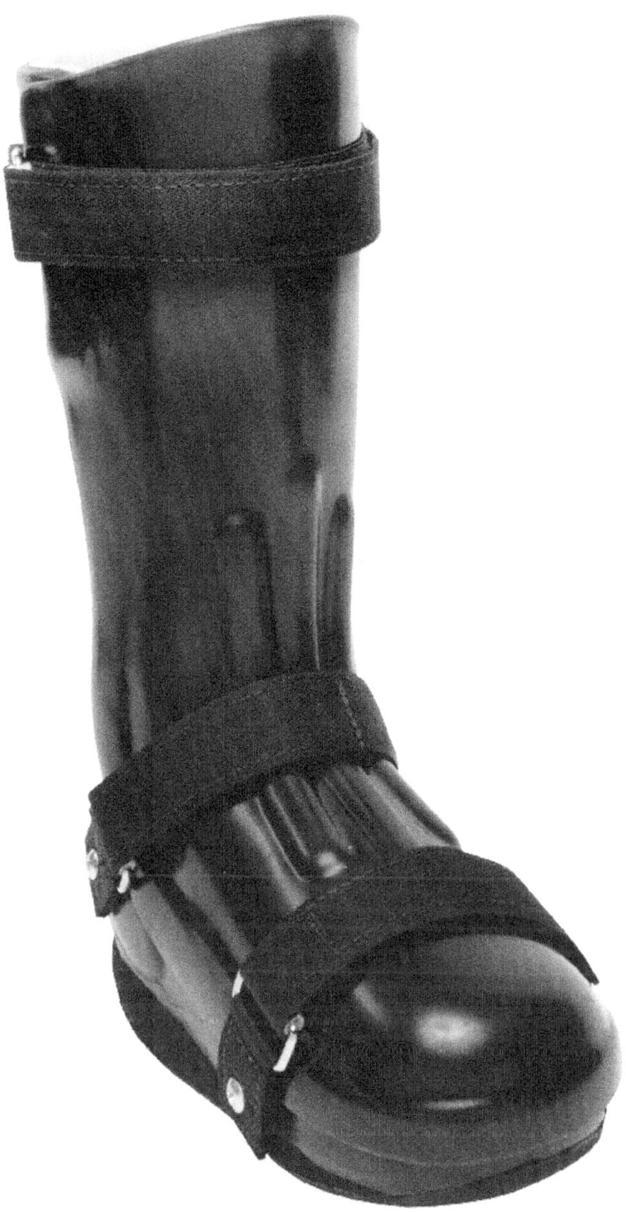

FIGURE 15 A custom boot called a CROW (walker) (by permission, Advanced Orthopro, Inc.).

PROBLEM-ORIENTED RECOMMENDATIONS

Forefoot Overload

The problem: Forefoot overload syndromes have been discussed many times in this book. They include plantar fasciitis, midfoot arthritis, sesamoiditis, metatarsalgia, and possibly fallen arches, bunions, and great toe arthritis. The underlying problem with these disorders is placing too much force on the front of the foot at the end of the step and wearing out the supporting structures.

The solution: Although it is possible to make recommendations for ways in which shoes can be used to reduce the pressure on the forefoot, many other things contribute to shoe comfort. Style is also a significant factor. Unfortunately, there is some aspect of trial and error in picking out comfortable shoes. Use the advice in this book along with recommendations from your physicians and shoe salespeople, and, even more importantly, your own experience to guide you. Try many different styles and brands as no one shoe works for everyone or every problem.

Rational shoe selection is centered on styles that reduce weight on the forefoot. The stiffness and shape of the rocker-soled shoe reduces midfoot motion, while reducing and dispersing force on the forefoot. This is done at the expense of increased motion and stress in the ankle and, to some extent, in the back, knee, and hip.

Many companies have suggested that these rocker-soled shoes help you get fit doing typical everyday activities. There is little scientific evidence for this claim. The changes in the way that you walk while wearing these shoes will alter the work in the hip muscles, giving you soreness in your buttock. It is not likely that they will improve the appearance of your body shape or lead to a measurable increase in your overall fitness or daily calorie usage.

All rocker soles are not the same. There are stable and unstable rocker soles. Unstable rocker soled shoes have a soft heel and may have a greater curve to the sole, especially the heel when seen from both the side and front. This may become a problem for people with poor balance. Falls may be more frequent. Stable rocker soles are stiff and have a curved contoured on the midfoot and toe region, but have a flat area in the heel that helps with stability.

Specific recommendation: Several companies make acceptable rocker-soled shoes ranging in price from under $100 to more than $300. MBT makes exclusively rocker-soled shoes and was one of the first companies to bring them to the commercial market. Others have followed.

All MBT styles, Skechers Shape Up®, Reebok Easytone®, and New Balance Rock and Tone® are unstable rocker-soled shoes. Dansko styles, Finn Comfort, and Mephisto Sano® make a more stable rocker-soled shoe. Other companies make many shoes that, while they are not exactly rocker-soled shoes, are firm and have many of the same properties such as Keen, Clark, and Ecco.

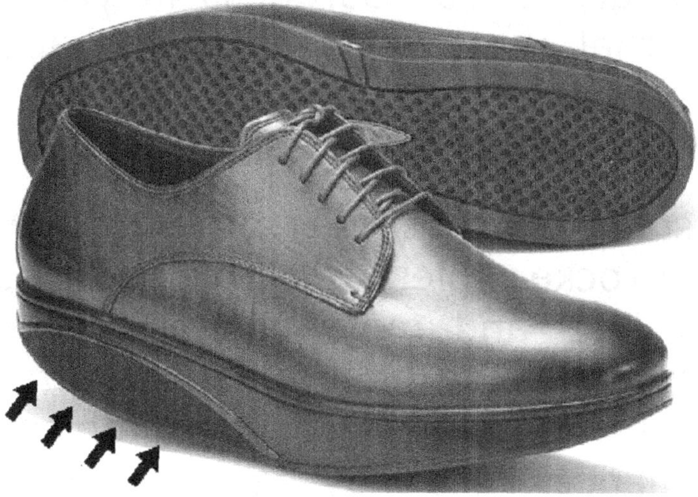

FIGURE 16 An unstable rockersoled shoe. (MBT Kabisa, by permission, the Walking Company)

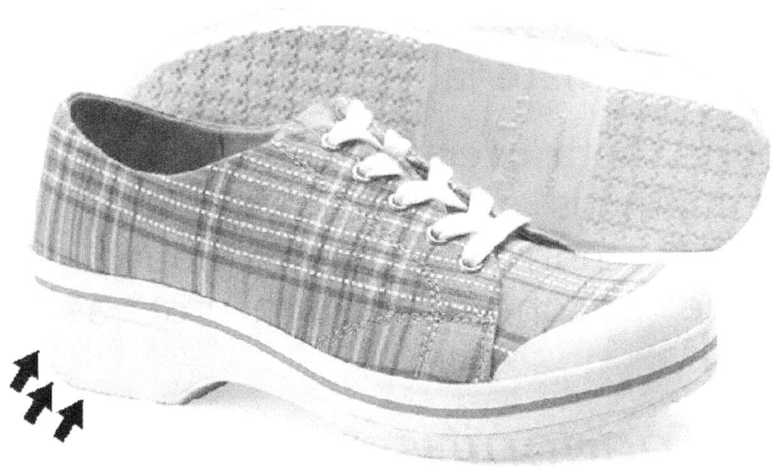

FIGURE 17 A stable rockersoled shoe. (Dansko Veda, by permission, the Walking Company)

MBT and Mephisto make a wide variety of styles including sandals and dress shoes, but are somewhat more expensive. Skechers is broadening their range of styles from tennis shoes into other types of casual wear and is less expensive. Reebok Easytone®, and New Balance Rock and Tone® are tennis shoe–style rockers. Dansko has an extensive women's shoe selection, but less extensive for men. Keen styles tend toward athletic wear and sandals, although they do have a few styles that would be appropriate for industrial/commercial settings. Ecco has a very wide selection of styles.

Midfoot spurs from arthritis can be approached either by using a compliant material for the upper such as a softer leather or Spandex or by using a sandal-type of shoe. Nearly all companies have some form of sandal, but Dansko has models with an upper made of very compliant oiled leather and Ecco makes some with a GoreTex® material.

Arch supports, both over-the-counter and custom, can be helpful methods of reducing load on the front of the foot and controlling arch motion. Heel pads including the silicone ones are not as helpful or effective.

Achilles Tendonitis

The problem: Achilles tendonitis is a scarring of a tendon in the back of the ankle that occurs from wear on the tendon. It causes problems both because the shoe can press on this area and because tension on the tendon perpetuates the damage to the tendon. Overload of the front of the foot can be a problem from poor flexibility.

The solution: Direct pressure on the back of the heel can be lessened either by wearing a backless shoe or by using a shoe with a soft heel counter. Backless shoes include clog styles and sandals. Soft padded heel counters can lessen friction and pain on prominences on the back of the heel.

Using a shoe with a slight heel elevation can reduce tension in the Achilles tendon. Even a one-half- to one-quarter-inch heel lift can be helpful, although many shoes are constructed with an elevation of the heel with respect to the toe area.

Specific recommendations: Many shoe companies (Keen, Ecco, Clarks, Abeo, Birkenstock, and many others) make clog or sandal styles for both men and women with a heel greater than one-half-inch in height. Some companies seem to essentially specialize in them. Many Raffini and Dansko shoes have a one- or two-inch heel lift. Mephisto makes several styles in varying heel heights. Many are backless or have straps to avoid sensitive areas on the back of the heel. With regard to heel height, more is not always better. A shorter heel is suggested before moving on to a higher heel with comfort being the important factor.

A heel pad can be placed in any shoe to elevate the heel. These heel pads are available in most drug stores. Hapad, a company that specializes in selling adhesive felt inserts among other foot-care products, makes an assortment of useful heel pads that are inexpensive and convenient. These pads have adhesive backing and can only be practically transferred from shoe to shoe if they are attached to a shoe liner or orthosis. It can be fixed to the top or bottom of the insert, or it can be placed under the insert on the sole.

If the pad is placed into a shoe, it is recommended that only a portion of the paper backing be removed from the adhesive on the felt. This is done by scoring the paper with an object such as the tip of a ball pointed pin. The pad can be adjusted this way or removed if it is found to be uncomfortable. The felt can then be easily removed by sliding a finger or other blunt instrument under the adhesive backing and teasing it away from the shoe. If the adhesive is completely removed, it can be difficult to remove completely without shredding the felt.

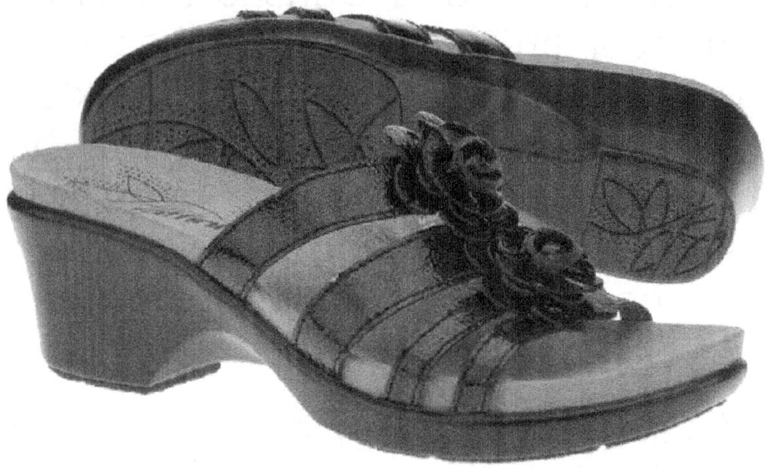

FIGURE 18 A shoe with a wide elevated heel such as this may be helpful in reducing the strain on the Achilles tendon. (Umberto Raffini Nina, by permission, the Walking Company)

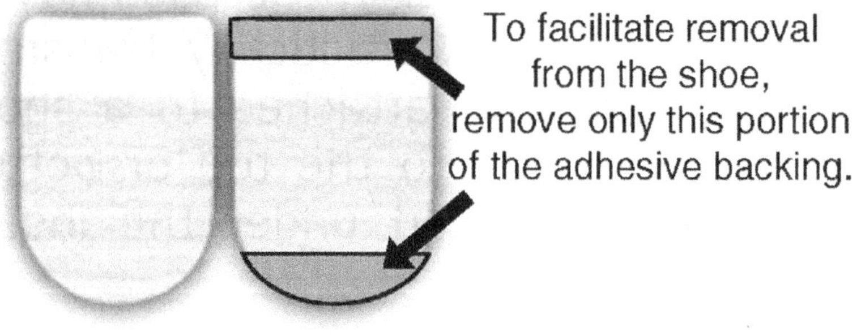

FIGURE 19 A useful and inexpensive heel lift. (By permission, Hapad)

Bunions, Hammertoes, Corns

The problem: The problem is fairly simple—the shoe often does not fit the foot. The heel is too wide when the forefoot fits. The toes ride against the top on the toe box because of their abnormal position. The bunion angles abruptly into the inside of the shoe causing intolerable pain.

The solution: Despite the simple problem, the solution of making a commercially viable shoe that fits every one of the sometimes-bizarre forefoot deformities that doesn't look awful is daunting. Making the toe box wide and high enough for the toes is possible by increasing the width selection. Custom shoes may be necessary for severe deformities or deformities that develop wounds.

Specific shoe recommendations: Nearly any high-quality sandal can be helpful in temperate weather. Keen, and Dansko make closed-toed shoes that have extra room and flexible uppers. Many companies have shoes with the upper of a compliant leather or synthetic mesh-like Gore-Tex® or Spandex®. These materials will decrease the pressure on sensitive bony edges.

A shoe stretcher is an inexpensive device that can help increase the volume of a shoe. Many can increase the amount of room within the shoe in length, width, and height. Small pegs can be added to loosen specific areas. Sometimes, the upper material of a shoe will recoil if the shoe is not worn for a time. A shoe stretcher can help resist this or can be placed into the shoe the night before using it to loosen it. A wide assortment of economical shoe stretchers for a variety of needs can be obtained at heelingtouch.com.

(A)

(B)

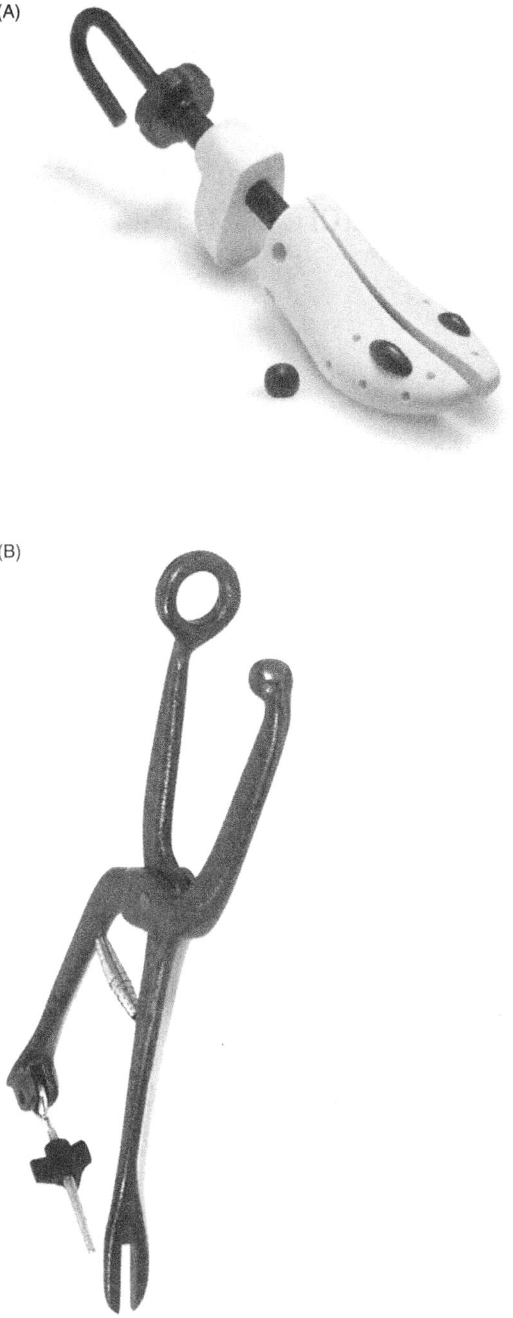

FIGURE 20 A commercially available shoe stretcher that is capable of increasing the volume of the shoe in several directions and loosening specific areas of

the shoe. (A) Two-way shoe stretcher that can increase length or width of the shoe. The pegs can be used to stretch small areas. (B) Ball-ring stretcher to loosen specific areas such as bunions. (By permission, heelingtouch.com)

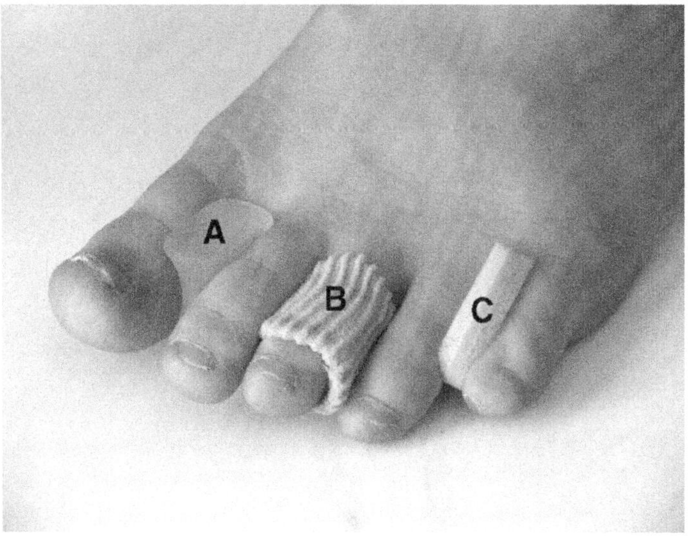

FIGURE 21 An assortment of toe pads (A) Silicone toe separator. (B) Silicone toe sleeve. (C) Foam toe separator.

Toe spreaders and corn pads can be helpful methods of reducing pressure in between toes or in between the foot and the shoe or ground. An adhesive pad in the shape of a doughnut can be placed around the corn to relieve the pressure on the hard tissue. For corns in between toes, a circumferential pad or toe sleeve may be more secure and easier to control within the shoe.

Diabetes and Other Forms of Neuropathy

The problem: Nerve damage is common in diabetes. When nerve damage occurs, protective sensation of the foot is lost. Damage to the circulation can compound the problem. Ulcerations can occur to the feet without any pain or other sense of the injury.

The solution: In addition to other forms of protection such as regular inspection and adequate control of blood glucose levels, shoe selection is very important. In recognition of this, Medicare provides partial reimbursement for shoe wear for eligible people with diabetes and nerve or circulatory damage, foot deformities, calluses, or a history of ulceration. The law requires that the shoes be a part of a comprehensive diabetes program, prescribed by a physician, and dispensed by a prosthetist, pedorthotist, podiatrist, or orthotist.

It is important that the shoes accommodate any deformities present. People with diabetes should avoid going barefoot, wearing sandals, or slippers to prevent foreign bodies such as rocks getting within the shoes and causing damage to the skin. Since an ulcer in a neuropathic foot can be a disaster, guidance from your doctor or other shoe specialist is advised.

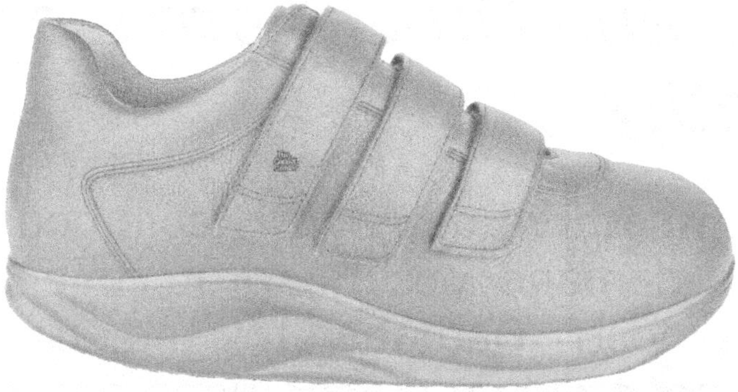

FIGURE 22 A commercially available shoe appropriate for diabetic neuropathy. (Finn Ortho, by permission, Kanner Corporation)

Specific recommendations: Proper fit is critical and it is highly recommended that shoes be examined and fit by a trained shoe-fitting professional. The feet should also be examined very closely every several hours after beginning use of new shoes. Closed-toed shoes are recommended and many manufacturers such as Keen, SAS, Ecco, and Dansko as well as many athletic shoes can be appropriate if custom or prescription shoes are not needed or desired. Several companies, including FinnComfort, make shoes designed specifically for diabetic people.

Ankle Instability

The problem: The ligaments along the ankle sometimes do not function properly after tearing during an ankle sprain and, as a result, irregularities of the ground or other sudden stresses on the ankle will roll the ankle on to its side.

The solution: One way of addressing this problem is to create a buttress along the lateral side of the heel and middle foot to make it more difficult to turn the shoe onto its side. A second way is to extend the upper around the ankle as in a high-topped athletic shoe or to use a brace, either premade or custom, to resist this instability. Another strategy is to minimize the heel height and to take advantage of foot flexibility to accommodate irregularities on the ground by using a low profile flexible shoe such as the newer "minimalist" shoe lines. These shoes may not be appropriate for all activities.

Specific shoe recommendations: Stirrup and lace-up braces are effective methods of providing stability. Some stirrup braces are too bulky or have uncomfortable edges to fit well into a sport shoe. The Active® ankle is a functional, low-profile brace that is appropriate for sports. A lace-up ankle brace does not contain rigid parts, but it can be inconvenient and time-consuming to put on. The choice of ankle brace is mainly a matter of personal preference. Taping is also an effective method of stabilizing the ankle if a well-trained athletic trainer or physical therapist is available.

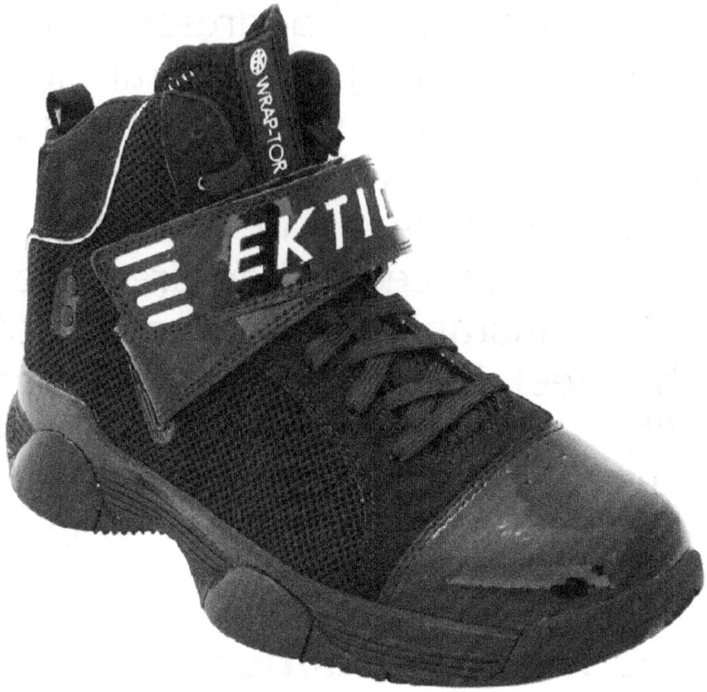

FIGURE 23 Athletic shoe designed to resist recurrent ankle sprains. (By permission, Ektio)

Shoes can be modified with buttresses along the outside to increase the resistance and leverage to rolling over. These can be applied by a pedorthotist. Ektio makes lateral stabilizing high-topped sports shoes with many features that should help to avoid recurrent sprains. Evaluation of this shoe for the prevention of ankle sprains has not yet been done.

Ankle Arthritis

The problem: Motion is restricted in ankle arthritis. Sometimes, it is painful to place the foot so that the heel contacts the floor when standing without shifting the leg. In addition, when the leg passes behind the body during gait, the ankle extends and this can be painful.

The solution: Elevating the heel in the shoe or choosing a shoe with a heel can tilt the foot and open up the front of the ankle so that pain is reduced. In addition, any form of immobilization through bracing will reduce and restrict motion, decreasing pain.

Specific recommendations: Shoe selection should revolve around finding a shoe with a slight heel. A wide variety of shoes fit this criterion. Rocker-soled shoes may be helpful, but stay away from shoes with an unstable or negative heel as this will increase ankle motion and may make the arthritis more painful.

Useful braces include various ankle-foot-orthoses (AFOs) that either restrict ankle motion or eliminate it. Posterior shell AFOs or a molded-leather AFO such as an Arizona brace may be useful. Although the Arizona brace may be more comfortable, it is expensive and many find the lace-up closure to be cumbersome.

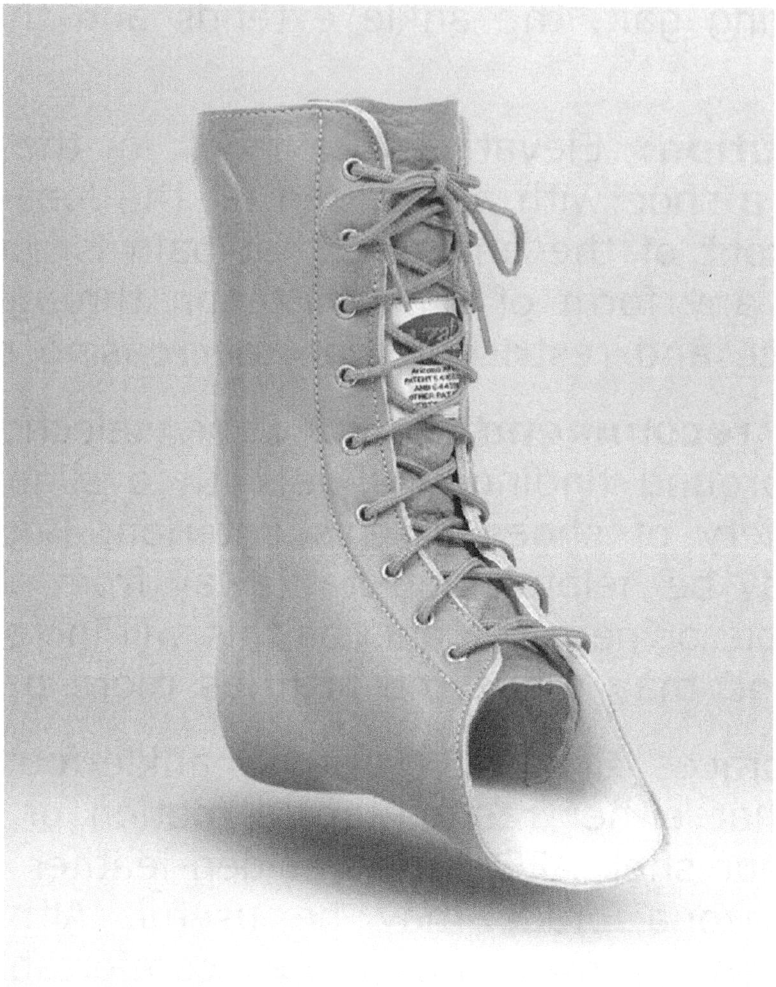

FIGURE 24 A molded ankle-foot-orthosis (AFO) that can be helpful for a number of ankle and hindfoot problems. (By permission, Arizona AFO)

Fallen Arches/Acquired Flat-Foot Deformity

The problem: In fallen arches, the arch flattens and the heel tilts inward, making the inside of the ankle appear bowed. The joints of the arch become unstable and the muscles become weak.

The solution: Fallen arches are treated by repositioning the foot so that it is aligned as close to normal as possible. Most of the time, it is impossible to reproduce the normal alignment of the foot in the brace because of stiffness that is often present in the foot and because it sometimes requires excessive pressure on the foot.

Specific recommendations: An over-the-counter or custom insert can be helpful if the foot is flexible and the degree of deformity is not marked. Sometimes a custom AFO is more reliably effective. Fallen arches are one of the most common conditions treated by an AFO. A short-articulated AFO is often the best choice for this problem. This is a type of AFO with a hinge along the ankle joint.

Shoe choice is based primarily on the shoe's ability to accommodate the brace or insert. The cut around the ankle should be loose enough to accommodate the extra bulk of the brace. Leaving the laces out of the top one or two eyelets may loosen the shoe enough. A medial buttress is sometimes helpful in particularly severe deformities because the ankle can break down and warp the inside portion of the liner. A medial heel wedge can also help to support the hindfoot if the deformity is not too stiff. These modifications would be done by a pedorthotist.

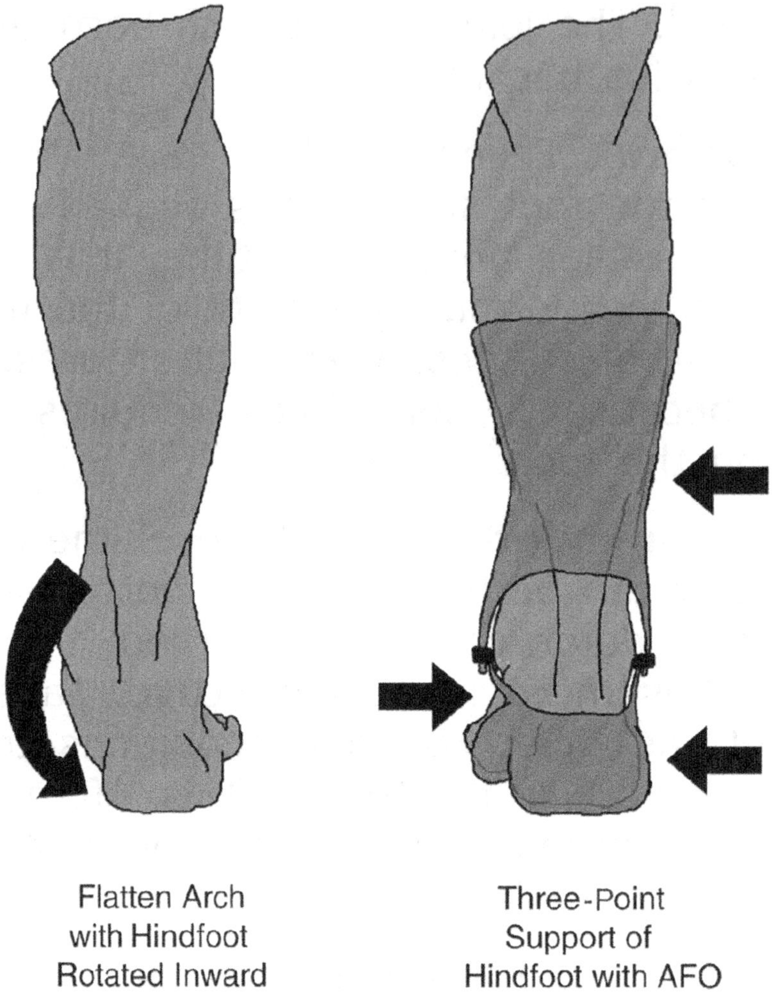

FIGURE 25 A foot with a flattened arch loses support and rotates in the ankle, hindfoot, and arch. A properly fitted short articulated AFO resists this rotation by applying an acceptable amount pressure against the leg using its increased leverage.

Common Medications for Foot Problems

Medications are commonly used in the treatment of foot and ankle disorders. While some may help to cure the problem, most are used to control pain. It is important to be familiar with your medication's mechanism of action and the common side effects.

ORAL PAIN MEDICATIONS

Nonsteriodal Anti-Inflammatory Drugs (NSAIDs)

This is a class of medications that interferes with the production of hormones called *prostaglandins.* The body uses prostaglandins for a wide variety of things including beginning labor, producing mucous to protect the stomach, and clotting blood. Different prostaglandins produce fever, adjust sensitivity to pain and mediate inflammatory responses after injury. Prostaglandins regulate the sensitivity of peripheral nerve pain receptors. NSAIDs are good pain medications that in many studies compare favorably with narcotics. In most clinical situations, they are used as pain medications and not as "anti-inflammatories" as the name implies. Although it is generally assumed that they treat swelling well, there is little evidence of this in most circumstances.

NSAIDs restrict prostaglandin production by inhibiting an enzyme called *cyclo-oxygenase* (COX). There are two or more versions of this enzyme and each is used by the body differently. Most NSAIDs inhibit all of the types of this enzyme. Celecoxib (Celebrex®) inhibits primarily COX-2. This decreases its effect on the stomach. However, stomach problems are still reported with the use of Celecoxib.

Side effects and precautions: Because prostaglandins are used by the body for many beneficial purposes, inhibiting the COX enzyme has fairly predictable side effects. These include:

- Stomach ulcer and bleeding
- Kidney damage and failure
- Asthma and respiratory problems
- Photosensitivity
- Bleeding problems

People taking NSAIDs have a higher rate of cardiac death especially when preexisting heart disease is present. Two COX-2 selective NSAIDs (Bextra® and Vioxx®) have been taken off the market over these concerns. NSAIDs should never be used in pregnancy or if you are breastfeeding.

Common NSAIDs:

- Aspirin (e.g., Bayer®)
- Ibuprofen (Advil, Motrin®)
- Naproxen (Aleve®)
- Diclofenac (Voltaren®)
- Sulindac (Clinoril®)
- Indomethacin (Indocin®)
- Celecoxib (Celebrex®)

Narcotic Analgesics/Opiates

Narcotic analgesics are commonly used to treat pain after surgical and traumatic injuries. They work by mimicking endorphins that help with pain naturally in the body. However, there are many important things to know about this class of medications.

Side effects and precautions: Normal side effects of these medications include nausea and vomiting, itching, sleepiness, wakefulness, vivid or bizarre dreams, and constipation. Sometimes these side effects are tolerable. Occasionally, they require treatment with other medications. True allergic reactions are rare.

All narcotics carry with them a risk of dependence or addiction if taken for a long time. Withdrawal symptoms such as agitation, nervousness, and tremors sometimes are felt after discontinuation of narcotics. Some forms of discomfort do not seem to respond very well to narcotics regardless of the dosage and should be managed using other methods.

Narcotic analgesics are controlled substances and it is against the law to alter or forge prescriptions for narcotics or to give them to anyone else but the person for whom they were prescribed. No person should receive narcotic prescriptions from more than one doctor at a time.

Narcotics are effective medications for the relief of pain. However, they should not be used longer than they are absolutely required and are not a particularly effective way of managing pain over the long term.

TABLE 1. COMMON NARCOTIC PAIN MEDICATIONS

Trade name	Narcotic medication	Other added medication	Anticipated relief
Ultram®	Tramadol	None	6–8hrs
Ultracet®	Tramadol	Acetaminophen	6–8hrs
Tylenol #3®	Codeine	Acetaminophen	4–6hrs
Vicoprofen®	Hydrocodone	ibuprofen	4–6hrs
Vicoden/Lortab®	Hydrocodone	Acetaminophen	4–6hrs
Percocet/Tylox®	Oxycodone	Acetaminophen	4–6hrs
Oxycontin IR®	Oxycodone	None	4–6hrs
Oxycontin ER®	Oxycodone	None	12hrs
Durgesic®	Fentanyl	None (transdermal/patch)	3 days

Steroids (Also Known as Cortisone)

Glucocorticoids or steroids are hormones produced by the adrenal gland that suppress the inflammatory system in response to physiological stress. They are produced from cholesterol and are closely related to sex hormones such as testosterone and estrogen. When released into the blood stream, they enter the cells and bind to a receptor protein. The effect of this is to promote the production of proteins that inhibit inflammation and stop the production of proteins that cause inflammation. Glucocorticoids reduce the production of many types of prostaglandin and closely related leukotriene and inhibit the activity of white blood cells. The result is a potent reduction of many types of pain.

Glucocorticoids can be administered orally, or IV. They can be directly injected into a joint or tendon sheath. Tendon rupture especially in weight-bearing tendons is sometimes seen after this. There is also a possibility that steroid injection into a joint may contribute to arthritis. Steroids can also be applied through the skin using creams.

Side effects and precautions: Side effects of glucocorticoids are numerous. Glucocorticoids increase glucose production and serum glucose levels and so can worsen diabetes. They cause immunosuppression so that infections in people taking them are more common. Longstanding use can cause skin fragility, mood changes, muscle and bone wasting (osteoporosis). The use of oral glucocorticoids should be tapered to avoid potentially dangerous withdrawal symptoms. Spontaneous death of portions of the bone and often the hip joint has occurred after even brief use of steroids, potentially leading to rapidly progressive arthritis.

Common steroids:

- Cortisone
- Hydrocortisone
- Prednisone
- Betamethasone
- Methylprednisolone
- Triamcinolone

Gabapentin/Pregabalin

Gabapentin (Neurontin®) and pregabalin (Lyrica®) were developed to treat epilepsy. Gabapentin has since been FDA-approved to treat epilepsy and post-herpetic neuralgia (shingles). Pregabalin is also FDA-approved for fibromyalgia and diabetic neuropathy. Much of the usage of these medications is off-label, which does not mean it is wrong or illegal. It means that the FDA has approved it for specific problems and is, in some cases, not able to say whether other problems may respond to the medications. It is illegal for the drug companies to market medications for purposes that have not been FDA-approved.

These medications were engineered to inhibit a chemical used by nerves for the transmission of nerve pain signals. However, it is not entirely known how this medication works to relieve pain.

Side effects and precautions: The most common side effects are drowsiness, dizziness, and swelling. There have been reports of suicide while on the medication, so any thoughts of suicide should be immediately reported to a doctor. It also should not be stopped abruptly as withdrawal symptoms can occur.

Duloxetine

Duloxetine (Cymbalta®) was initially developed as an anti-depressant that acts on the neurotransmitters (chemicals that allow signals to go from nerve to nerve) serotonin and norepinephrine. It inhibits the reuptake of these chemicals that are as a result depleted within the nerves. It is thought to modulate pain through its effect on nerves in the pain pathways in the brain and spinal cord. It is currently approved for the treatment of diabetic peripheral neuropathy, fibromyalgia, and chronic pain. The pain relief seems to be an effect that is separate from the medications antidepressant properties.

Side effects and precautions: The most common side effects encountered include dizziness, fatigue, and nausea. There have been reports of withdrawal effects after discontinuing the medication and so it is recommended to taper off it. There have also been reports of suicide while taking duloxetine.

Tricyclic Anti-Depressants (Amitryptaline, Nortryptaline)

Tricyclic antidepressants have been in use for nearly 50 years in the treatment of depression. They have found a use in the treatment of pain although this is not FDA approved. They also inhibit the reuptake of serotonin and norepinephrine within the nerves involved in the transmission of pain. Nortryptline has been recommended as a first-line medication in the treatment of neurogenic pain.[1] They have also been used in fibromyalgia off-label with some reported success.

Side effects and contraindications: Common side effects include dry mouth, blurred vision, urinary retention, constipation, and dizziness. Confusion and delirium are also seen. The medication should be discontinued gradually as withdrawal symptoms have been reported.

Common tricyclic antidepressants used to treat pain:

- Amitriptyline

- Nortriptyline
- Desipramine
- Clomipramine
- Imipramine

MEDICATION USED FOR GOUT

Colchicine

Colchicine is a chemical produced naturally in a plant, the meadow saffron. It acts by retarding the production of microtubules, structural proteins that make up the skeleton of cells and are important in cell reproduction and movement. This is important in white blood cells. Inhibiting this migration keeps the white blood cells from traveling to gouty joints and contributing to inflammation. It also lowers the pH of joints and keeps gout crystals from forming.

Side effects and precautions: The most common side effect is diarrhea. This usually limits the amount that can be taken. It can also suppress bone marrow production and decrease white blood cell production as well as red blood cell and platelet production. Colchicine should not be taken by people with limited, or no kidney function.

Probenecid

Probenecid interferes with the resorption of uric acid and a number of other chemicals by a transport protein in the kidneys. It helps to increase the elimination of uric acid and lowers the concentration of uric acid level within the serum. It may also interfere with the way that the kidneys handle other medications such as NSAIDs and penicillin antibiotics.

Side effects and precautions: Salisylate NSAIDs such as aspirin should not be taken with probenecid. Probenecid should not be taken until the acute stage of gouty joint inflammation has stopped to avoid aggravation of the gout attack. People who have had uric acid kidney stones should not use probenecid.

Allopurinol/Febuxostat (Uloric)

Allopurinol is similar in structure to a precursor of uric acid and inhibits the enzyme that metabolize this precursor into uric acid. Febuxostat also inhibits this enzyme in a slightly different way. Both therefore inhibit the production of uric acid. Because of the considerably higher price of febuxostat, its use should probably be reserved for people that cannot take allopurinol or do not achieve the desired reduction of uric acid levels with allopurinol. Neither should be used to treat acute gout attacks, but they can decrease the serum level of uric acid so that uric acid deposits resorb over time (often a period of months).

Gout is a chronic disease and usually treatment continues throughout the lifetime once started.

Side effects and precautions: Side effects with allopurinol are rare. In rare cases a serious skin allergic reaction can occur.

ANTI-FUNGAL MEDICATIONS

Anti-fungal antibiotic medications are effective against onchyomycosis or fungal infections of the foot. They can also be useful in severe athlete's foot. For fungal infection of the toenail, the medication must be taken over a prolonged period of time and be incorporated into the growing nail.

Side effects and precautions: As a class, these medications as very similar. Many troublesome complications are possible, but the medications are usually well tolerated. Liver irritation (about 3% of people), potentially progressing to liver failure (very, very rare), is probably the most worrisome and is usually monitored with blood tests during the treatment. Some people notice changes in taste or smell, and occasionally develop depression.

Examples of antifungal medications:

- Terbinafine (Lamisil®)
- Itraconazole (Sporonox®)
- Griseofulvin (Grisovin®)

TOPICAL MEDICATIONS FOR SKIN

Topical Medications for Pain

Capsaicin (*Zostrix®*)

Capsaicin is the chemical that makes hot peppers hot. It works by stimulating the pain nerves within the skin specifically those that use a special neurotransmitter (a chemical that nerves use to communicate) called *Substance P.* If the nerve is stimulated frequently, the nerve's supply of Substance P becomes depleted and it cannot transmit pain signals as well.

Capsaicin is an over-the-counter cream or ointment that can be applied up to four times a day. It can cause the skin to burn after the first few applications. Apply it to the skin overlying the painful area and rub in.

Cautions: Allergic reactions to Capsaicin are possible. Wash the hands thoroughly after applying Capsaicin as contact with mucus membranes such as the eyes can cause painful burning.

Topical Nonsteroid Anti-Inflammatory

Many preparations are available with topical nonsteroidal anti-inflammatory medications within them. The mechanism of action for the topical medication is the same as above. The most popular medications use tolamine salicylate (Aspercreme®) and diclofenac (Flexorpatch®, Pennsaid®, and Voltaren® gel). In most studies, it is equivalent or superior to taking NSAIDs by mouth. Although the amount of medication that gets into the body system is still quite small, it is not approved for use in people that are pregnant or nursing.

Side effects and precautions: Allergic reactions or skin problems to the medication or parts of the topical carrier are the primary side effects.

Anesthetics (Lidoderm®)

Lidocaine accumulates in the cell membranes of nerves and reduces their ability to conduct signals temporarily. Topical Lidocaine (Lidoderm®) in patch form is approved by the FDA for the treatment of painful postherpetic neuralgia (shingles), but is sometimes prescribed by doctors for other painful problems. It may not be effective for pains arising from problems deep under the skin. The patch is applied for up to 12 hours and absorption into the body's circulation is low. If used as directed, toxicity is unlikely.

Side effects and precautions: Primarily allergic reactions and application site rashes.

Steroid Creams

The mechanism of glucocorticoid or steroid action has been mentioned previously in this section. Topical administration of glucocorticoids, cortisone, or steroids have the same effect, but absorption and side effects relating to its effect on body structures other than the skin is greatly reduced. Steroids are used in the treatment of many rashes relating to reactions from the immune system such as allergic rashes and psoriasis.

Side effects and precautions: Many reactions are possible but primary concerns are atrophy or thinning of the skin, stretch marks and decreasing the resistance to infection.

Examples of steroid creams:

Over-the-counter:

- Hydrocortisone (0.5% and 1.0% preparations)

Low potency:

- Alclomethasone (Aclovate®)
- Triamcinolone (Kenalog®)

High potency:

- Betamethasone dipropionate (Diprolene®)
- Fluocinonide (Lidex®)
- Clobetasol propionate (Temovate®)

Anti-Fungal Creams

Anti-fungal creams are an important method of treating fungal infection of the skin, most commonly Athlete's foot. In less severe cases, oral medication is usually not necessary. These medications are applied two to four times per day according to the package and your doctor's instructions.

Side effects and precautions: Side effects are mostly allergic and other skin reactions. Occasionally, numbness on the treated area can occur, which usually resolves after usage is discontinued.

Examples of anti-fungal creams include:

- Clotrimazole (Lotrimin®)
- Miconazole (Monistat®)
- Fluconazole (Diflucan®)
- Tolnaftate (Tinactin®)

NOTE

[1] Robert H. Dworkin et al. (2010). "Recommendations for the Pharmacological Management of Neuropathic Pain: An Overview and Literature Update." *Mayo Clinic Proceedings 85* (3): S3–S14.

Ten Important Rules for Weight Control

This book is not meant to be a weight-loss guide. However, there seem to be some simple basic principles that often get forgotten when discussing weight loss. If they are followed closely, they are the keys to reducing and maintaining a healthy weight.

1. COMMIT!

A solid mental commitment needs to be made prior to beginning healthy lifestyle habits. If your goal is to lose 10 pounds, get into that dress or suit for your son's wedding, and then go back to your normal routine, you might as well stop here. These tips will not get you there. The odds of your keeping that weight off are low. A healthy lifestyle is a commitment for life, every day, every meal, and every food and activity choice. You must commit to avoid foods that are high in salt, fat, and simple carbohydrates and choose foods that are flavorful in other ways. So stop dieting and start making healthy decisions.

Do not try to solve all of your problems at one time. Smoking and alcohol abuse are even more dangerous problems than being overweight. Tackle these first. Success at any one of these is a major accomplishment.

Begin by weighing yourself. Get a notebook and keep it in your purse, briefcase, or pocket. Make reasonable obtainable goals for exercise and weight loss. Determine that before you sit down for a meal what you're going to eat and stick to it. Don't starve yourself, but control and pace yourself. Then write down what you ate. This is absolutely crucial as it provides you accountability and a way to evaluate yourself. Write down when you fail and why. One important principle is to analyze the causes of failure and develop strategies to solve these problems.

2. PRACTICE WILL POWER!

Will power is not a gift that some have and some don't. It is a skill or strength that requires practice to develop. Giving in to a sweet treat that you eat on impulse is a bad habit that must be broken. Yielding to temptation makes it difficult to have will power the next time and, before you know it, your whole program is down the drain. Sitting on the couch all night watching TV is also a routine that can sabotage your health and fitness. Be proud of yourself when you make the right choices.

There will be times when you fail and there will be times when you get something special that is out of bounds, but limit the damage by controlling the amount you take and get back on the program right away. Limit these special times to a few per month. It's more than the extra calories. Giving in to these things develops habits that get you off track. It is a lot like giving a reformed alcoholic just one drink. It nearly always leads to more.

One way to minimize these lapses is to understand when you are vulnerable. Stress, confusion, frustration, and fear will lower your guard. It is important to understand this and to find ways of minimizing the opportunities to stray from your plan.

3. GET A HOBBY!

Food stimulates pleasure sensors within the brain that also control many other important behaviors (sex, parenting, drug and narcotic addiction). Find something else to take food's place in your life. If work takes 40 hours per week and 56 hours of sleep, that leaves another 82 hours per week that you must fill. Look for something rewarding that you can be proud of. Start a project such as cleaning up the yard or working on your house. Remember those household projects that need tackling? How about that garden that you want to replant? Just find something that gets you out from behind the computer, TV, or magazine.

Volunteer! Work at your church, synagogue, or mosque. Go have some fun in the park with your spouse or pet.

4. CONTROL STRESS!

Stress is a waste-line killer. Stress changes the way that our body uses nutrients by storing more fat. Stress and dieting seems to provoke behaviors that lead to binge eating. Deep in the wiring within our brains, we have developed tactics to help us survive. When our ancestors were exposed to periodic starvation (similar to modern-day dieting) and stress, things weren't probably going too well. Binge eating was a way of ensuring that we got nutrition when it was available. Animals that are exposed to these pressures in laboratory studies[1] do the same thing. In modern culture, it is adaptation that is not necessary, yet it persists within our brain.

The first step is to identify the stress and realize the effect that it has on behavior. Anticipate the problems that it might cause and look for solutions to avoiding temptations during those times. Evaluate the problems in your life, financial, marital, social, and see if you can find a way to decrease the stress or find resources around you that can help you find other ways to cope with it. Counselors, friends, and physicians can be good sources for help, but you need to ask.

5. CHOOSE THE RIGHT FOODS!

We all know what they are. Fresh fruits, vegetables, lean meats, and legumes and there are hundreds of cookbooks out there that show us how to make them delicious. So get the other stuff out of your house. Don't wait until you've eaten it. If you feel bad about throwing it away, give what you can to the food pantry. Eating it is just as much a form of waste as throwing it away. Then stop buying more. Always avoid shopping for groceries while hungry.

Stay away from salty, fatty, or sweet foods as much as possible. However, it is even more important to stay away from these foods before meals or when you are very hungry. The habit of binge eating is much easier to slip into when the eating and pleasure centers within your brain are highly stimulated by these foods. Begin with fresh vegetables and salads with light dressing, before going on to heavier courses.

Alcohol also contains a lot of calories and lessens inhibitions. After a few drinks, you will be much more impulsive. Avoid overindulging as much as possible. Stay hydrated with water, but avoid sweet (even artificially sweet) drinks.

Other than this, a key word is fiber. Fiber slows the digestion and gives you a prolonged satisfied feeling. Learn about it and buy foods that contain it.

6. SAVOR YOUR FOOD!

People who eat slowly, eat less. Pace yourself. It takes time for your stomach to react to the food within it by sending the appropriate hormones to signal that you've had enough. Food is made to enjoy and you should choose delicious foods that make eating a pleasure. A meal should take 30 to 60 minutes without second helpings, but do not sit with the food in front of you after you are done. Clear it away so that you are not tempted to pick at it. Enjoy the conversation of your family and friends around you.

7. PORTION CONTROL!

For people who are serious to lose weight, this can be a major source of failure. Portions that are on side of the box of cereal can be surprisingly small. However, they may be the appropriate amount for you. It takes some time to get used to pushing yourself away from the table after a smaller portion, but you may find that you are just as satisfied.

8. EXERCISE!

Lack of exercise is perhaps the most important reason that most of us put on weight. Make a commitment to exercise one hour or more five days a week, more if you can. Be sure that at whatever level you start, it's something that is sustainable. Too many exercise programs eventually burn out from enthusiasm that is not maintained and goals that are not realistic. Consistency is the key. If you just have to watch that TV program, get an exercise bike or treadmill in front of your TV and exercise while you watch.

9. GET A COACH!

It's hard to stop overeating without help. There are going to be times when you're going to get away from your goals and begin to slip back into your old ways. This is where a coach is critical. Ideally, it is someone who is as interested and excited about your success as you are. When you choose your coach, find:

- Someone with whom you have a stable relationship.
- Someone who cares about your success.
- Someone whose opinion is important to you.
- Someone from whom you can take criticism.
- Someone who has enough self-confidence to tell you to shape up.
- Someone who sees you enough to check up on you. Your coach should evaluate your foot and activity diary periodically and discuss improvement.

If you are going to choose your wife, husband, son, daughter, mother or father, you need to take a close honest look at your relationship. People have a lot of baggage in these relationships. It is the exceptional close family relationship that fulfills all of these points.

To the coach: Your job is to keep your friend on track. Your friend is counting on you to keep him or her honest and achieve your goals. It is a long-term commitment.

Don't:

- Be mean.
- Accept the same excuses.
- Give up.

Do:

- Be encouraging.
- Be patient.
- Look over your friend's diary.
- Make suggestions.
- Offer solutions.
- Help make realistic goals.
- Stay in touch.
- Find ways to celebrate the victories.

10. REEVALUATE!

Keep a diary of your food and exercise. In the best circumstances, count calories. If you don't think that you can commit to the time required to do this indefinitely, then just keep a list with the number of portions and the types of food you eat. Also, record your workout activities. Weigh yourself weekly. Make goals for weight loss and working out. Review them with your coach periodically.

Look at your progress and if you are not achieving the results you want, look for reasons why. If the amount of energy you use is larger than what you are consuming, you will lose weight. That is a Law of Thermodynamics. Find out what is wrong. It usually isn't that hard to figure out if you are honest with yourself.

NOTE

[1] Boggiano MM, Chandler PC. Binge eating in rats produced by combining dieting with stress. *Curr Protoc Neurosci.* 2006 Aug;Chapter 9:Unit9.23A.

Care of Your Cast or Dressing

Casts are used in the treatment of many different conditions including various forms of tendonitis, sprains, and other soft tissue injuries as well as fractures. Proper care of your cast is important for the successful treatment of your problem and for your safety.

Although casts can be uncomfortable and the conditions that they treat can be painful, the cast itself should not be painful. If your pain increases or if the cast feels too tight, you should elevate the cast above the level of your heart. If this does not quickly alleviate the problem, contact your physician immediately.

Itching is also quite common. Over-the-counter antihistamines such as diphenhydramine (Benadryl®) and the nondrowsy antihistamine, loratadine (Claritin®) can help stop this. Never stick anything into the cast to scratch an itchy area, because it can damage your skin and cause potentially serious infections and wounds. Commercially available vacuum devices have been introduced that suck air through the cast, decreasing some of the itching and drying the perspiration within the cast (www.castcooler.com).

Protect your cast when in the rain or in damp places. If the cast gets slightly damp, it can be dried with a blow dryer on low heat. If it gets wet, the cast should be changed because it can damage the skin.

If a cast rubs on your skin, wounds and blisters can occur. This should be immediately reported to your doctor. Any drainage from the cast not related to a surgical wound or ulcer should also be immediately reported to your doctor. These areas are most common at the ends of the cast, especially the top of the foot, and the front of the shin. Other danger areas are more difficult to check such as on the front of the ankle, along the bony prominences on the inside and outside of the ankle, and at the back of the heel. They are easily and quickly treated with replacement of the cast and simple wound care if they are caught early. If you are experiencing discomfort or rubbing in any of these places, it needs to be checked out right away.

Fiberglass cast surfaces can be abrasive. It is advisable to wrap the cast with an ace wrap at night to avoid damaging your sheets, your other leg, or partner. This is especially dangerous when you have nerve damage from diabetes or another disorder or if you have circulatory problems.

Cast odor is a common problem and can be helped by regular cast changes usually every three or four weeks. Avoiding heavy physical activity and exercising, anything that makes you sweat, also will help. Do not pour powder down the cast as it can cake and damage the skin.

SHOWERING/BATHING WITH YOUR CAST

It is impossible to guarantee that your cast will remain completely dry during a shower or bath, but most people are unwilling to forgo showering or take a "sponge bath" for the entire time that they will be wearing a cast. Safely showering with a cast is possible with some preparation.

The first step is to ensure that you have a safe place to rest while you are in the shower. If there are restrictions on the weight that you can place on your leg, ensure that you have a seat on which to rest. Even if you can place full weight on the leg, a prepared cast can be very slippery. A shower chair should be obtained if the shower does not have a bench. Nonslip adhesive shower strips can also make slick shower surfaces safer.

Prepare the cast by taking a washcloth or hand towel and rolling or fold it into a roll. Tape or ace wrap this above the cast. An ace wrap should be wrapped around the weight-bearing portion of the cast to avoid abrasion and tearing of the plastic bag by the cast. Place the cast and towel completely within a heavy plastic bag and secure the bag with a rubber band. If there are significant circulatory problems in the leg, avoid very tight rubber bands.

Commercially available cast protectors can be substituted for the plastic bag and can be obtained at most medical supply stores or online. The cost is about $30. Many find them more convenient than plastic bags, but they also can leak. Many of the designs seem to be made out of a flimsy plastic and can tear easily. Securing them in the way that is described earlier can prevent problems. The Dry Pro™ cast protector does an excellent job in preventing leaks and is very durable, but is also slightly more expensive.

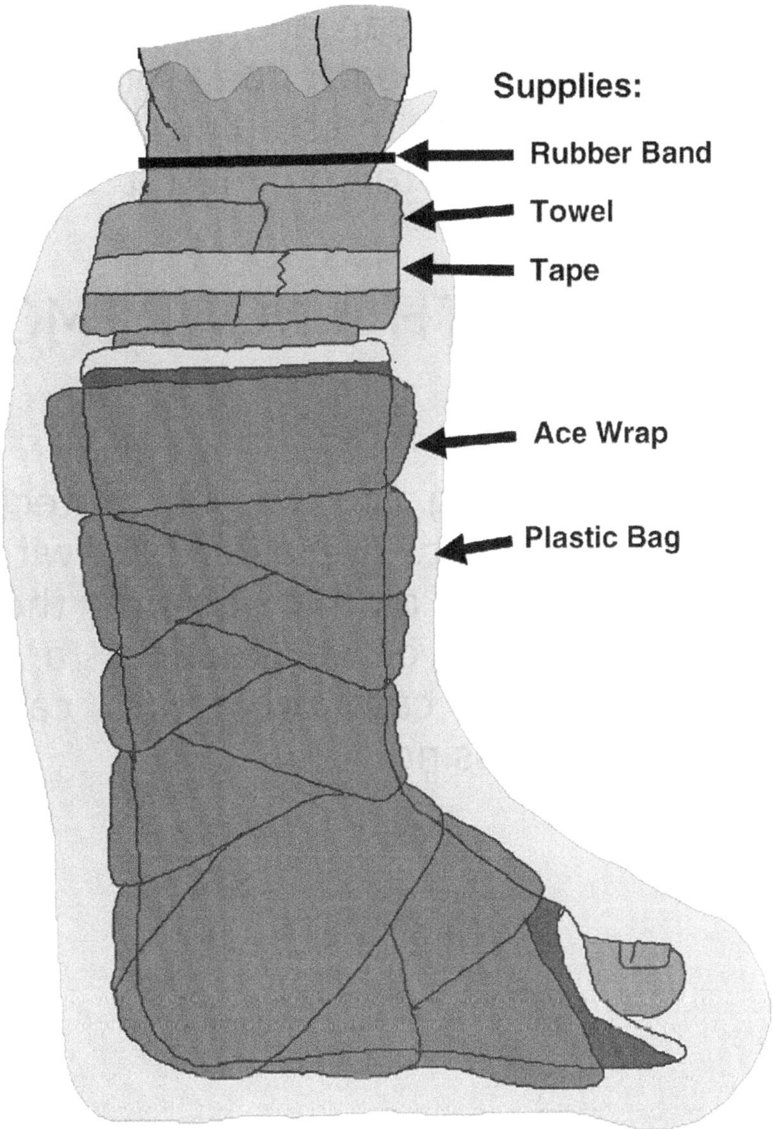

FIGURE 1 A cast secured for a shower with commonly available household items.

While showering, avoid directing the showerhead at the cast or leg. A hose attachment to a faucet with a nozzle is very effective at accomplishing this and can be obtained at most department stores. Ideally, you should wet your body and hair for a short period.

Turn the shower off and soap and lather appropriately. Then turn the shower back on for rinsing. This minimizes the chance of moistening the cast. Never submerge the cast in water no matter how well it is protected.

SHOWERING WITH A NONREMOVABLE DRESSING

A nonremovable dressing can also be protected in the shower similar to a cast. A plastic bag with a towel barrier between the top of the bag and the dressing is an effective way of protecting a dressing. Commercially available cast protectors can also be used to protect a dressing.

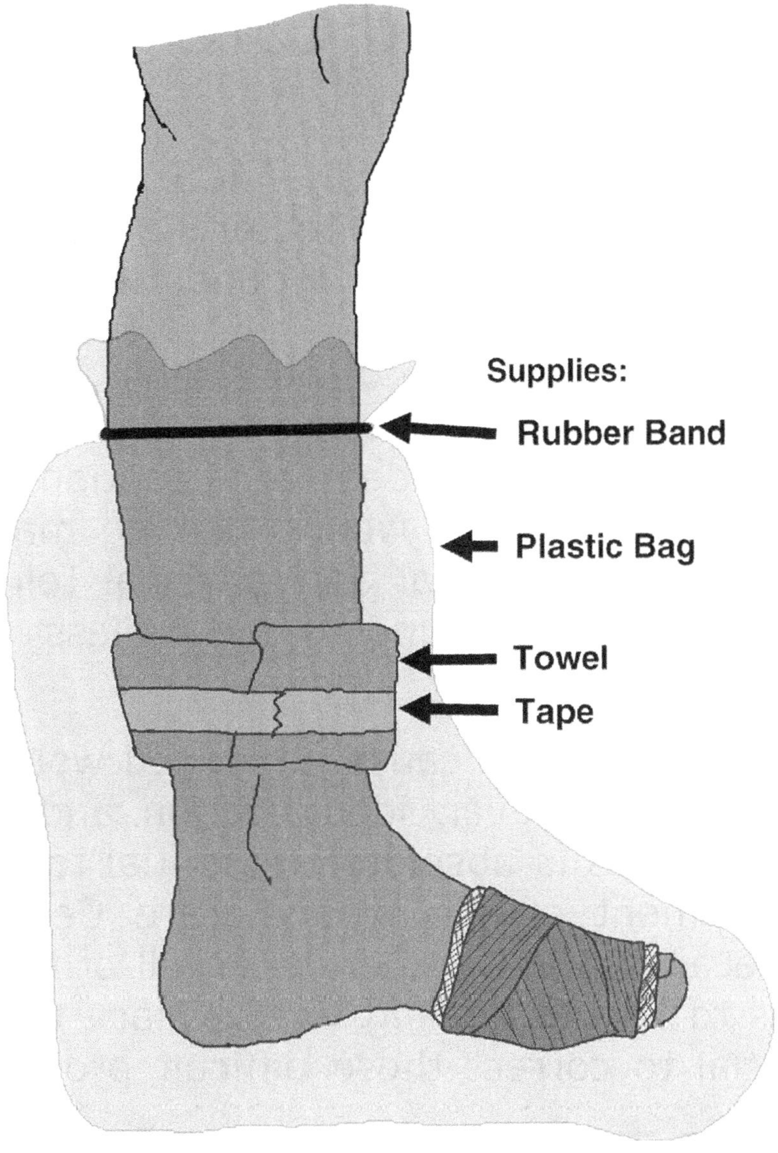

FIGURE 2 Safe preparation for showering for a foot with a nonremovable dressing.

Wound Care

S. Campbell Gabrielsen M.D. FACS CWS FACCWS
Medical Director
Hancock Center for Wound Healing

Injuries such as cuts and abrasions are common experiences in life. We are accustomed to these issues healing without a great deal of attention. However, in certain circumstances, wound healing may become a problem. The emotional and physical toll that this extracts is difficult to understand unless you have experienced it.

The problems that may cause prolonged wound healing are numerous. However, identification and correction of these problems is absolutely essential to treatment. The development of the Wound Care Center in the last two decades brings expertise on all of the different challenges to wound healing to one place to maximize the potential to correct these difficult problems.

FACTORS THAT INTERFERE WITH WOUND HEALING

To heal, a wound requires nutrition. Nutrition involves providing the nutrients that the body needs to build tissue. These factors are the energy- and tissue-building blocks, oxygen, sugar, and protein.

Oxygen is probably the single most important factor. If the wound does not have enough oxygen, it will not heal. Adequate oxygen cannot enter the injured tissue through the wound or the skin. Contrary to popular belief, wounds do not need direct contact with air to heal. Oxygen is carried by the blood on the hemoglobin molecules within the red corpuscles. Tobacco smoke exposes the hemoglobin to carbon monoxide, which binds to the hemoglobin much better than oxygen. Smoking is a major cause of poor wound healing.

The circulation is important because it carries the nutrients within the serum, the oxygen within the red blood cells, and white blood cells that fight off infection to the wound. The arteries can be thought of as the roads entering the wound. Arteriosclerosis or "hardening of the arteries" clogs the arteries by narrowing them with cholesterol deposits until they are blocked. Factors that might cause arteriosclerosis are age, hypertension, smoking, diabetes, and cholesterol and lipid diseases. Other substances in our environment and diet can also affect the circulation. The most common is nicotine, again, in cigarette smoke. Nicotine activates small muscles within the small blood vessel walls cell to contract, further limiting blood supply. High levels of caffeine in the diet can also have similar effect.

The veins return blood to the circulation. In the feet, the blood pushes toward the heart against gravity. The pressure resisting the blood's return is called hydrostatic pressure. The reason that the water comes out of the faucet in a home at a significant pressure in many cities is because the water is pumped into a water tower. The vertical height of the column from the top of the water in the water tower to the faucet is the pressure of the water as it comes out of the faucet. This is often measured in millimeters of mercury (like blood pressure is measured), but it could just as well be measured in millimeters or feet of water.

In the body, the water tower with its pump is the heart. The vertical distance from your heart to the foot is the possible pressure on your veins. If there were no valves in the veins, this pressure would directly push the fluid in your blood into your tissues. The valves in your veins help to decrease this pressure by dividing up the pressure column into small segments and using the muscle action within the legs to help pump the blood in small increments, reducing the hydrostatic pressure on the legs.

One of the most common problems with this system is damage to the vein valves, commonly called varicose veins. When clots within the veins or too much pressure over a long period of time damages the valves, the pressure in the veins increases. The increased pressure causes the veins to dilate, which damages the valves further. The increased pressure also pushes fluid from the circulation, across the vein walls into the tissue, resulting in swelling. Small bleeds cause a dark discoloration around the ankles called venous stasis dermatitis. This discoloration comes from the iron within the blood depositing into the tissue. The iron deposits, swelling, and the resistance to blood flow all make the skin prone to wounds that may be difficult to heal.

When fluid gets out of the circulation and in between the tissue cells, it is recovered by a series of vessels that are difficult to see with the naked eye called lymphatic vessels. Lymphatic vessels collect fluid and transport it into the chest where it drains into the veins. Blockage of these vessels either through external pressure on the lymphatic vessel or damage from surgery and other trauma will also cause swelling. Sources of external pressure causing blockage may be abdominal obesity, swelling in the hip or knee, or infections and tumors anywhere from the foot to the chest.

The damage or overload of the lymphatic vessels, causing the swelling, can result from severe infections, trauma, and congenital defects in the formation of the lymphatic system, heart disease, and kidney problems. The high water and protein concentration within a swollen leg promotes bacterial growth possibly, causing an infection within the skin called cellulitis. The distended tissue also does not allow nutrients and oxygen to get to the tissue cells as well.

Nutrition is absolutely crucial while healing a wound. In a person with a long-standing wound, the drainage from the wound contains important proteins that may be lost so fast that the body is not able to replace them. Protein malnutrition may be discovered in a significant number of people experiencing severe chronic wounds. Malnutrition is also fairly common in the elderly and people with multiple chronic diseases including cancer and diabetes.

Keeping the cut clean is very important in wound healing. Caustic substances will retard metabolism and reproduction of the cells that heal a wound including the skin cells and connective tissue cells. Although bacteria produce some of these substances, the source can be the body itself. The inflammatory process creates chemicals that kill bacteria. The white blood cells that fight infection excrete proteins that digest other proteins. These proteins are meant to destroy bacteria, but like any weapon, it can cut both ways. These substances also can damage the fragile repair cells in the process. Infected or dead tissue should be removed to encourage healing.

The substances that people place on the wound in the misguided effort to clean it may also become part of the problem. Hydrogen peroxide, concentrated iodine solutions and Dakin's solution, bleach and baking soda have been used for many years as wound cleansers. Although each of these is somewhat toxic to the bacteria on a wound, they are perhaps more damaging to the repairing tissue and should be avoided.

Mechanical pressure, abrasion, or tension on the wound can also inhibit healing. These factors are a common cause of repeated tissue injury. If it is not reduced, it will perpetuate the wound. Tension on the skin from unstable joints can also produce a wound that will not heal.

TREATMENT OF WOUNDS

Many times, bad personal habits need to be addressed and eliminated if you need help healing a prolonged wound. Smoking is perhaps the worst. Although any reduction in smoking can help, quitting is the best way to promote healthy healing. Cutting down on sweets and alcohol is also helpful. These foods replace nutritious food and lead to reductions in vitamin and protein in your diet. Finally, drinking large quantities of caffeinated beverages can affect wounds and should be limited to no more than two cups of coffee or two soft drinks per day.

Proper wound care is perhaps the next most important step. A healing wound should be kept moist at all times. Skin cells must migrate from the edge of the wound and form new skin over the old wound. Dryness or desiccation damages these immature cells. In certain wounds, special dressings or ointments can help maintain this moist environment.

An ideal dressing for all wounds should:

- Remove the excess fluid and toxic materials.
- Maintain a moist wound healing environment.

- Provide thermal insulation.
- Provide protection from infection.
- Be free from contaminants.
- Be able to be removed without sticking to or otherwise injuring the wound bed.
- Absorb wound odor.
- Be easy to use.
- Require a reasonable changing frequency.
- Come in a variety of sizes and shapes.
- Be cost-effective and is covered by most health plans.

Cleaning is the first step. Some wounds have infected or dead tissue. If this is not removed, dead tissue provides an environment where the bacteria can exist that is protected from the immune cells within the body and the antibiotics that are used to treat infections and promote a damaging prolonged immune response. Removal of this dead tissue may require surgery or cleaning by a professional wound care specialist in an outpatient clinic.

The area should be rinsed by a cleanser such as saline, mild soap, or dilute, iodine-based products. An effective cleanser should not disrupt healing and should not have antibacterial properties that kill the normal skin organisms. Saline has no inherent anti-microbial properties, but it has a salt concentration that is similar to body fluids and so is not toxic to the wound. More sophisticated wound cleansers like Allcleanz® and Dermagram® are water-based and contain mild detergents along with a salt concentration that is similar to that of the body. These products soften the tissue, making it easier to remove the debris and keep the wound clean.

Antibacterial soaps have been marketed to increase the effectiveness of common soaps, but, in scientific study, have not been found to be more effective and can induce drug resistance.

Dressing options have undergone a bit of a revolution in the past decades. Simple gauze dressings, while inexpensive and readily available, do little to improve the wound environment and can stick to the wound if allowed to dry, injuring fragile regenerative cells. Gauze can be used as a primary dressing, wet or dry, or as a secondary dressing over another product.

The petroleum dressings such as xeroform, scarlet red, and Unna® boots were introduced in the early 1980s and helped to reduce the adherence of gauze dressings. Foam dressings, and hydrocolloids were subsequently introduced in the late 1980s. Foam dressings such as Allevyn®, Reston®, and Polymem® are absorbent and do not form lint. They absorb water and so are good when wounds have continuous drainage. In general they do not work well for dry wounds or in very moist wounds, the moisture in the dressings can make the surrounding skin irritated and wet.

Hydrocolloids such as Duoderm®, Restore®, and Replicare® are dressings made of cellulose, pectin, and gelatin. This allows the dressing to absorb wound fluid and creates a gel-like substance that pulls the fluid into the dressing and wicks it away from the wound and skin. They help clean wounds to heal and wounds with debris to clean themselves. They are useful in some, but not all wounds.

More recently, other sophisticated dressings have been introduced including alginates, hydogels, and collagen dressings. These new dressings, although more expensive, often do not need frequent changing. Alginates such as Maxsorb®, Sorbsan®, and Algisite® are dressings that are made from brown seaweed. The products are soft, highly absorbent and conform well to the shape of the wound. Alginates are suited for wounds that drain a moderate to large amount and can absorb up to 20 times their weight in fluid.

Hydrogels such as Curasol®, Curagel®, and Solosite® re-hydrate the wound. They are soothing and decrease pain and can also be used with infection in place. They are good for partial or full thickness wounds, radiation injuries, deep wounds, and some wounds with dead tissue.

Collagen dressings such as Fibracol® and Purachol® are made from the most abundant protein in the body.

By placing collagen in the wounds this encourages the deposit of new collagen fibers and promotes tissue healing. They are very versatile dressings. Due to cost, however, specialists primarily use these dressings. They have a nonadhering layer can be removed from the wound without trauma.

Although some swelling is unavoidable, excessive swelling impairs circulation and nutrition within the tissue. Elevation is an effective method of controlling edema and should be used to reduce severe swelling. Do not ice the leg to decrease swelling. Your foot should be kept warm to improve the circulation of the leg and speed the metabolism of the tissue, but never use heating pads or immerse the extremity in hot water. Compression is the key, along with elevation, and exercise. Since most wounds associated with severe swelling tend to be wounds with copious drainage, absorptive dressing under compression-changed daily or twice a day, alginates changed daily, or foams are excellent choices.

Concentrations of pressure on certain parts of the foot are the most common cause of a wound formation on the foot. This is especially difficult when the tissue damage is difficult to sense because of nerve damage. Relieving this pressure is important in its treatment. The most effective way of relieving pressure is by eliminating weight bearing on the leg, using crutches or a walker. Unfortunately, because of problems with strength, endurance, and balance, many people cannot absolutely avoid weight bearing on one of their legs.

If you are able to use a walker, it is preferable to unprotected full weight bearing. Pressure relief shoes, pads, or casts can also help. In some instances, surgery may be necessary.

Antibiotics are sometimes prescribed for foot ulcers when they are infected. Any advantage of long-term use of these medications should be balanced by the possibility that it may help induce antibiotic resistance in the bacteria or cause other infections and problems. Ulcers take weeks or months to heal and long-term antibiotics for uninfected ulcers may not shorten healing time and can possibly have negative effects. Antibiotics attack bacteria, not only in the wound, but also throughout the entire body. Many bacteria, such as those that are naturally in your intestine, are actually beneficial. Destroying these natural bacteria can lead to overgrowth of harmful micro-organisms that can cause serious diarrhea, nausea, skin rashes, mouth sores, and, in women, vaginal yeast infections. However, prudent use of topical anti-microbial medications either in ointments and creams or impregnated into the dressing and systemic antibiotics for cases of infected wounds is sometimes effective in reducing the quantity of bacteria on a wound.

Daily protein requirements increase by 50% to 100% during wound healing depending on the size of the wound. Good sources of protein include lean meat, eggs, dairy, beans, peas, and nuts.

Other vitamins and nutrients play a key role in healing. Vitamin C is important in collagen formation, a key protein formed by your body during wound healing. About 500 IU per day is required in someone with a chronic wound. Taking more that the recommended allowance of this vitamin is not beneficial. This is more than is in the typical multivitamin and, if your diet is low in such things as raw leafy green vegetables, fruits, and potatoes, you should consider supplements. Daily ingestion is necessary to maintain an adequate supply.

Zinc is necessary to repair wounds also. Zinc deficiency can lead to delayed wound healing. Zinc is found in most meat. In addition, beans and nuts are sources of zinc. An adequate dietary intake is necessary to maximize wound-healing potential, but it is not necessary to take more than the recommended daily requirement. A multivitamin with a vitamin C supplement is adequate if your diet is deficient in these nutrients. Maintaining adequate hydration is also very important to circulation.

Proper control of other medical problems can promote healing of ulcers. Perhaps central to this is proper control of diabetes mellitus. Tight control of blood sugar can reverse a portion of the nerve damage that diabetes causes. It can also promote a healthy immune system, because white blood cells work better when blood sugars are as close to normal as possible. Migratory healing cells such as connective tissue and skin repair cells function and grow better when sugars are well controlled.

Optimal function of the heart and circulation improves blood flow to ulcers and decreases swelling. If your blood circulation is impaired, surgery in the form of an arterial bypass or stenting may be necessary.

Negative pressure therapy is a method of managing wounds that is especially helpful in large wounds. It involves attaching a machine to the spongy dressing trimmed to the wound. The machine draws the air out of the dressing. The vacuum created decreases wound swelling, pulls the wound together, and improves the circulation. The wound can become very smelly during treatment, and many people dislike this. The machine also can be noisy and disturb sleep. Applying the dressing is sort of an art form that takes wound care specialists some time to perfect.

Hyperbaric oxygen therapy is available in many different wound care centers across the country. The disadvantage is that repeated daily treatments are necessary for several weeks. The oxygen chambers can be cramped so that claustrophobic people may have difficulty tolerating them without sedation. The high pressure can bother people who have difficulty with their ears adjusting to pressure.

Skin graft substitutes have replaced the use of surgical skin grafting in some circumstances. These are interesting tools in the treatment of severe, extensive, or resistant wounds. Some contain skin that has been treated to remove the cells and so is basically a mesh of skin connective tissue. Others contain live cells in a protein mesh.

Successful treatment of wounds and ulcers is a partnership between you and your wound care team. Although wound care is very important, taking care of the rest of your health is as crucial. Look to improve your diet and take the medicines prescribed for all your health problems. With this in mind, regular evaluation and aggressive wound care will get any problem wound healed as quickly as possible.

Imaging of the Foot and Ankle

X-RAYS

Often when evaluating a foot problem, x-rays are obtained. This test uses high-energy electromagnetic waves (x-rays) from a radioactive source within the machine to expose a photographic film. The images created are based on the body tissues' ability to block these x-rays. It gives great detail of tissues that block a lot of these x-rays such as bone- and other calcium–containing materials and metallic structures, but less definition of soft tissues. A high-quality x-ray can differentiate between air, water, or soft tissue, bone and fat, but not much more.

X-rays are helpful in identifying fractures and bone tumors. They give little information on tendon and ligament problems or nerve problems. X-rays can identify arthritis and other joint disorders only indirectly because signs of arthritis on x-rays are mainly changes in the bone that often accompany arthritis such as spurring along the margins of the joint, cyst formation under the surface of the joint into the bone, thickening of the bone under the joint, or irregularity in the space separating the bones underlying the joint. When any pressure is placed across the joint such as with standing, the joint surfaces are compressed, giving a clear picture of the amount of tissue holding the joint surfaces apart, which is the thickness of the cartilage. This thins in joints with arthritis.

Although the test does not give a great deal of information about soft tissue structures, it is widely available, relatively inexpensive, and often answers the most important questions. If the diagnosis is clear clinically beyond a reasonable doubt, then nothing else needs to be done. Otherwise, radiographs are usually routinely obtained.

It is helpful to have an appreciation for what is normal when looking at your radiographs. There are basically two x-ray series obtained, the ankle and the foot series. Although other views are helpful, they are usually only ordered in special circumstances.

Bones and joints are identified. The width of a typical joint is demonstrated by the black arrows. The contours of these joints are even from side to side and are about two to four millimeters in width when healthy. (1) Anterioposterior (AP) view of the foot, or a view from the top or bottom. (2) Lateral or side view of the foot. (3) Mortise or view from the front of the ankle.

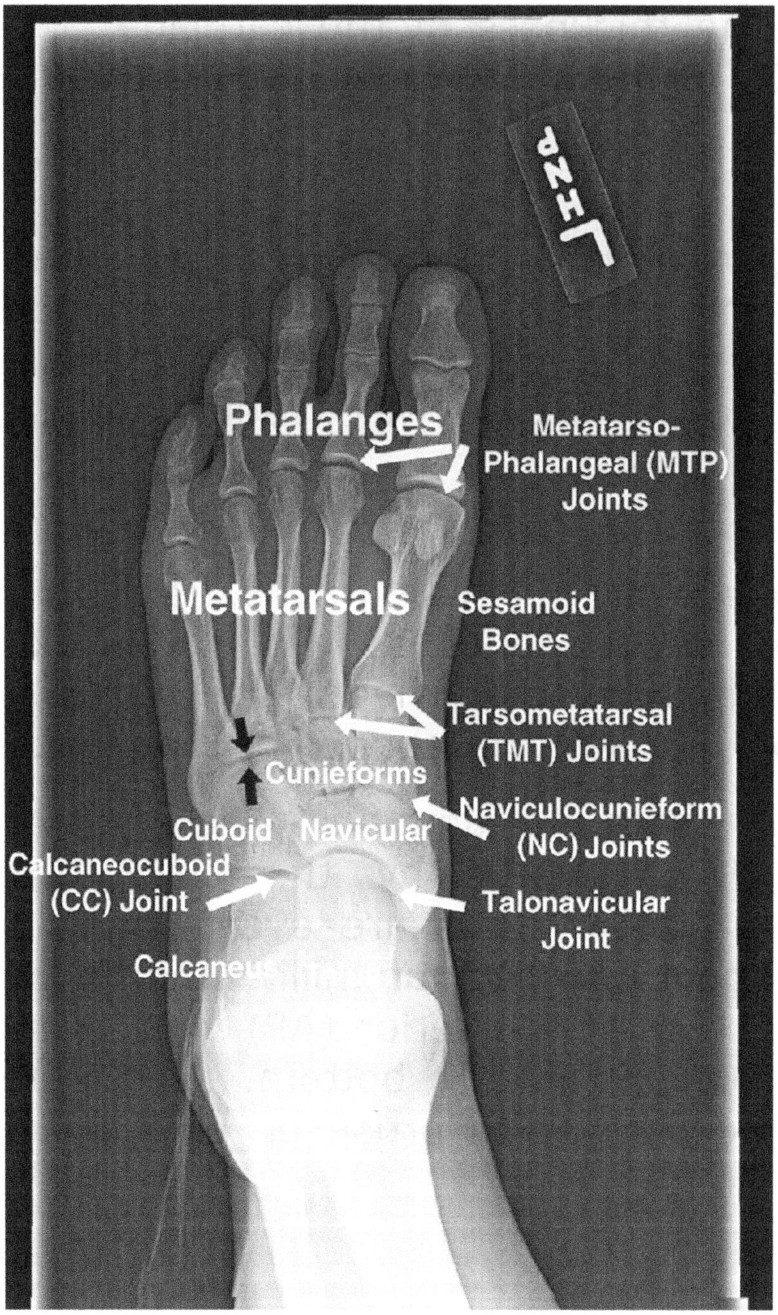

Phalanges
Metatarso-Phalangeal (MTP) Joints
Metatarsals
Sesamoid Bones
Tarsometatarsal (TMT) Joints
Cunieforms
Naviculocunieform (NC) Joints
Cuboid
Navicular
Calcaneocuboid (CC) Joint
Talonavicular Joint
Calcaneus

FIGURE 1

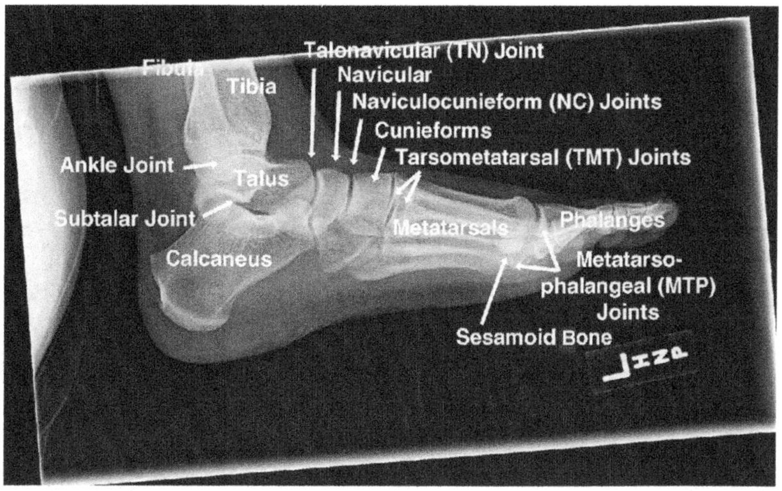
Talonavicular (TN) Joint
Fibula
Tibia
Navicular
Naviculocunieform (NC) Joints
Cunieforms
Ankle Joint
Tarsometatarsal (TMT) Joints
Talus
Subtalar Joint
Metatarsals
Phalanges
Calcaneus
Metatarso-
phalangeal (MTP)
Joints
Sesamoid Bone

FIGURE 2

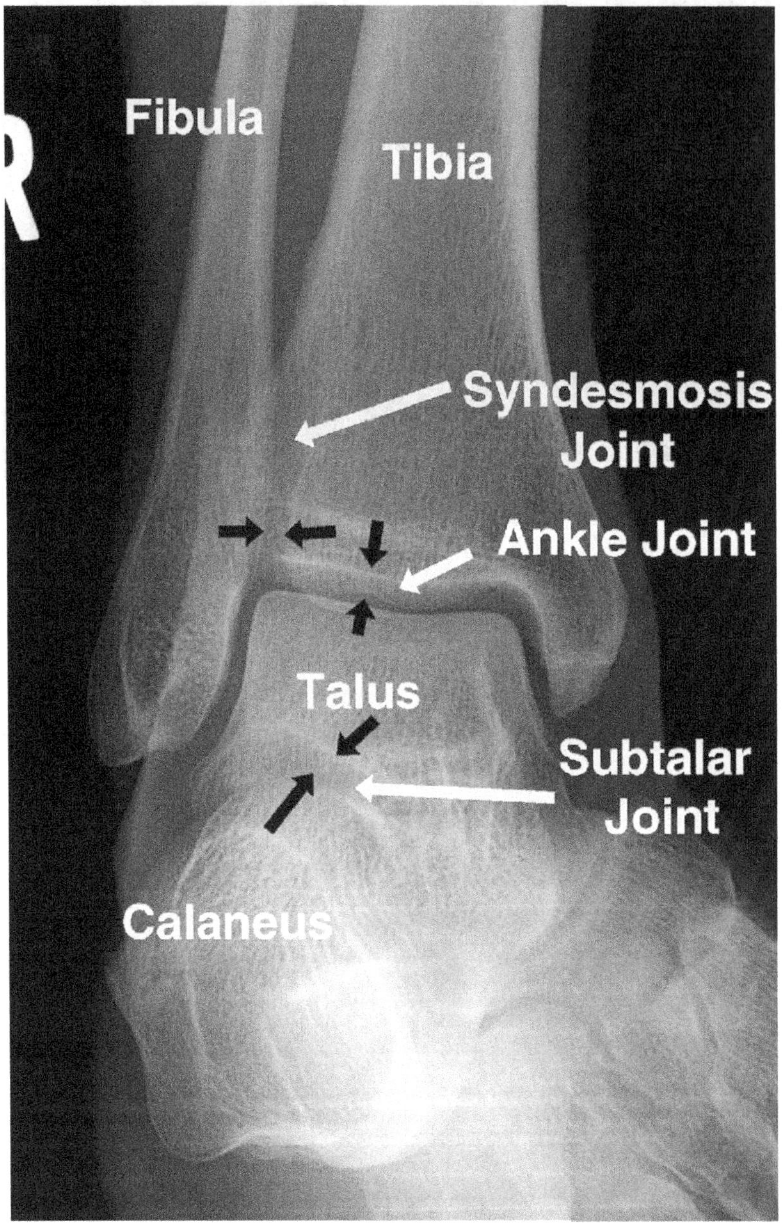
R
Fibula
Tibia
Syndesmosis
Joint
Ankle Joint
Talus
Subtalar
Joint
Calaneus

FIGURE 3

COMPUTED TOMOGRAPHY (CT OR CAT) SCAN

Computed tomography (CT) is a sophisticated technique that uses x-rays and computers to develop a detailed 2-D or 3-D view of the body. It can identify fractures and other bony abnormalities much easier than plain x-rays. The amount of radiation that the body is exposed to in CT scanning is considerably greater than that used in x-rays. The risk of developing a cancer as a result of the radiation received during this test is considerably less than the lifetime risk of cancer. However, a number of cancers in the population are caused by repeated x-ray and CT tests, but it is very small in relation to the overall number of cancers diagnosed. Nonetheless, it is important to use these tests sparingly.

CT scanning is extremely useful in determining the displacement and pattern of fracture. This can be useful to quantify the change in alignment of fracture fragments after an injury and can help in deciding whether surgery is necessary. It can also help a surgeon plan for surgical realignment so that surgical tissue damage can be minimized. Like x-rays, the amount of information about the soft tissue is limited.

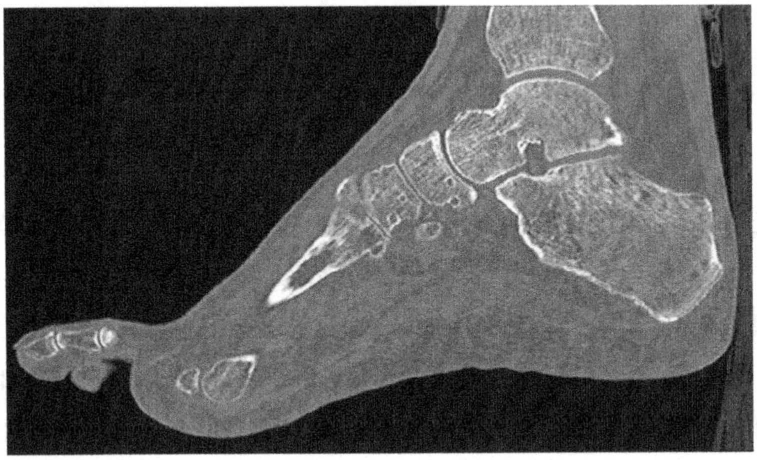

FIGURE 4 An image of the foot using CT scanning. Detail in the bones is excellent. The Achilles tendon and the muscles in the bottom of the arch are identifiable but there is little definition between many soft tissue structures.

MAGNETIC RESONANCE IMAGING (MRI)

MRI has truly revolutionized medicine and foot and ankle radiographic evaluation. The MRI uses strong magnets to align all the molecules in your body electomagnetically. Many of the molecules in your body have a positive and a negative pole including water and can be thought of as tiny magnets. When a strong magnet is placed around the body, these tiny magnets will align with the magnetic field. When the magnetic field is turned off, the molecules will return to a random alignment. This gives off radio waves that are detected by the MRI scanner. The MRI scanner makes millions of measurements of these radio waves and processes them with a computer to create an image. This helps not only image the anatomy, but to some extent can detect various ways that the chemical composition of the tissue has changed or is different than normal.

An MRI is not painful, but it takes some time to complete and many scanners have a small area for the examined person to lie while taking the test. People with claustrophobia or fear of close spaces and anxiety attacks will have difficulty with this test. The powerful magnets will destroy most electronic devices and cards with magnetic information such as credit cards. People with implanted devices such as pacemakers, automatic defibrillators, and spinal cords stimulators cannot have an MRI. Most orthopedic devices such as joint replacements and plates and screws do not affect an MRI, but if the metal is near the area that is going to be scanned, then it will ruin the image so that the test will be difficult to interpret.

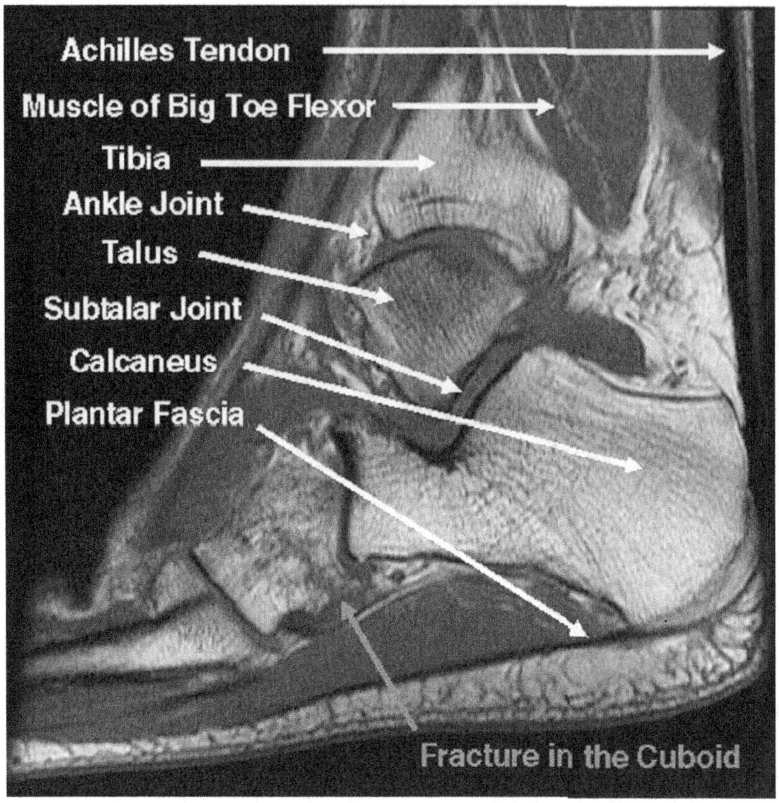

FIGURE 5 Exquisite detail is seen in this MRI of the ankle. In this case, an undisplaced fracture of the cuboid is detected (gray arrow).

Although MRI is an amazing medical breakthrough, it is an expensive test and needs to be used only when it is appropriate. The rational for getting such a test needs to be closely thought out before ordering it. It is rarely necessary unless surgery is being contemplated.

TECHNETIUM BONE SCAN

A technetium bone scan is a test that requires injecting a radioactive material, technetium, into the blood stream. Technetium circulates through the blood stream and is taken up by bone cells along with nutrients. The more active the bone cells, the more of the radioactive tracer is taken up. The amount of radioactivity that the person is exposed to is quite small. The resulting image is a fuzzy picture of the skeleton that shows areas of increased metabolism in the bone as intensely prominent. The intense uptake is commonly caused by arthritis and fractures although tumors and infections can also cause this.

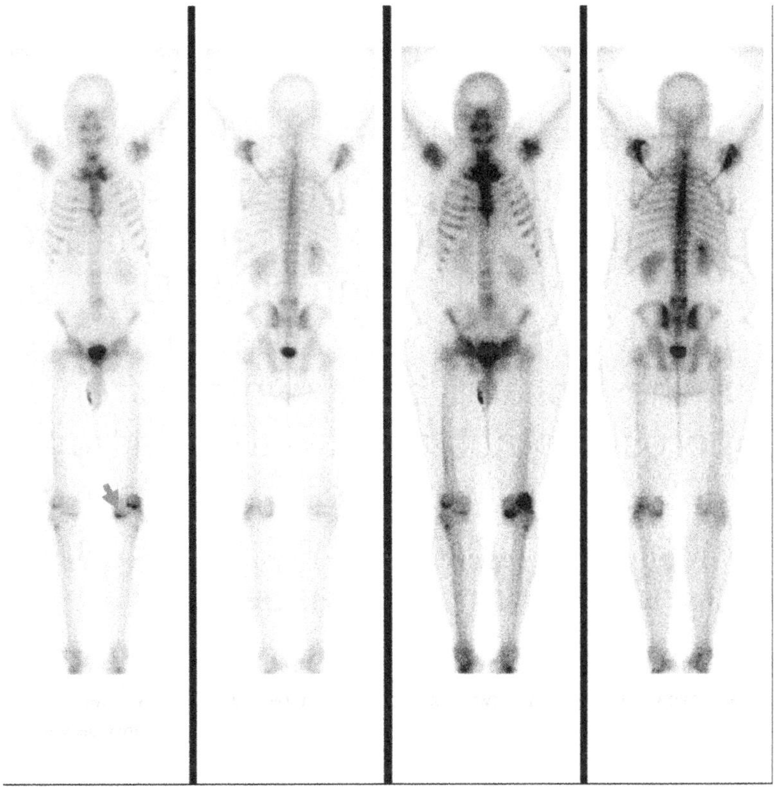

FIGURE 6 Whole body bone scan. The only significant abnormality in this scan is uptake in the knee along the inside of the joint and kneecap due to osteoarthritis.

Technetium bone scans can be helpful when you are looking at the whole body or need to evaluate a large part of the body. This sometimes comes up with trauma or cases of domestic abuse. It is extremely helpful to screen for metastatic bone cancer throughout the body. It is also used in the evaluation of certain tumors if there is a question as to whether the lesion is new or growing. Although there are some exceptions to this, if the bone scan shows normal uptake, a tumor or bone lesion is old or inactive.

BONE DENSITY SCAN

Bone density scans are used to identify osteoporosis. This test is very different from the technetium bone scan or, commonly, *bone scan,* although it is understandable why it is confusing. Osteoporosis is a decrease in density and strength of the bones especially in the hip and back, which often occurs with age. Osteoporosis is not a painful condition, but it can increase the probability and ease of fracturing a bone including bones of the foot and ankle. Loss of bone density is common with age especially in women and people of white or oriental race, who smoke, are thin, or have a family history of osteoporosis.

Bone density scans measure the density of bone by precisely determining how it absorbs x-rays as they pass through the bone. The density is then compared to the density of a population of people who are 20 to 40 years of age to determine a T score. Three percent of people will have a T score less than −2, which indicates osteoporosis. A T score below −2.5 is considered to indicate a high risk for an osteoporotic fracture and medication to treat this should be strongly considered. An age-matched bone density score or Z-score is not as useful.

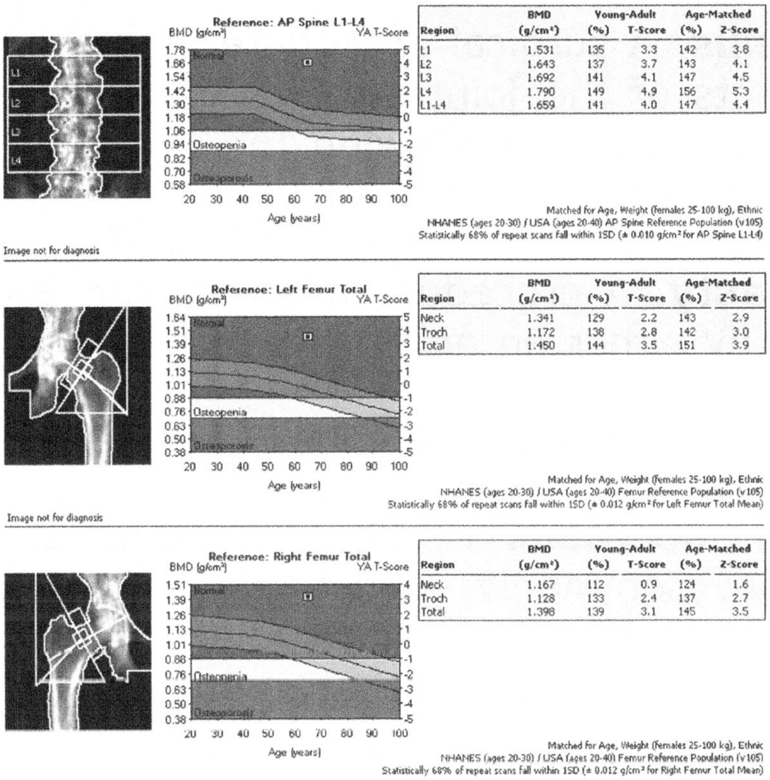

Region	BMD (g/cm²)	Young-Adult (%)	Young-Adult T-Score	Age-Matched (%)	Age-Matched Z-Score
L1	1.531	135	3.3	142	3.8
L2	1.643	137	3.7	143	4.1
L3	1.692	141	4.1	147	4.5
L4	1.790	149	4.9	156	5.3
L1-L4	1.659	141	4.0	147	4.4

Region	BMD (g/cm²)	Young-Adult (%)	Young-Adult T-Score	Age-Matched (%)	Age-Matched Z-Score
Neck	1.341	129	2.2	143	2.9
Troch	1.172	138	2.8	142	3.0
Total	1.450	144	3.5	151	3.9

Region	BMD (g/cm²)	Young-Adult (%)	Young-Adult T-Score	Age-Matched (%)	Age-Matched Z-Score
Neck	1.167	112	0.9	124	1.6
Troch	1.128	133	2.4	137	2.7
Total	1.398	139	3.1	145	3.5

FIGURE 7 A normal bone density scan. As noted in the text on the scan, the scan is compared to a population of females aged 20 to 40 years.

Glossary

Arthritis. Literally, inflammation of a joint. Most commonly used to refer to a painful condition when the cartilage on the joint is worn away.

Arthrodesis. A surgical procedure involving removing components of the joint such as cartilage and the underlying bone and allowing the area to bridge across the joint.

Arthroplasty. A procedure in which the joint is replaced by either an artificial or a biological material.

Articular. Pertaining to a joint.

Avascular necrosis. Tissue death from lack of circulation. Commonly used to describe death of bones. This can be caused by glucocorticoid usage, trauma, or other causes that sometimes are never identified.

Avulsion fractures. A ligament or tendon injury that removes a usually small portion of bone as the tendon or ligament tears away from it. Although technically these are fractures, the treatment is more similar to the treatment of the ligament or tendon injury. Some people worry that these fragments have the capacity to move out of place, which is very rarely the case.

Cartilage. A tough elastic connective tissue. There are several types. Articular cartilage covers the bones in the joints, forming a low fiction surface. Fibrocartilage is a gristly tissue found in cartilage that has been damaged and in certain stiff bony linkages such as coalitions.

Chevron. V shaped. Sometimes used to refer to a cut made in the shape of a V. This shape has better stability than a flat surface. Most often this refers to a type of bunionectomy.

Coalition. A condition in which two bones that are normally only loosely joined by ligaments have become tightly united by direct bony, fibrous, or cartilaginous linkages.

Connective tissue. Any nonbony tissue that functions to connect and control structures.

Distal. Away from the center of the body.

Dorsal. Toward the top of the body.

Dorsiflexion. Rotation of the foot or toe toward the top of the body, extension.

Eversion. A rotation of the hindfoot in which the sole of the foot points toward the outside of the body.

Fracture. A break in the bone. To doctors, a fracture and a break in a bone are the same thing.

Fusion. A surgical procedure removing the components of a joint such that the underlying bone is removed and, after healing, the joint is bridged with bone.

Gangrene. An infection that results in clotting of the nearby blood vessels, leading to death of a significant quantity of tissue. This can make the infection more difficult to control.

Glucocorticoid. A family of steroid hormones used by the body to react to stress. These include cortisol, cortisone, prednisone, and hydrocortisone among others. These substances are chemically similar but have different effects on the body from sexual steroids such as testosterone and estrogen.

Hallux. The big toe or great toe.

Inversion. A rotation of the hindfoot in which the sole of the foot points toward the inside of the body.

Lateral. Away from the midline of the body.

Ligament. A connective tissue that crosses one of more joints and functions to control the joints' motion.

Medial. Toward the midline of the body.

Osteotomy. A surgical cutting of the bone.

Phalanx (plural: phalanges). Small bones that make up the toes. Two are found in the big toe and three in each of the smaller toes.

Plantar. Toward the bottom of the foot.

Plantarflexion. Rotation of the foot or toe toward the sole of the foot, flexion.

Prophylactic. An action of treatment done in the effort to prevent a future problem.

Proximal. Toward the center of the body or thorax.

Spur. A bony projection usually as the result of arthritis around the joint or chronic traction of a tendon or ligament.

Tendon. Connective tissue that connects a muscle to a bone.

Valgus. A deformity in which the end of an extremity deviates away from the midline of the body and the apex toward the midline of the body.

Varus. A deformity in which the end of an extremity deviates toward the midline of the body and the apex away from the midline of the body.

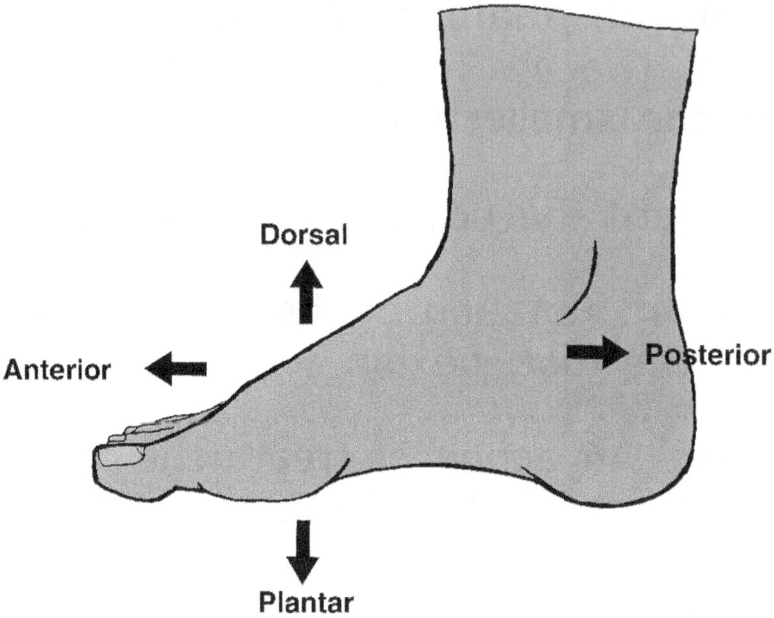

FIGURE 1 Words describing direction in the lateral view.

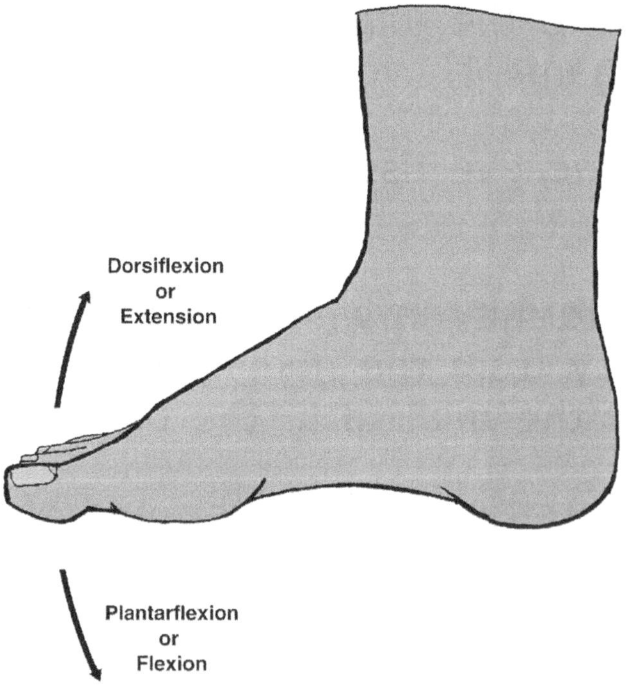

FIGURE 2 Words describing direction in the frontal view.

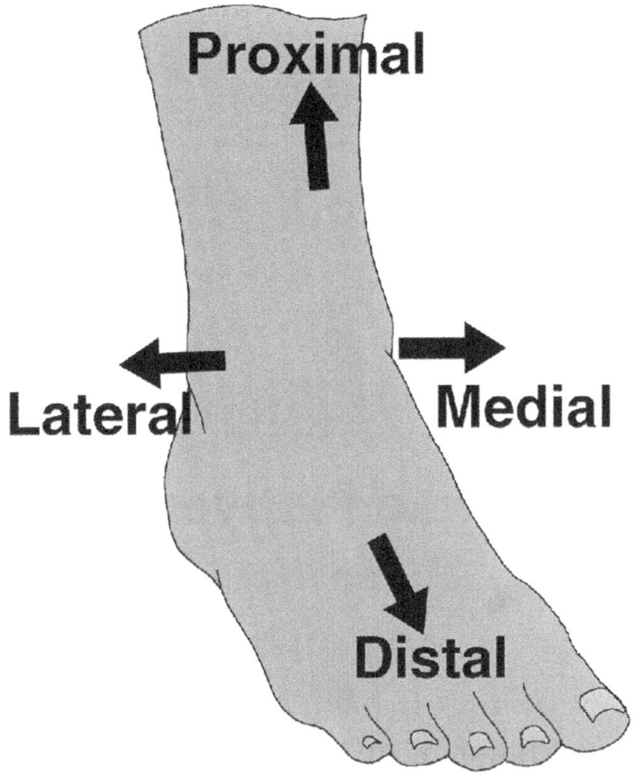

FIGURE 3 Words describing the direction of motion from the lateral view.

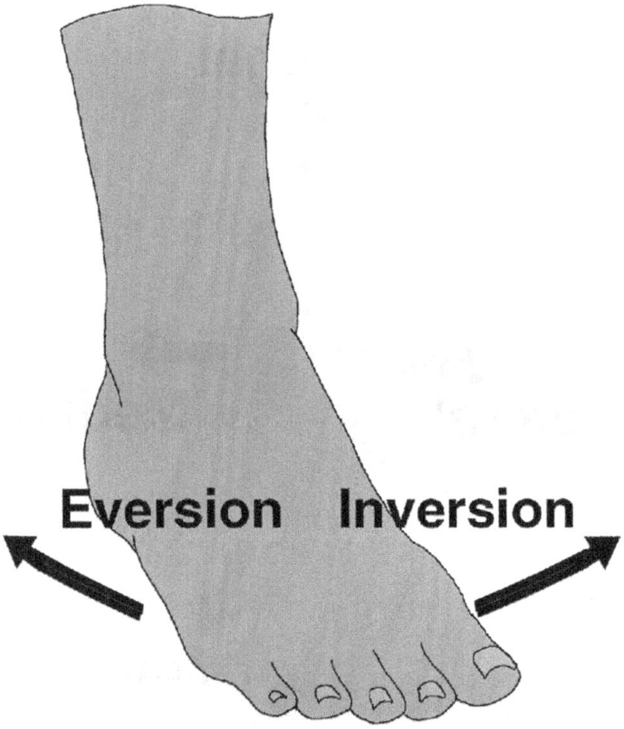

FIGURE 4 Words describing the direction of motion from the frontal view.

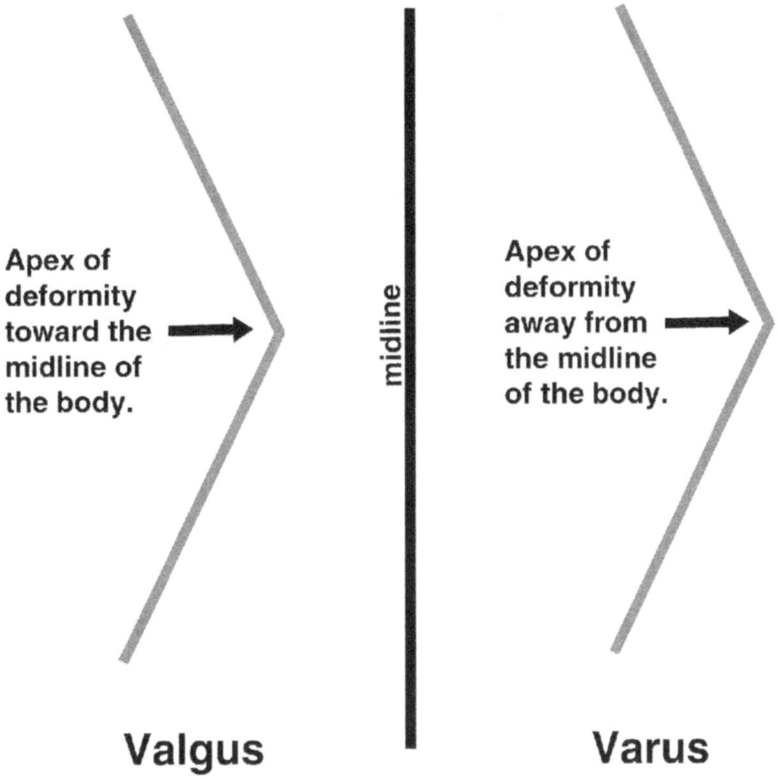

FIGURE 5 Varus/valgus.

Back Cover Material

"This book is impressive! It is written not only to be very useful for people to understand their condition, but as a primary care physician, I see direct application to my practice with respect to addressing my patients' foot and ankle concerns."

—Michael L. Baach, MD,
Parkside Internal Medicine, Carmel IN

"*The Whole Foot Book* is a comprehensive unbiased guide that will help people better understand their specific foot condition. *The Whole Foot* is an excellent tool..."

—Brian G. Elliott DPM, FACFAS,
American Health Network Foot and Ankle Surgeons, Greenfield, IN

"Today's society demands information that helps one make informed decisions concerning their own or families' health care. And this book does just that for foot and ankle health problems. In an era of fitness and need to be informed, this book is a must read for the active person or individual with chronic foot ailments."

—Richard Alvarez, MD,
Professor and Chair, Department of Orthopaedic Surgery,

College of Medicine Chattanooga, University of Tennessee

About the Authors

Brett Ryan Fink, MD, is an orthopedic surgeon currently in private practice in Indianapolis, IN, for the last eleven years and is President of the Indiana Orthopedic Center. He is a graduate of the University of Wisconsin and Washington University School of Medicine. He is a veteran of the U.S. Navy and the Persian Gulf War.

Mark Stuart Mizel, MD, has been a practicing foot and ankle specialist for over twenty-five years. He is a graduate of Columbia University and Tufts University. He is a veteran of the U.S. Navy and former naval aviator. He has held academic positions at the University of Miami and Tufts, Johns Hopkins, and Boston University. He is the editor of five scholarly orthopedic books and author of over seventy research and review articles.

B

F

G

H

P

T

U

Made in the USA
Monee, IL
13 September 2026

62976971R00319